Medical
Office
Procedures

Medical Office Procedures

FOURTH EDITION

Karonne J. Becklin
Edith M. Sunnarborg

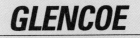

GLENCOE
McGraw-Hill

New York, New York   Columbus, Ohio   Woodland Hills, California   Peoria, Illinois

Library of Congress Cataloging-in-Publication Data

Becklin, Karonne J.
   Medical office procedures / Karonne J. Becklin, Edith M.
Sunnarborg. — 4th ed.
        p.   cm.
      Includes index.
      ISBN 0-02-802531-8 (PB)
      1. Medical assistants. 2. Medical offices—Management.
   I. Sunnarborg, Edith M. II. Title.
      [DNLM: 1. Office Management. 2. Practice Management, Medical.
   3. Medical Secretaries.   W 80 8397m 1996]
   R728.8.B44   1996
   651'.961—dc20
   DNLM/DLC
   for Library of Congress   95-35495
                                                                 CIP

Photo Credits: p. 1: Will & Deni McIntyre/Photo Researchers, p. 3: Yoav Levy/
Phototake, p. 7: Dick Luria/Photo Researchers, p. 11: M. Dwyer/Stock,
Boston, Inc., p. 18: Will & Deni McIntyre/Photo Researchers, p. 22: Leslie
O'Shaughnessy/Medical Images, p. 25: Crest Uniform Co., p. 28: *l* Tab
Products Co., *r* White Office Systems, p. 30: Ann Chwatsky/Phototake, p. 31:
C. C. Duncan/Medical Images, p. 49: C. C. Duncan/Medical Images, p. 53:
Werner Bertsch/Medical Images, p. 55: David R. Frazier/Photo Researchers,
p. 59: James Prince/Photo Researchers, p. 61: Jon Riley/Medichrome, p. 63:
Hewlett Packard, p. 80: Panasonic Company, p. 103: Blair Seitz/Photo
Researchers, p. 104: *l* Rolodex Corp., *r* Esselte Pendaflex Corp., p. 105: *t* Esselte
Pendaflex Corp., *b* White Office Systems, p. 108: Tom Tracy/Medichrome, p.
109: Colwell Systems, p. 125: Jon Riley/Medichrome, p. 137: Colwell Systems,
p. 142: C. C. Duncan/Medical Images, p. 173: Yoav Levy/Phototake, p. 176:
International Business Machines Corporation, p. 195: Medical Arts Press, p.
211: Hewlett Packard, p. 215: Hewlett Packard, p. 218: Werner Bertsch/
Medical Images, p. 224: Minnesota Mining & Manufacturing Co. (3M).

This program has been prepared with the assistance of Chestnut Hill
Enterprises, Inc.

Medical Office Procedures, Fourth Edition

Imprint 1998

Send all inquiries to:
GLENCOE/McGraw-Hill
936 Eastwind Drive
Westerville, OH 43081

ISBN 0-02-802531-8
Printed in the United States of America

4 5 6 7 8 9 10   024   02 01 00 99 98

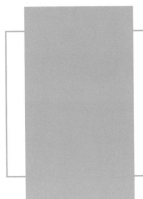

Contents

Preface

The fourth edition of Medical Office Procedures is a revision of a well-known and widely used textbook and includes additional use of computerized tasks. The administrative responsibilities of the medical assistant are emphasized in this text. The term *medical assistant* denotes any medical assistant who performs administrative tasks.

The medical profession is complex and demanding; therefore, the typical physician rarely has time to attend to the administrative responsibilities of the office. The medical assistant requires continuing education to keep up to date with office technology, including computer skills and new computer software. These requirements put more demands on the medical assistant of today than in the past.

The job opportunities in the medical field continually change with varying degrees of education and specialization. This textbook allows for the integrated application of office procedures skills and knowledge in the classroom through the use of simulation techniques. The student learns to perform the duties of the medical assistant under realistic conditions with input from a variety of sources, with access to a variety of records, through the use of different equipment, and with realistic pressures that require the student to organize the work and set priorities.

The fourth edition is divided into five parts. Part 1 introduces the administrative medical assistant's career, defining the tasks that an assistant performs, describing the various available work environments, and introducing medical ethics and medical law as they apply to the medical assistant. Specific administrative responsibilities are introduced and applied in Part 2. These include handling the telephone, scheduling patients, filing records, and writing medical correspondence. The use of the computer is emphasized in each of these aspects. In Part 3, procedures for preparing and organizing patients' charts and bills are discussed. Part 4 concerns financial records in the office. Methods for reviewing and completing health insurance forms are covered. Also discussed is the handling of daily journals, banking tasks, and payroll records. Part 5 includes meeting preparations, travel arrangements, and professional reports, then ends with a computer simulation using acquired skills from Parts 1–5.

■ PROJECTS

Within each chapter, integrating projects occur at frequent intervals so that students can immediately put into practice the procedure just studied. Records and correspondence that students create in these individual projects are used later in the simulations, where they illustrate the complexity of the medical assistant's responsibilities. The scheduling and financial projects can be completed on the computer using the program *MediSoft*. The written correspondence and charts can be completed using any word processing software.

■ SIMULATIONS

Two-day simulations appear at the end of Parts 2 and 3. A three-day simulation appears at the end of Part 4. The computerized project is available at the end of Part 5. In each of these four simulations, students listen to taped conversations between Linda Jenson (the doctor's medical assistant, with whom the student will identify) and Dr. Mark Newman, various patients, and other office callers. (*Note:* The simulation cassettes may be used by students individually or by the class as a whole.) A complete transcript of the material appears in the *Instructor's Manual and Key*.

■ WORKING PAPERS AND FORMS

A master form is supplied for those projects needing multiple copies. Some forms, medical histories, handwritten drafts, incoming correspondence, and other communications needed to complete the projects and the simulations are provided in the Working Papers in the back of the book.

Karonne J. Becklin
Edith M. Sunnarborg

To the Student

You have chosen a truly fascinating, challenging profession—one that you will find gratifying and rewarding. The field of health care is growing at a rapid pace, providing many opportunities for the trained professional. We welcome you to an educational program designed to prepare you for immediate and long-range success as an administrative medical assistant. In this course, you will use *Medical Office Procedures* not only as a source of practical information but also as an instrument for realistic practice in applying what you have learned.

■ PRACTICAL INFORMATION

Every topic that you will study in this course is directly related to one or more of the many administrative tasks that you will be performing as a medical assistant. In Part 1 of this textbook, you will learn about specific career opportunities available to you and the qualifications you need in order to succeed. After studying and absorbing this information, you should be better able to set your sights on the job that is best suited to your interests, qualifications, and ambitions.

In Part 2, you will learn how to work with patients in an efficient, effective manner. Since dealing with patients is a responsibility that you will encounter immediately and continually in a medical office, all the information concerning handling telephone calls, scheduling appointments, greeting patients, and preparing effective written communications is vitally important.

As an administrative medical assistant, you will be required to perform a variety of financial and records management tasks in a medical office. Parts 3 and 4 will help you to become thoroughly acquainted with medical records, patient billing, health insurance, and the financial records of the medical office.

The physician is frequently involved in a variety of professional activities outside the office. Part 5 will provide you with information about meeting preparations, travel arrangements, and professional reports.

At the end of the text, you will use the acquired skills in Parts 1 through 5 in a simulation. If your instructor so directs, you will use the computer software, Medisoft, to work with this simulation.

■ REALISTIC JOB TRAINING

At frequent intervals throughout each chapter, you will be asked to *apply* your newly acquired knowledge—not simply to tell how or why you would use the information on the job. Just as in a medical office, you will apply the information repeatedly throughout the course.

As you complete the projects within the text, you will accumulate many of the medical records and much of the correspondence needed in the simulations that occur at the end of Parts 2 through 5. You will be asked to assume the role of Linda Jenson, a medical assistant. During each of the simulations, you will handle various requests made by the doctor, the patients, and other office callers.

During the simulations, you will be expected to listen carefully to recorded conversations between Linda Jenson and the doctor, the patients, and other office callers and to perform your duties in the manner you think appropriate. (Your instructor will make the recorded conversations available to you; the medical forms, medical histories, correspondence, and other materials needed for the simulations are in the Working Papers at the back of the text and in the projects you will complete.)

Just as in the medical office, you will be performing a variety of closely related tasks in these simulations: transcribing dictation, answering the telephone, scheduling appointments, filing, opening mail, greeting office callers, preparing bills, and so on. You will have occasion to refer to various reference materials—dictionaries, reference books, medical references, and the like—just as you would in an office. Thus, you will gain proficiency in performing a wide range of administrative activities and in coping with a variety of problems and pressures in the medical office. All these activities will help you overcome some of the common problems of beginning office workers: difficulty in organizing work, setting priorities, relating one task to another, and managing time. After completing these simulations, you will find that you are well prepared for the transition from classroom to office.

You will also find a variety of personal development projects at the end of each chapter. The Key Terms and Medical Vocabulary will help you review important terms and concepts used in the chapter. The discussion problems will involve you in thought-provoking questions and situations that will help you better understand your chosen profession and its responsibilities. The role-playing situations will assist you in developing the tact, graciousness, and understanding needed to deal with patients, physicians, and other coworkers.

■ SUPPLIES

Starting with Part 2, you will be "working" for Dr. Mark Newman, a family practitioner. All the work you do in the chapter projects must be saved. This work will form the basis for your "office files." You will use and add to the information in these files as you complete the simulations.

The preprinted medical forms needed to complete the simulation are supplied as Working Papers in the back of the book. You will find specific instructions for removing and using them in the textbook directions. Because a large quantity of letterhead paper and clinical data sheets is required for the projects and the simulations, you will need to photocopy these Working Papers as you come to them. If you prefer, you may design your own letterhead or use plain paper. You will also need the following supplies:

- File folder labels and 35 file folders.
- A ring binder or a file folder to serve as your appointment book.
- An expandable portfolio to serve as your file cabinet. All your working materials should be stored in this portfolio.
- A box of paper for printing and envelopes.
- Miscellaneous supplies—rubber bands, a note pad, pens, pencils, papers clips, and so on.

You will need two additional file folders before you begin Part 2. Label one of these folders "Supplies." In it, you will store your letterheads and the supplies you remove from the Working Papers section of the textbook. Label the other folder "Miscellaneous." This folder will contain work that does not pertain to Dr. Newman's patients.

Karonne J. Becklin
Edith M. Sunnarborg

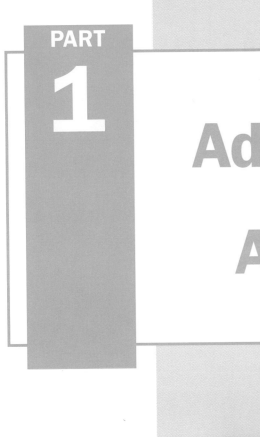

PART 1

The Administrative Medical Assistant's Career

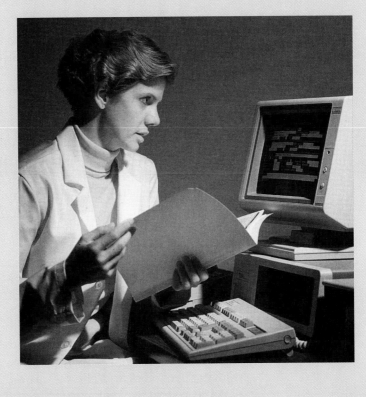

Medical Office Opportunities

OBJECTIVES

Upon completion of this chapter, you should be able to:

■ Discuss ten possible job settings available to a person with medical office skills.

■ List ten tasks that are performed by an administrative medical assistant and ten tasks that are performed by a clinical medical assistant.

■ State the limits of a medical specialty when the type of the specialist is given.

■ Discuss the advantages of a professional affiliation.

As new technology, new medications, and new treatments are introduced into the health care industry, the opportunities for a rewarding career in a medical office increase.

At the same time, sophisticated technology poses new challenges for health care professionals. Legal and ethical issues also are constantly being raised. A greater degree of specialization is required of physicians and medical assistants alike. Just as the physician must choose a field in which to specialize, the medical assistant must also select a particular career path and setting in which to work. In addition, increasingly sophisticated computer technology for the medical office makes continuing education a must for the successful medical assistant.

■ DESCRIPTION OF A MEDICAL ASSISTANT

The term **medical assistant** describes medical office professionals working in a broad range of jobs and settings. The responsibilities of the medical assistant can typically be divided into two categories: administrative tasks and clinical tasks.

Administrative tasks are those procedures used to keep any kind of office running efficiently. **Clinical tasks** are those procedures the

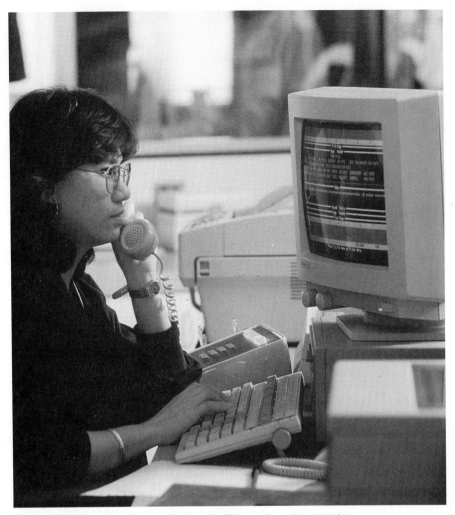

The medical assistant is a professional office worker who must be proficient in a number of skills.

medical assistant may perform to aid the physician in medical treatment of a patient. The assistant may specialize in either administrative or clinical responsibilities, or he or she may perform a combination of the two. However, the number of large incorporated medical practices is increasing, and in such settings it is likely that the medical assistant will specialize in a particular area, whether it be managing records, greeting patients, or assisting the physician with examinations and procedures.

In this text we will concentrate on administrative responsibilities, which involve valuable skills required in most medical office careers.

Important Skills for the Medical Assistant

The medical assistant is a professional office worker dedicated to assisting in the care of patients. To effectively perform all the required tasks, the medical assistant must be proficient in a number of skills.

Written Language Skills. The medical assistant must be proficient in English grammar, punctuation, style, and spelling in order to handle correspondence, filing, and other written work.

Oral Language Skills. Knowledge of correct pronunciation and the ability to speak clearly and correctly are essential skills for the medical assistant to communicate with patients, staff members, and other medical personnel.

Math Skills. The medical assistant must have sufficient math skills to maintain financial records, to bill patients, to order supplies, and to perform a variety of other office tasks.

Equipment Skills. The medical assistant must be able to operate and keep current with office equipment. Computers are used in all phases of the medical office to improve the level of care and to run the office more effectively. Computers can handle:

- Scheduling of patients' appointments.
- Billing of patients for office visits and treatments.
- Updating of patients' accounts.
- Maintaining office financial records.
- Transcribing and keying medical records and correspondence.

Correspondence and documents such as release of information or reports of special tests can be sent to another medical facility using a facsimile machine (fax machine) when quick action is required. A fax machine is a device that transmits a copy of a document via telephone lines to another location.

Many hospitals, clinics, and offices also have electronic mail systems, by which messages are sent through a computer network to other staff members or physicians.

Some of the training needed to use this equipment will take place on the job through equipment manuals or vendor-training sessions. Other new skills in using technology can be acquired in continuing education classes and seminars. Whatever the source, the ability to use the latest office technology will ensure success on the job and will enhance the possibility of promotion.

Organizational Skills. In order to manage the sometimes hectic pace of work in the health care field, the medical assistant must have intelligent, systematic work habits and a willingness to take care of details. Scheduling appointments and maintaining an office routine require strong organizational skills.

Interpersonal Skills. Above all, the medical assistant must possess excellent interpersonal skills and a genuine desire to work with people. As the physician's representative, the medical assistant is usually the first person to have contact with patients. How the assistant welcomes patients, talks to them, and attends to their requests will influence the patients' attitudes toward the doctor and the treatment and will affect the entire atmosphere in the office.

Many Functions Performed by the Medical Assistant

One attractive characteristic of the medical assistant's job is the variety of tasks to be done. In a large setting such as a hospital, the medical assistant may specialize in one job function. In a small setting such as a doctor's office, however, the assistant may perform many functions. These may include the following:

- **Receptionist:** Answers the telephone, schedules appointments, and greets patients.
- **File clerk:** Pulls patients' charts, files information in the charts, and returns the charts to the files.
- **Transcriptionist:** Prepares the transcription of the doctor's dictation and correspondence.
- **Accounting clerk:** Keeps records of patients' visits, fees, and payments.
- **Insurance clerk:** Handles insurance forms.

The health care industry is continually undergoing change. New technology and a more competitive environment for both hospitals and physicians have made it necessary for the medical assistant to be skilled in many areas. A comprehensive list of those skills appears in Figure 1-1 on page 6. Depending on the career path you choose, you will be responsible for many or all of the tasks shown.

A Day in the Office

What is it like to be a medical assistant? The work in a medical office is interesting and varied. A typical day might be described this way.

The assistant arrives before the start of office hours so that the first patient will be greeted by a composed, organized, and properly dressed representative of the physician. Being on time means being able to attend to the routine of preparing the office before the arrival of patients.

The morning mail, especially reports concerning patients, is sorted and distributed, and charts for patients who have appointments on that day are taken out of the files and organized for the physician.

Shortly after the start of office hours, the telephone starts ringing as patients call to schedule and cancel appointments. In response, appropriate notations are made on the calendar and in patients' charts. Perhaps a patient who has been awake all night with pain calls to speak with the doctor. There may also be calls for refills of medications and for emergencies.

As patients arrive for appointments, the medical assistant attends to each patient personally. New patients need to complete forms. Addresses, telephone numbers, and insurance information must be updated for established patients.

As the day progresses, the physician may give the assistant correspondence and medical histories to be prepared from transcription or other kinds of work. For example, if the physician is active on a medical committee, the assistant may have items to prepare for a meeting.

Administrative Duties

- Handling the telephone.
- Scheduling appointments.
- Greeting patients.
- Maintaining financial records.
- Reconciling bank statements.
- Quoting fees to patients.
- Maintaining payroll records.
- Recording patients' charges and payments.
- Handling petty cash.
- Preparing bills.
- Collecting bills.
- Coordinating patient's care.
- Operating office equipment.

- Coding diagnoses and procedures.
- Transcribing medical dictation.
- Composing and processing correspondence.
- Planning travel for physician.
- Arranging hospital admissions.
- Maintaining dates for license renewals, premiums due, membership fees, meetings, subscriptions.
- Checking medical journals for items of interest to physician.

- Ordering, handling, and storing supplies.
- Maintaining the office in physician's absence.
- Procuring nurses for patients.
- Preparing records for use in court.
- Proofreading physician's articles, lectures, and manuscripts.
- Filing medical records.
- Completing insurance forms.
- Scheduling surgery.

Clinical Duties

- Obtaining and recording patients' data.
- Performing routine diagnostic tests.
- Taking patients' temperature, height, weight, and pulse.
- Operating and maintaining clinical equipment.

- Sterilizing instruments.
- Assisting with examinations, treatments, and office surgery.
- Administering medications specified by physician.
- Preparing patients for examinations and tests.
- Taking X rays.

- Administering electrocardiograms.
- Changing dressings and bandages.
- Preparing sterile examination and treatment areas.
- Collecting and processing laboratory specimens.

Figure 1-1   Administrative and Clinical Duties of the Medical Assistant

At some point during the day, the medical assistant will need to take care of financial records—preparing bills, reconciling bank statements, and completing insurance forms. For these and other tasks, the assistant may have to use a computer, a photocopy machine, or other office equipment.

The assistant may also have some managerial tasks to perform. Perhaps supplies need to be ordered or deliveries checked. Service for equipment might need to be scheduled. If the physician is out of the office, the assistant will have to manage the office work.

Although the routine of office work may follow a familiar pattern from day to day, the medical assistant must be prepared for emergencies and for special requests by the physician and by patients. Indeed, there is no routine in working with patients. Patients represent a cross

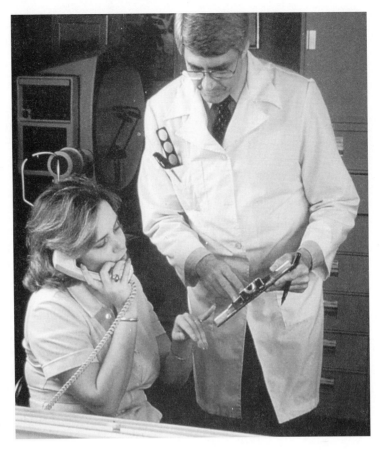

During the course of the workday the medical assistant may be asked to handle special requests by physicians and by patients.

section of humanity; each patient is different from the others. The assistant is constantly required to be tactful, gentle, understanding, firm, and patient.

At the end of the day, the assistant makes sure that the office is orderly and ready for the next day's work.

PROJECT 1 Choosing a Medical Career

You have decided to become a medical office assistant. Explain why you chose the medical area. State your goals in terms of these time periods: one year from now and five years from now. Use plain paper. Be prepared to discuss your opinions in class. Beginning with this project, you should set up a folder marked "Personal" in which you will keep all nonmedical assignments.

■ MEDICAL CAREER OPPORTUNITIES

A thorough training in office skills, as well as the art of getting along with people, will ensure the assistant a successful career in almost any field. Moreover, because the health care industry is booming, a well-trained medical assistant will have a wide variety of opportunities from which to choose. Following is a description of the various environments in which a skilled assistant may find employment.

Physician's Office

In a small, one- or two-physician practice, the assistant acts as the doctor's right hand, handling all administrative tasks and perhaps assisting with clinical duties. This setting provides the medical assistant with an opportunity to perform a wide variety of tasks and to develop close ties with patients and with the physician. There also may be an office nurse who looks after patients. In such a setting, responsibility for work may at times overlap.

A **group practice** might include an internist, a cardiologist, an endocrinologist, and a specialist in infectious diseases. Each specialty has its own patients, but patients are often referred to other specialists within that practice. Group practices are becoming more prevalent because they allow physicians to control spiraling costs better by sharing overhead costs for the office. Such practices also give new physicians the opportunity to join an established practice and to acquire a clientele. Because of the high volume of patients, the assistant may specialize in a particular area, such as greeting and scheduling patients, or may perform a variety of duties. Group practices also offer advantages to patients since they can receive the services of several physicians in one office. Figure 1-2 describes medical specialties and subspecialties.

PROJECT 2 **Medical Specialties**

Working Paper 1 (WP 1 in the Working Papers section at the back of this book) lists various kinds of medical specialists. Match the specialist to its definition. Be prepared to discuss your answers in class.

Clinics

A **clinic** may specialize in the diagnosis and treatment of a specific disorder (for example, a scoliosis clinic, a mental-health clinic, a back-pain clinic), or it may be composed of many specialties within one building where patients move from one department to another for completion of an extensive examination with specialty consultations.

Hospitals

It is possible for medical assistants to find positions in the following departments of hospitals:

- Admitting
- Emergency room

Allergy
Diagnosis and treatment of adverse reactions to foods, drugs, and other substances.

Anesthesiology
Maintenance of relief from pain and of stable body functions during medical procedures.

Critical Care Medicine
Treatment of patients in intensive care units.

Dermatology
Diagnosis and treatment of diseases of the skin and related tissues.

Emergency Medicine
Immediate treatment, usually in the emergency room of a hospital, of accidents or illnesses.

Family Practice
Total health care of the family.

Internal Medicine
Diagnosis of a wide range of nonsurgical illnesses. Subspecialties include:

    Cardiovascular Medicine
    Diagnosis and treatment of diseases of the heart, blood vessels, and lungs.

    Endocrinology
    Diagnosis and treatment of diseases of the endocrine glands, which secrete vital chemicals into the bloodstream.

    Gastroenterology
    Diagnosis and treatment of diseases of the digestive tract and related organs.

    Hematology
    Diagnosis and treatment of diseases of the blood.

    Infectious Disease
    Diagnosis and treatment of all types of infectious diseases.

    Nephrology
    Diagnosis and treatment of disorders of the kidneys and related functions.

    Oncology
    Diagnosis and treatment of all types of cancer.

    Pulmonary Disease
    Diagnosis and treatment of disorders of the lungs.

    Rheumatology
    Diseases of the muscles, joints, bones, and connective tissues.

Neurology
Diagnosis and treatment of disorders of the nervous system.

Obstetrics and Gynecology
Care during pregnancy and childbirth and diagnosis and treatment of diseases of the female reproductive system.

Ophthalmology
Care of the eyes and the vision.

Orthopedics
Treatment of the musculoskeletal system.

Orthopedic Surgery
Preservation and restoration of the spine and the extremities through surgical means.

Otorhinolaryngology
Diagnosis and treatment of illnesses of the nose, ears, and throat.

Pathology
Investigation of the causes of disease through laboratory techniques.

Pediatrics
Comprehensive treatment of children. Subspecialties include:
    Allergy, Cardiology, Neonatology (care of the newborn), **Nephrology,** and **Oncology**

Physical Medicine and **Rehabilitation**
Evaluation and treatment of all types of disease through physical means, such as heat.

Plastic Surgery
Repair and reconstruction of body structures through surgical means.

Preventive Medicine
Overall health of individuals. Defined areas include:
    Aerospace, Occupational, and **Public Health**

Psychiatry
Diagnosis and treatment of mental, emotional, and behavioral disorders.

Radiology and **Nuclear Medicine**
Use of radioactive materials to diagnose and treat disease.

Thoracic Surgery
Use of surgery to diagnose or treat diseases in the upper body cavity.

Urology
Diagnosis and treatment of diseases of the urinary tract.

Figure 1-2   Medical Specialties and Subspecialties

- Clinics (such as cardiac rehabilitation or chronic-pain clinics)
- Insurance billing
- Laboratory or pathology
- Medical records (including filing, coding, and transcription)
- Operating room
- Patient education
- Physical therapy
- Radiology
- Social services

Institutions

Institutions such as nursing homes, convalescent homes, sanatoriums, and homes for people with mental or physical disabilities all require experienced medical assistants. Such facilities provide long-term care for patients with chronic, or prolonged, illnesses as well as short-term care for patients recovering from a hospital stay.

Insurance

As the health care industry changes, insurance companies have a greater need for medical assistants who are experienced in handling medical documents and procedures. Places of employment might include Blue Cross and Blue Shield; Medicare or Medicaid; any of the growing number of health maintenance organizations (HMOs) or preferred provider organizations (PPOs); or any of the private plans operated by organizations, clubs, unions, and employee associations. HMOs and PPOs require clients to pay a set rate for which they receive as many health care services as they require, thus encouraging care that maintains good health and reduces costly treatment after an illness occurs. The operation of any of these plans requires a vast amount of clerical work such as completing and checking reports received from doctors, coding medical diagnoses and procedures, adjusting claims, mailing out payments of claims, and renewing contracts.

Foundations

Foundations that direct fund-raising and research efforts in various medical fields also need office workers familiar with the medical environment. Foundations may be concerned with a particular disease (for example, the National Heart Foundation), with standards of professional health care (for example, the Professional Standards Review Organization), or with a variety of other research.

Public Health Departments

Each state and many municipalities have their own health departments. Enforcement of proper sanitation, supervision of public eating places, and maintenance of a clean water supply are a few of the activities that concern public health departments. As with insurance companies and foundations, there usually is little direct contact with patients. Most of the assistant's duties involve clerical and support tasks.

Research Centers

Research centers conduct programs that seek to increase medical knowledge. University medical centers, hospitals, foundations, pharmaceutical firms, and other private businesses have special departments devoted entirely to finding cures for diseases and solutions to health care problems. As such, this can be a rewarding field for the medical assistant.

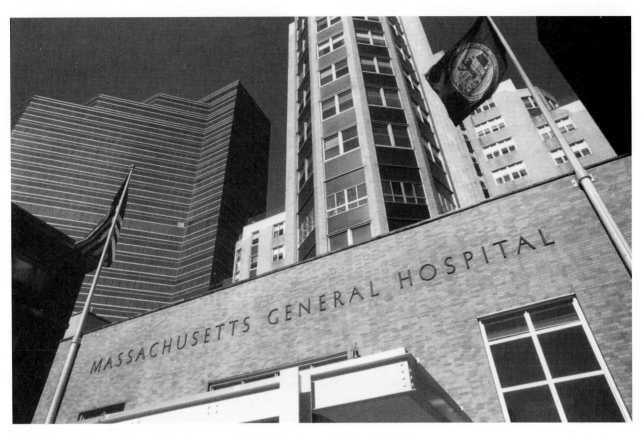

Hospitals provide a wide variety of career opportunities for medical assistants.

Private Industry

Private businesses manufacture and distribute pharmaceuticals, surgical instruments, hospital supplies, and other products associated with the health care industry. Some also engage in medical research. All such firms need office workers with medical experience.

Publishing

Those assistants with a flair for writing and an interest in editorial work can find positions as medical editorial assistants. Many doctors publish books and articles and employ full-time editorial assistants; others hire assistants on a freelance basis to help with a specific book or article. Specialized editorial training is required for such work. It is necessary to know how to use a library, prepare a manuscript, compile a bibliography, create an index, and proofread. One advantage of working on a freelance basis is having a more flexible schedule than someone who holds a regular office job.

Some publishing companies specialize in publishing medical books, while others have a medical department as part of their operation. Other companies publish medical journals. These firms need the experience of medical editorial assistants to help produce medical publications.

Teaching

Perhaps the best teacher of medical assistants is someone who has been employed in a medical office. Formal training in education and experience as a medical assistant are necessary for a teaching career.

Laboratories

Laboratories are facilities that have been equipped to conduct scientific testing, whether for medical evaluation, research, or product development. Laboratories need medical assistants skilled in clinical procedures as well as in clerical support.

Other Fields of Medicine

Medical assistants can find rewarding opportunities in any of the following medical practices. Duties in such practices are often the same as those in a medical physician's office. The assistant would need to learn terminology specific to the particular practice and to become familiar with procedures common in that area.

Dentistry. Dentists are concerned with the care and treatment of the teeth and gums. Subspecialists in dentistry include the following:

- Endodontist: Specializes in root canal work.
- Oral surgeon: Specializes in jaw surgery and extractions.
- Orthodontist: Specializes in straightening teeth.
- Pedodontist: Specializes in dental care for children.
- Periodontist: Specializes in gum disease.
- Prosthodontist: Specializes in dentures and artificial teeth.

Optometry. Optometrists examine eyes, detect visual problems, and prescribe corrective lenses. Unlike ophthalmologists, optometrists cannot prescribe drugs or perform surgery.

Osteopathy. Osteopaths use physical manipulation of the spine and muscles along with other therapeutic measures to treat disorders.

Podiatry. Podiatrists are concerned with the prevention, diagnosis, and treatment of disorders of the feet.

PROJECT 3   Selecting a Medical Area

Consider the variety of work environments described in this chapter. Select three areas in which you would prefer to work. Write a short paragraph stating at least three reasons for each choice. Be prepared to discuss your selections in class.

Successful medical assistants enjoy an enviable professional status. Upon completion of specific requirements, they are eligible to join several professional associations and to seek national **certification** (an indication of having met certain qualifications) through examinations. These organizations provide medical assistants with opportunities to grow as office professionals and, in turn, to advance in their careers.

The American Association of Medical Assistants (AAMA) and the Council on Allied Health Education and Accreditation (CAHEA) of the American Medical Association (AMA) accredit formal educational programs for medical assistants, outlining the curriculum requirements for accredited programs. In addition, the AAMA and the National Board of Medical Examiners develop the national certification examination for medical assistants. An assistant who passes this examination and completes certain educational and work experience requirements earns the designation of Certified Medical Assistant (CMA). Special certifications such as the CMA and CPS (Certified Professional Secretary) show that the assistant is a top employee and increase chances for advancement. The AAMA also establishes the guidelines for continuing education through its national, state, and local societies.

In order to provide a comprehensive description of the job responsibilities of medical assistants, the AAMA has developed the chart shown in Figure 1-3 on pages 14-15. The DACUM (which devises its name from **D**eveloping **A** Curricul**UM**) describes the qualifications of a successful assistant. It can give you an idea of the qualities necessary to become successful and what the job will entail.

Another professional organization, the American Medical Technologists (AMT), serves as a registry of clinical laboratory personnel. The AMT also develops and administers a national registry examination for medical assistants. Assistants who pass this examination can earn the title of Registered Medical Assistant (RMA).

The American Association of Medical Transcription (AAMT) is an organization whose goal is to promote the professionalism of medical transcription. It provides members with continuing education, professional publications, and information on new products. It also works with legislators to promote and improve the profession. The AAMT has developed a model curriculum for medical transcription available from AAMT.

Professional Secretaries International (PSI) is a professional organization for administrative support personnel. PSI keeps members in touch with the latest trends in office technology and provides members with opportunities for continuing education and personal and professional development. Also, PSI develops and administers the CPS examination. Passing this comprehensive exam earns the designation Certified Professional Secretary, which often is a first step to promotion.

1.0 DISPLAY PROFESSIONALISM
1.1 Project a Positive Attitude
1.2 Perform Within Ethical Boundaries
1.3 Practice Within the Scope of Education, Training, and Personal Capabilities
1.4 Maintain Confidentiality
1.5 Work as a Team Member
1.6 Conduct Oneself in a Courteous and Diplomatic Manner
1.7 Adapt to Change
1.8 Show Initiative and Responsibility
1.9 Promote the Profession
Enhance* Skills Through Continuing Education

2.0 COMMUNICATE
2.1 Listen and Observe
2.2 Treat All Patients With Empathy and Impartiality
2.3 Adapt Communication to Individuals' Abilities to Understand
2.4 Recognize and Respond to Verbal and Non-verbal Communication
2.5 Serve as Liaison Between Physician and Others
2.6 Evaluate Understanding of Communication
2.7 Receive, Organize, Prioritize, and Transmit Information
2.8 Use Proper Telephone Techniques
2.9 Interview Effectively
2.10 Use Medical Terminology Appropriately
2.11 Compose Written Communication Using Correct Grammar, Spelling, and Format
Develop* and Conduct Public Relations Activities to Market Professional Services

3.0 PERFORM ADMINISTRATIVE DUTIES
3.1 Perform Basic Secretarial Skills
3.2 Schedule and Monitor Appointments
3.3 Prepare and Maintain Medical Records
3.4 Apply Computer Concepts for Office Procedures
3.5 Perform Medical Transcription
3.6 Locate Resources and Information for Patients and Employers
3.7 Manage Physician's Professional Schedule and Travel

4.0 PERFORM CLINICAL DUTIES
4.1 Apply Principles of Aseptic Technique and Infection Control
4.2 Take Vital Signs
4.3 Recognize Emergencies
4.4 Perform First Aid and CPR
4.5 Prepare and Maintain Examination and Treatment Area
4.6 Interview and Take Patient History

4.7 Prepare Patients for Procedures
4.8 Assist Physician With Examinations and Treatments
4.9 Use Quality Control
4.10 Collect and Process Specimens
4.11 Perform Selected Tests That Assist With Diagnosis and Treatment
4.12 Screen and Follow-up Patient Test Results
4.13 Prepare and Administer Medications as Directed by Physician
4.14 Maintain Medication Records
Respond* to Medical Emergencies

5.0 APPLY LEGAL CONCEPTS TO PRACTICE
5.1 Document Accurately
5.2 Determine Needs for Documentation and Reporting
5.3 Use Appropriate Guidelines When Releasing Records or Information
5.4 Follow Established Policy in Initiating or Terminating Medical Treatment
5.5 Dispose of Controlled Substances in Compliance With Government Regulations
5.6 Maintain Licenses and Accreditation
5.7 Monitor Legislation Related to Current Health-care Issues and Practice
Develop* and Maintain Policy and Procedure Manuals
Establish* Risk Management Protocol for the Practice

6.0 MANAGE THE OFFICE
6.1 Maintain the Physical Plant
6.2 Operate and Maintain Facilities and Equipment Safely
6.3 Inventory Equipment and Supplies
6.4 Evaluate and Recommend Equipment and Supplies for a Practice
6.5 Maintain Liability Coverage
6.6 Exercise Efficient Time Management
Supervise* Personnel
Develop* Job Descriptions
Interview* and Recommend New Personnel
Negotiate* Leases and Prices for Equipment and Supply Contracts

7.0 PROVIDE INSTRUCTION
7.1 Orient Patients to Office Policies and Procedures
7.2 Instruct Patients With Special Needs
7.3 Teach Patients Methods of Health Promotion and Disease Prevention
7.4 Orient and Train Personnel
Provide* Health Information for Public Use
Supervise* Student Practicums
Conduct* Continuing Education Activities
Develop* Educational Materials

* Denotes advanced-level skills.

8.0	**MANAGE PRACTICE FINANCES**	8.4	Manage Accounts Receivable
8.1	Use Manual Bookkeeping Systems	8.5	Manage Accounts Payable
8.2	Implement Current Procedural Terminology and ICD-9 Coding	8.6	Maintain Records for Accounting and Banking Purposes
8.3	Analyze and Use Current Third-Party Guidelines for Reimbursement	8.7	Process Employee Payroll Manage* Personnel Benefits and Records

*Denotes advanced-level skills.

The medical assistant should be able to perform all other skills after completing a CAHEA-accredited program and starting a first job.

Developed by The American Association of Medical Assistants, Inc.

Figure 1-3   The 1990 DACUM Analysis of the Medical Assisting Profession

PERSONAL DEVELOPMENT PROJECTS

Key Terms

The following terms appear in **boldface** type in this chapter. Do you recall what they mean? Refer to the chapter for definitions you need to review.

accounting clerk
administrative tasks
certification
clinic
clinical tasks
file clerk

group practice
insurance clerk
medical assistant
receptionist
transcriptionist

Topics for Discussion

1. Bring help-wanted ads from local newspapers into class. Discuss the job possibilities.
2. Compare the advantages and disadvantages of working in a medical office with those of working in a business office.

Role-Playing

1. Your friend Laura works as a medical records clerk in a large hospital, and she tells you about a job opening in the same medical records department. Explain to her why you might prefer a job that involves contact with patients.
2. Karl, a colleague, works as a medical assistant in an orthopedic office. He does not have the Certified Medical Assistant (CMA) designation. Explain to him the importance of becoming a CMA.

Qualifications for Success

Upon completion of this chapter, you should be able to:

■ List six personality characteristics essential to a medical assistant.

■ List and explain eight positive work attitudes.

■ Describe the appropriate appearance of a well-groomed assistant.

■ Discuss how to handle the following situations:
A talkative patient or coworker
An inquisitive patient
Requests for advice
Communications barriers
Office gossip
A patient with a complaint

■ Discuss social relationships between the assistant and office staff, and discuss social relationships between the assistant and patients.

■ PERSONAL ATTRIBUTES

In addition to a mastery of essential office skills, the success of the medical assistant is based on a positive attitude toward work and a cheerful personality. **Personality** is defined as the outward evidence of one's character, and certain aspects of an assistant's personality are important in dealing with patients and other medical professionals.

Most patients consider a friendly, pleasant personality to be the most important attribute in a medical assistant. Because so much of the medical assistant's time is spent helping patients, the following qualities are essential tools of the trade.

Genuine Liking for People

One key to the success of the medical assistant is genuinely liking people and wanting to help them. Smile and greet patients by name when they enter the doctor's office. This shows them that you like dealing with patients and care enough to give each of them personal attention.

Cheerfulness

Patients' spirits are lifted by a cheerful assistant, and this helps build goodwill between the patient and the physician. Not even a well person wants to see a gloomy face or deal with a gruff, uncaring person. No matter what cares or irritations you may have in your personal life, you must know how to suppress them and to present a calm and pleasant manner. A pleasant, friendly assistant can help avoid potential difficulties that may occur when patients are worried, anxious, and irritable.

Example

It is five o'clock, normal closing time for the office. The doctor is behind schedule because of several difficult cases, and there are two patients yet to be seen in the waiting room. One of the patients approaches the assistant.

PATIENT: I've been waiting a long time to see the doctor. How much longer will I have to wait?

Despite possibly feeling tired at the end of the day and ready to go home, the assistant must remain cheerful and explain the situation without frustration.

ASSISTANT: Dr. Newman has had several difficult cases today that have caused this delay. He will see you next, but it may be another 20 to 30 minutes.

Understanding and Patience

Sometimes patients may be irritable and difficult to deal with, but it is important for the assistant to remember that patients' irritability may be caused by concern for their health. The assistant must never argue with a patient or lose his or her temper, no matter what the situation. It is important to deal with any situation in an understanding and tolerant manner. Calmly repeating instructions to an uncooperative patient may be difficult, but it may prevent having to ask a patient to redo a procedure or task or having to repeat the instructions later.

Example

ASSISTANT: Peter, here are the instructions for the X ray you are going to have on Monday. Let me go over them with you again to make sure you understand them and to see whether you have any questions. If you think of any at a later time, you may call me. I have written my name and telephone number here and will be happy to help answer your questions.

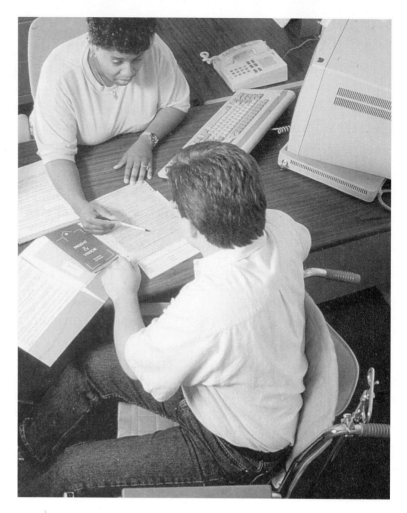

One of the best guides to conduct in dealing with patients is to remember your own experience with an illness and to ask yourself how you would like to be treated in a similar situation.

Helpfulness

The assistant should be aware of situations in which extra help can be offered to the physician, to patients, or to fellow employees. An unsolicited offer of help makes you a valued employee, one who goes beyond the job's regular responsibilities. For example, offering to stay late to help the physician or coworkers finish extra work is always appreciated. To give patients additional help, you may offer to complete insurance forms, telephone for a taxi after an appointment, obtain a wheelchair when needed, write out instructions, or send a reminder card before the next appointment.

Example

ASSISTANT: Mr. Larson, if you sign this insurance form now, I will enclose today's bill and put it in an addressed envelope for you. Then, all you need to do is put a stamp on it and put it in the mail.

Empathy

Almost everyone has been a patient at a medical facility at one time or another. One of the best guides to conduct in dealing with patients in the office is to remember your personal experience with an illness and to ask yourself how you would like to be treated in a similar situation. The ability to understand how a patient feels by mentally putting yourself in the patient's situation is called **empathy**. Having empathy for patients enables you to treat them with kindness.

Example

ASSISTANT: Mr. Strauss, I realize you are not feeling well after your surgery yesterday. Would you feel more comfortable lying down while you wait?

■ QUALITIES OF A GOOD MEDICAL OFFICE WORKER

Because the work in a physician's office often has life-or-death implications, having a reliable assistant is imperative to the physician. Even the slightest error on the part of the assistant may have consequences for a patient's health. Among the many requirements for a good medical assistant, most physicians stress that accuracy and dependability are the most important.

Accuracy and Dependability

The physician in a medical office depends on the medical assistant to know the responsibilities of the job and to perform them with little supervision. The physician issues exact instructions to the assistant but may not be present to oversee their completion. The physician counts on the assistant to perform tasks with complete **accuracy**, including constant attention to detail, especially if the assistant is responsible for clinical duties. Negligence may harm a patient or even endanger a life. If a patient is harmed during treatment as a result of an assistant's carelessness, the physician is legally responsible.

Dependability means finishing assigned work on time and doing unpleasant jobs without complaint. A dependable assistant does not need to be reminded to complete work or to follow up on assignments. The dependable assistant always:

■ Asks questions and repeats instructions to avoid making mistakes.
■ Asks for assistance with unfamiliar tasks.
■ Enters data such as lab values and information on patients carefully.
■ Takes clear and complete messages.

Judgment

The assistant must be able to evaluate a situation in a logical manner and use good **judgment** in making a decision.

Honesty

Trustworthiness and **honesty** are required of the medical assistant in all situations and at all times. Because of the serious nature of the physician's work, even the slightest indiscretion can involve the doctor and the assistant in a lawsuit. If you make a mistake, do not try to cover it up or blame another employee. Such behavior will inevitably ruin an assistant's career. Remember that using office supplies for personal business is dishonest.

Punctuality

An important part of being a dependable medical assistant is **punctuality**. If the office opens at 9 a.m., you should be there and ready to start work at 9 a.m. Allow a few minutes before the start of office hours to pull patients' charts from the file and to attend to other routine duties before patients start arriving. Patients anxious to see the doctor may arrive even before the start of business hours, so it is important to be at the office a little early to greet them. Traffic delays, missed trains or buses, and last-minute interruptions at home are not excuses for being late. Take only the allotted time for breaks and for lunch.

Thoroughness

The practice of medicine is filled with many details that must be checked to ensure accuracy. Proper care of patients is founded upon the accuracy of information used in treatment. Attending to details may seem to be a waste of time at the moment, but making an extra note or saving a printed statement may save time and effort later. The successful medical assistant knows **thoroughness** means:

- Listening attentively.
- Taking ample notes.
- Paying attention to details such as who, when, why, where, and how.
- Verifying information.
- Following through on details without having to be reminded.
- Always doing work that is neat, accurate, and complete.

Efficiency

Doing a job with a minimum of cost, waste, and effort means doing a job with **efficiency**. A well-organized medical assistant plans the day's work in advance, develops a schedule for its completion, and does not waste time. Large tasks are often completed most effectively by being divided into smaller, more manageable components. The efficient assistant also keeps the office well organized by returning items to their proper place after using them.

Flexibility

Even the plans of the most highly organized medical assistant will be sidetracked by changes, interruptions, and delays. **Flexibility** is the key to calmly dealing with such situations. The flexible assistant is able to meet deadlines under pressure and to complete several tasks at the same time.

The assistant must be prepared to perform additional assignments at a moment's notice without becoming frustrated or angry. An important technique for keeping flexible in such situations is to make notes about the work you were doing when you were interrupted. Such notes serve as timesaving reminders when you resume the interrupted task.

Tact

Much of the medical assistant's work with patients and medical staff requires **tact**, which is the ability to speak and to act skillfully and considerately in difficult situations or with difficult people. This ability can be developed by being sensitive to the reactions of others. Using tact enables you to achieve the purpose at hand in a manner that will not give offense but will create goodwill with the patient or staff member.

Accepting Criticism

No matter how capable and efficient you are, the doctor may prefer things done in a different way than you know from your training or previous employment. **Criticism** should be accepted gracefully as a constructive way of helping you do a better job or avoid mistakes. Emotional outbursts are out of place in any office, especially in an office full of patients.

Getting Along With Others

Learning the unwritten rules of the office is an important step toward getting along with the physician and fellow employees. Observe the accepted procedures in your office for the following situations:

- Sitting at another employee's desk.
- Eating or drinking at your desk.
- Timing a break and determining how long it should be.
- Conversing with coworkers.

Never waste the employer's time by conducting personal activities during work hours or by making personal phone calls. Always knock before entering an office, whether the door is open or closed.

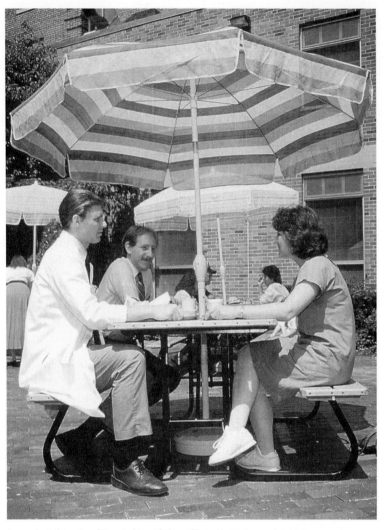

Learning the unwritten rules of the office is an important step toward getting along with the physician and fellow employees.

Exercise good judgment when contributing to a conversation or sharing personal aspects of your life with coworkers. It is not appropriate to discuss your feelings about patients or other coworkers with members of the staff. In addition, work is not the place to develop intimate relationships. Dating a coworker may cause gossip and jealousy, thus becoming a detriment to staff harmony and to your career.

Be cooperative with other staff members by performing your share of the workload. Refrain from asking others to cover for you.

It is important to respect office practices that are already in place. Establish good working relationships with other staff members before suggesting changes you feel would improve the office. Be assertive in offering new ideas and in working with others, but do not be aggressive. **Assertiveness** is stepping forward to make a point in a confident, positive way; **aggressiveness** involves taking a hostile tone.

A doctor assumes the assistant knows how to act in a professional manner—doing and saying the right thing at the right time, not the wrong thing at any time. Remember that as a medical assistant you are part of the professional staff of the hospital or the doctor's office and must act accordingly.

Poise

A person who chooses a career as a medical assistant must realize from the beginning that the hours may be as irregular and hectic as those of the doctor. For example, patients may become upset when they cannot choose a convenient appointment time. Even when office hours are regular, unexpected events are quite likely to occur, causing delays. Delays are frustrating for the patient, the doctor, and the assistant. Patients are sensitive to the assistant's mood, so it is important to be calm in every situation. An assistant must possess considerable **poise** to be able to remain calm, gracious, and pleasant in the face of the most troublesome situations.

Personal and Professional Growth

The assistant should feel motivated to take advantage of seminars, in-service workshops, and professional organizations to keep up to date with new developments. Maintaining an awareness of the latest developments in office and medical technology, as well as a solid base of technical skills, is the mark of a true professional. As computer software evolves, it is likely that new **applications software** will be included in your job responsibilities. Software is the program used to run a computer and to instruct it to perform specialized tasks, or applications, such as word processing. Your learning must keep pace with these changes.

Sound knowledge of medical terminology and abbreviations is also an important requirement for work in a medical office. In addition, proficiency in office skills such as keyboarding, transcribing, and records management are essential.

Participation in community activities is another part of being a responsible office professional. One way to participate is to assist your employer at community functions such as health fairs or fund-raising events.

Maturity

Emotional **maturity** is not dependent upon age. Maturity is made up of many characteristics. The mature person is able to work under authority and under pressure, in conditions that may be frustrating or unpleasant. The mature person possesses the ability to stick with a job and give more than is asked. Maturity means making your own decisions and following through with them, being independent, and having the ambition and determination to be a success.

PROJECT 4 | **Professional Conduct**

On WP 2, match each of the professional conduct terms shown in Column 2 with the proper definition in Column 1. Be prepared to discuss your answers in class.

PROJECT 5 | **Evaluating Your Qualifications**

A checklist of qualities needed by a medical assistant appears on WP 3. Evaluate yourself on the qualities listed by checking Column 1 under the appropriate category for each quality. At the end of the course, your instructor will rate you using Column 2. You will also have an opportunity to re-evaluate yourself in Column 3 and compare the ratings.

■ PERSONAL APPEARANCE

In addition to the qualities just discussed, personal appearance is also very important. Because you will be working in a medical office, your appearance should present to patients the picture of health. Good health is the result of taking proper care of yourself—maintaining good posture, eating a healthy diet, getting proper rest, and exercising regularly.

Good Grooming

Good **grooming** implies more than just cleanliness. A daily bath or shower, use of deodorant, and good dental care are indispensable, but so is a neat appearance. Nails must be manicured so that hands look cared for and presentable. Gaudy, vividly painted or stenciled fingernails are not appropriate in a medical office.

Hair requires frequent shampooing and should be styled in a conservative, appropriate style. Hair should not look unkempt. For women, cosmetics may be used to help you look better and healthier, not to make you conspicuous. Perfumes and colognes are acceptable if the fragrance is light; strong fragrances may be noxious to a patient who is ill.

Clothing

Clothes should be freshly laundered and neatly pressed, with no ripped seams, open hems, or loose buttons.

Some offices require staff members to wear a uniform. Uniforms have a psychological effect: Patients may have more confidence in a

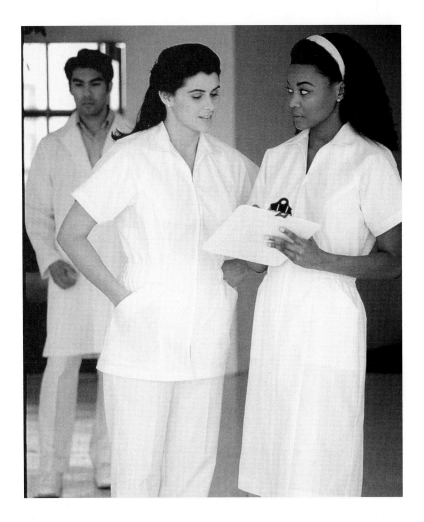

Uniforms give the medical assistant a professional appearance that inspires confidence in the assistant's ability.

uniformed assistant's ability to perform a test; also, patients may be less embarrassed to disrobe in front of or to give personal information to a uniformed assistant. If the uniform is white, it must be kept snow white and should not be worn over dark underclothes.

Street clothes are preferred in practices such as pediatrics, psychiatry, and oncology. Street clothes should be simple and appropriate, without elaborate ornamentation, lacy flounces, low necklines, or short hemlines. Sweat shirts and jeans are inappropriate. Shoes should be comfortable and kept well polished. White shoes worn with a uniform should be kept white. Jewelry and hair ornaments do not go well with uniforms, and they should be kept to a minimum with street clothes in the office. Some necklaces and bracelets get in the way when you are working, while rings are exposed to soaps and lotions with the frequent hand washing done in a medical office.

■ INTERACTING WITH PATIENTS

As a rule, the assistant is the first person that patients meet when coming to the doctor's office. The way the assistant receives and welcomes the patient will influence the patient's attitude toward the doctor and the treatment.

When the office is busy, the assistant may be called upon to do many things at once. Both the doctor and patients may want to speak to the assistant at the same time; the telephone may be ringing; a patient may be waiting for treatment. In such situations the efficient assistant remains calm. No matter how many demands there are on the doctor's and the assistant's time, each patient must be made to feel important and to believe that sufficient time is available to attend to treatment.

Patients should be greeted by name, if possible. If a patient enters while you are away from the desk, you should acknowledge the patient's presence by a smile or a hello.

Every patient should be offered the same respect and concern regardless of age, race, or socioeconomic background. In every doctor's office, there are patients who receive medical care for a nominal fee or even completely free of charge. The amount a person pays should have no bearing on the quality of treatment received. The physician's aim is to make that person well in the shortest time possible. Indigent patients require the same amount of attention and sympathy as patients paying a fee.

Familiarity

Theoretically, it should make no difference to patients whether the doctor and the assistant are related to each other or friends. Nevertheless, regardless of the degree of **familiarity**, or intimacy, between the physician and the assistant, nothing in their conversation in front of patients should indicate anything other than a professional relationship. The doctor should be referred to by title and last name. The assistant may be referred to by first name only or by title and last name, if that is preferred. For example, "Doctor Newman will see you now."

The assistant should ask patients whether they prefer to be called by their first or last name ("Mrs. Haynes," for example). This relationship promotes goodwill and gives a personal touch.

Example

ASSISTANT: Mrs. Haynes, Dr. Newman is ready to see you now.

PATIENT: Thank you, Linda, but please call me Margaret. I'm not used to being called Mrs. Haynes.

Social Relationships

In the course of work, the assistant will meet men and women who come to the office frequently and with whom the assistant becomes friendly. A real liking may develop, and patients may invite the assistant to go out with them. Under no circumstances should a social engagement be made with a patient without first checking the office policy and discussing the situation with the employer. Many physicians have a strict rule on this point, feeling that a social relationship between patient and assistant is not consistent with a professional atmosphere and may interfere with the proper medical management of the patient's case.

Conversation

If the assistant has to spend considerable time with a patient, the patient should be the one to decide whether to start a conversation. If the patient wishes to talk, let the patient choose the subject. The assistant should listen and respond courteously. Safe, general subjects such as the weather, motion pictures, or books are ideal topics for conversation. Avoid matters that may be controversial, such as politics and religion.

Never argue with a patient or try to persuade a patient that a certain view is right. Never, under any circumstances, offer a patient medical advice. The patient identifies the assistant with the doctor and thus believes the assistant carries the doctor's authority. Very few patients have a substantial knowledge of medicine, anatomy, or physiology, and so they may easily misunderstand a remark made by an assistant.

Example

PATIENT: I've been having these spasms in my back occasionally. Should I take Motrin or Flexeril?

ASSISTANT: That is a question the doctor should answer for you. Be sure you ask about that during your examination.

Confidentiality

The medical assistant must understand the importance of maintaining the **confidentiality**, or secrecy, of patients' medical information. In fact, it is a legal requirement. A doctor who divulges information about a patient without permission from the patient, except to another doctor, can be prosecuted under the law, and the doctor's license may be revoked. This also applies to employees in the doctor's office.

Employees will learn many things about the personal affairs of patients and doctors alike, but these should not become topics for conversation and gossip. The medical histories of patients yield much confidential information, not only regarding the patients themselves but also about other members of their families and perhaps their friends as well. Employees may not disclose any details of a patient's illness, personal history, or matters relating to the family.

Example

COWORKER: Have you heard the latest about Mr. Jefferson?

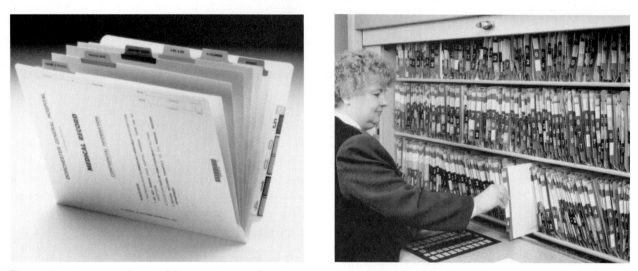

The assistant must understand the importance of maintaining the confidentiality of patient medical records.

ASSISTANT: No, I haven't. I don't think that information about a patient should be discussed with anyone.

A patient may question the assistant about an illness, hoping to learn more than the doctor has told. It is not the assistant's place to tell the patient the doctor's opinion in regard to either the diagnosis or the prognosis of the case, even when the assistant knows it. The doctor has medical reasons for giving or withholding information and is the judge of what the patient should know about the condition. The assistant should firmly refuse to discuss the patient's case, refer the patient to the doctor for information, and limit the conversation to general topics.

Patients are often curious about other patients, especially those who have an obvious deformity or illness. Friends or relatives of a patient may inquire about the doctor's opinion, the method of treatment, or the length of illness. Patients may try to obtain personal information about the doctor, the staff, or other patients. Without giving offense, the assistant must make it clear that such information will not be revealed. A tactful, courteous, but firm refusal will prevent further questioning.

Example

PATIENT: How long has Mrs. Berg been taking that medicine?

ASSISTANT: I'm sorry, but that information is confidential.

Office papers should be carefully guarded from prying eyes. Patients' histories, laboratory tests, letters, and other data should not be left lying on a desk while the assistant is out of the room. A person may innocently be standing at the front desk to fill out a form and casually glance at a paper that contains information of a most personal and private nature. Patients may ask to see their own medical records. However, refer this request to the doctor, who will then explain the data to the patient to avoid possible misunderstandings.

Be aware of the location of the front desk and the various work areas in relation to the lobby or waiting room. Conversations between a patient and an assistant or among employees can easily be overheard, whether the conversation is over the telephone or face-to-face.

Special care must be taken never to mention a patient's name outside the office. For example, there may be a good reason that a patient wishes not to tell family members or business associates that medical care is required. The doctor's specialty may be an indication of the disease for which the patient is being treated, and the patient may not wish this to be known.

Nothing that happens in the office should be repeated at home or to friends because a patient can sometimes be identified from the circumstances of a case, even if the patient's name is not mentioned.

Remember the adage: What you see here, what you hear here, must remain here when you leave.

Difficult Patients

The best test of good interpersonal skills is being able to handle the difficult, unreasonable, or unpleasant patient.

At times, the patient's power of self-control may be undermined by the pain and worry that accompany an illness, causing the patient to be short-tempered or disagreeable. Dealing with such patients requires a great deal of understanding and restraint. It is difficult not to show signs of anger or frustration in such circumstances, but the assistant must maintain an air of calm professionalism.

A patient who has to wait a considerable time before being seen by the doctor may become restless or impatient. In such instances, some gesture of attention, such as a brief, friendly conversation, may be helpful. An inquiry about a person's health is usually appreciated, but it is sometimes resented, especially if the patient has not felt the expected relief from the treatment given or prescribed by the doctor. This topic may also lead to a long conversation that takes up the time of a busy assistant. Safe, general topics such as the patient's interests or hobbies or the weather are preferable.

The patient's time is important too. When the assistant knows there will be a long delay, one option is to call the patient ahead of time to suggest that the patient come to the office later than scheduled, if possible. If the patient is already at the office, mention that there is time for the patient to run an errand or go for a cup of coffee and return in 20 minutes. Either of these options goes a long way toward recognizing the patient's inconvenience and promoting goodwill.

If a patient continues to complain about a situation, it may be wise to take the complaining patient into a private office away from the other patients. The assistant should maintain a calm and pleasant manner at all times and speak in a quiet, soothing voice. This may have a calming effect on the patient.

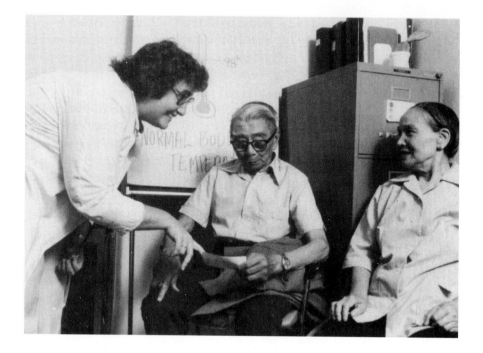

Language barriers between patients and office staff can be overcome by using good communications skills.

Example

ASSISTANT: I can understand that you are upset about your insurance payment, Mrs. Sanchez. If you will come with me, you can explain the situation to me and we will see what we can do.

Never argue with a patient. Politely offer to help correct the situation in any way you can. Such an offer will help eliminate the patient's anger.

The patient should leave the medical office with a feeling of goodwill. Frequently, the assistant will have an opportunity to talk with the patient when the doctor is through with the examination and before the patient leaves the facility. A pleasant good-bye from the assistant will have beneficial effects, whatever the results of the visit. A satisfied patient will spread the word about the good relationships in the doctor's office.

Language Barriers in the Office

If the office staff does not have sign language skills, an ideal way to communicate with deaf patients is to write notes with a pad and pencil. A greater barrier to office communication occurs when the patient and staff do not speak the same language. Ideally, an accompanying friend or family member can act as an interpreter. Another solution is to have several foreign language phrase books on hand in the office. Using models, illustrations, and hand signs may be the only alternatives in certain situations. Remember these guidelines for communicating with patients who do not speak English:

- Speak slowly and clearly.
- Do not raise your voice. Speaking louder does not increase understanding.

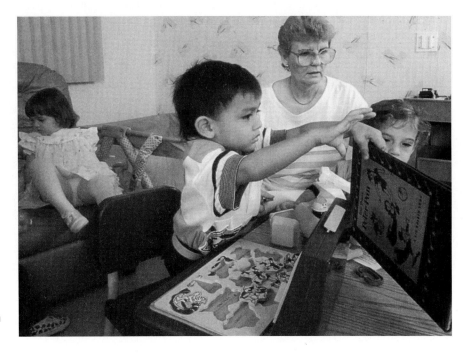

It may be necessary for parents to leave children unattended while being examined by the doctor; the medical assistant should help by suggesting suitable activities for the children while they wait.

- Use simple words, not technical terms.
- Be brief.

Terminally Ill Patients

If a terminally ill patient chooses to start a conversation with you, try to steer the conversation to general topics or subjects of interest to the patient, such as hobbies. Do not discuss the patient's health or ask the question, "How are you?"

Nonpatients

All visitors to the doctor's office should be greeted courteously. Often, a patient's friends or relatives will accompany the patient to the office. A parent may leave children in the waiting room unattended while being examined by the doctor. In such cases, the assistant may have to help children by suggesting alternatives to disruptive behavior.

Example

ASSISTANT *(TO NOISY CHILDREN)*: Your father should be back soon. While you are waiting, here is a puzzle for you to do.

Sales representatives of firms such as medical supply companies, pharmaceutical companies, and book publishers will visit the office for business reasons. The doctor's schedule may not permit the doctor to see these people, and the doctor may ask an assistant to talk with the representatives, gather information about the products, obtain samples, and keep the business cards on file. Some offices schedule a definite time each month for representatives to present materials to the doctor.

Example

SALES REPRESENTATIVE: I'm here to see Dr. Newman about ordering a new antibiotic from my company.

ASSISTANT: Dr. Newman has scheduled the first Monday of each month from noon to 2 p.m. as the time he will see sales representatives. Shall I enter your name on the calendar for next month?

There may be other visitors who take up the doctor's time unnecessarily, and most doctors appreciate an assistant who screens them. For example, if the assistant has been told that the doctor is not interested in the particular material a sales representative is showing, the assistant should tell the salesperson firmly and politely that the doctor is not interested.

PROJECT 6   Interactions With Patients and Coworkers

On WP 4, circle the best answer for each situation described. Be prepared to discuss your answers in class.

PERSONAL DEVELOPMENT PROJECTS

Key Terms
The following terms appear in **boldface** type in this chapter. Do you recall what they mean? Refer to the chapter for definitions you need to review.

accuracy	flexibility
aggressiveness	grooming
applications software	honesty
assertiveness	judgment
confidentiality	maturity
criticism	personality
dependability	poise
efficiency	punctuality
empathy	tact
familiarity	thoroughness

Topics for Discussion
1. Relate to the class any good impressions or bad impressions you received from your personal experience of visits to medical offices.
2. Different kinds of jobs require people with different types of personalities. Discuss the type of personality needed by a medical assistant in various kinds of medical offices as well as in business offices.
3. Visit a clinic or medical facility to observe the medical assistant as if you were a patient. Be prepared to discuss your observations with the class. (*Caution*: Do not identify the facility.)

Role-Playing
The following situations are occurring in your office. Discuss with the class how you would handle them.

1. Two children in the lobby are taking pebbles out of the plant containers and tossing them. No parent is in attendance.
2. Mrs. Phillips, a patient, tells you that her prescribed medicine costs too much, so she stopped taking it.
3. Bob Jones, a patient, complains because he has to return the next day for another blood test.
4. During the holiday season, your neighbor brings candy into the office to sell for a fund-raising event.

Medical Ethics and Law

Upon completion of this chapter, you should be able to:

- Define *ethics*, *etiquette*, and *medical liability*.

- Discuss the principles of medical ethics as they apply to both physicians and medical assistants.

- Discuss the general requirements for the licensing of a physician.

- Explain the physician's liability for employees.

- Explain what is meant by *implied, informed, expressed*, and *written consent*.

- Determine appropriate behavior when asked for information about a patient and when a patient requests treatment advice.

- Identify situations requiring a release-of-information or a consent form.

- Select and prepare the proper forms for procedures requiring consent or release of information.

- Discuss the patient's rights and responsibilities in receiving medical care.

- Give the definitions of legal terms used in this chapter.

- Discuss the physician-patient relationship.

- Summarize safeguards for preventing malpractice litigation as they apply to employees.

■ MEDICAL ETHICS

Every profession is governed by certain standards, known as **ethics**, which are the principles of right and wrong conduct for members of that profession. These are not laws, but they are principles developed to maintain a high degree of competency among the members of a profession. Medical ethics concern the conduct of the physician regarding the patient and society. Laws are established by elected local, state, and national officials as rules for proper conduct, but they may be less strict than medical ethics.

Etiquette

Ethics is defined as a "standard of conduct"; **etiquette** is defined as "manners and customs." These two areas complement each other, and at times they overlap.

Etiquette forms a basis for all communications in a medical office and includes using good telephone techniques, greeting office visitors with a smile, expressing consideration in medical correspondence, and being courteous in all situations. Professional courtesy is shown when another physician visits the office. For example, rather than have the visiting physician wait in the reception area, the medical assistant asks the visitor to wait in the doctor's private office. In addition, doctors typically do not charge a fee when providing medical care to another doctor or the doctor's family.

The Hippocratic Oath

Medical ethics are based on the Hippocratic oath. Hippocrates, a Greek physician who lived in the fourth and fifth centuries B.C., is called "the Father of Medicine." The principles he devised governed the conduct of physicians toward their patients, other health professionals, and the public.

Principles of Medical Ethics

The basic principles behind the Hippocratic oath remain the foundation for modern medical ethics. To accommodate the rapid changes of the modern world, the American Medical Association (AMA) has developed the Principles of Medical Ethics, which serves as an accepted code of conduct for physicians. This code, shown in Figure 3-1, outlines the relationship between the physician and the patient, the physician and other members of the profession, and the physician and society at large.

Bioethics

The development of new medical technology and procedures has raised many new moral and ethical questions that fall within the realm of bioethics. The field of bioethics deals with issues that present many questions but few answers. Issues include the time of viability of a fetus; fetal rights; genetic engineering; artificial insemination; surrogate motherhood; paternal responsibility; maternal obligations; use of fetal tissue; allocation of organs for transplantation; and regulation of health care, euthanasia, and life support.

With the advancement of technology in sustaining life, more and more people are concerned with living wills and durable power of attorney. Simply stated, the living will is made by a competent person stating the intent to refuse certain life-sustaining measures at some future time should that person become unable to make that decision. This document becomes invalid upon the incapacity or death of that individual.

The durable power of attorney, given by a competent person, delegates the authority to act on the patient's behalf if the patient becomes incapacitated. As with the living will, its purpose is to make the patient's wishes regarding life support known. A patient may wish this document to become part of the medical record. The physician

Figure 3-1 American Medical Association Principles of Medical Ethics
Reprinted with the permission of the American Medical Association.

will discuss this with the patient, and a notation is then made in the patient's record. Life-support measures may be documented in the chart as "do not resuscitate"(DNR) or "do not intubate "(DNI).

In situations where these issues have not been discussed or family members disagree, the case may require settlement through a court of law.

It is important to understand that the ethical decisions of a physician may not coincide with your own feelings. If, in such cases, your feelings differ very strongly from those of the doctor, it may be wise to seek employment with another practice. Because research and technology increase the scope of medical treatment daily, new bioethical issues are certain to arise.

The Assistant's Responsibility

The underlying principle of the physician's devotion to the profession is evident in the AMA's Principles of Medical Ethics. While performing within the scope of employment, the medical assistant is considered an agent of the physician. The American Association of Medical Assistants (AAMA) has developed the Code of Ethics and Creed to provide assistants with guidelines for ethical conduct. This code is based on the AMA principles; it is shown in Figure 3-2 on page 36. A competent assistant plays an important role in the office by aspiring to these same standards of conduct in his or her professional life.

Remember to respect human dignity by treating each patient with the same respect and concern regardless of the patient's race, age, nationality, or socioeconomic background. The assistant plays an important role in maintaining a good rapport with the patient and the hospital or clinic.

AMERICAN ASSOCIATION OF MEDICAL ASSISTANTS
CODE OF ETHICS AND CREED

CODE OF ETHICS
The Code of Ethics of AAMA shall set forth principles of ethical and moral conduct as they relate to the medical profession and the particular practice of medical assisting.

Members of AAMA dedicated to the conscientious pursuit of their profession, and thus desiring to merit the high regard of the entire medical profession and the respect of the general public which they serve, do pledge themselves to strive always to:

A. Render service with full respect for the dignity of humanity;
B. Respect confidential information obtained through employment unless legally authorized or required by responsible performance of duty to divulge such information;
C. Uphold the honor and high principles of the profession and accept its disciplines;
D. Seek to continually improve the knowledge and skills of medical assistants for the benefit of patients and professional colleagues;
E. Participate in additional service activities aimed toward improving the health and well-being of the community.

CREED
I believe in the principles and purposes of the profession of medical assisting.
I endeavor to be more effective.
I aspire to render greater service.
I protect the confidence entrusted to me.
I am dedicated to the care and well-being of all patients.
I am loyal to my physician-employer.
I am true to the ethics of my profession.
I am strengthened by compassion, courage and faith.

Figure 3-2 American Association of Medical Assistants Code of Ethics and Creed

Also keep in mind that a promise or commitment made by an assistant can be legally binding upon the doctor. Keep to yourself everything you hear, see, and read about doctors or other health professionals. However, if you believe a doctor or other health professional is acting unethically or unprofessionally, discuss your feelings with your employer or another physician. A physician has the medical background to determine whether questionable conduct should be referred to the AMA or to another regulatory organization.

MEDICAL PRACTICE ACTS

The primary responsibility of the physician is the welfare of his or her patients. The practice of medicine means the diagnosis; the treatment; and the prescription for prevention or cure of a disease, ailment, injury, or deformity of a physical or a mental condition. It encompasses physicians, nurse practitioners, physicians' assistants, and other health professionals who are held to the standards of care required by their state licensing organizations. These standards are stated in the Medical Practice Act and are regulated by each state. Exact provisions of this law vary slightly from state to state, but the general principles prescribe who must be licensed to perform various procedures, the requirements for licensure, duties imposed by the license, grounds on which a license may be revoked, statutory reports that must be made to the government, and similar matters.

Licensing

Each state has a board that grants the license to practice medicine. Licenses are issued after completion of the required education, upon examination, as a result of **reciprocity** (one state's recognizing another state's requirements for licensure), or by endorsement (passing the exam of the National Board of Medical Examiners). Periodic relicensure (registration) is required either annually or biennially. This is accomplished by paying a fee and providing evidence of continuing education requirements.

The Medical Practice Act in each state prescribes penalties for practicing medicine without a valid license. Suspension or revocation of a license may result from conviction of a felony (for example, insurance fraud), unprofessional conduct (for example, sexual misconduct with a patient), personal or professional incapacity, inappropriate personal use of drugs or narcotics, or overprescribing such drugs.

Specialization

Additional education is required to become a specialist. Specialties vary from state to state and have different lengths of hospital residency. For example, dermatology may require five years; obstetrics, four years; and family practice, two years. Specialists may then choose to become board-certified by the American Board of Specialties. This board determines the competency of a candidate in accordance with requirements for academic in-hospital training, in which the student, known as a "resident," concentrates on learning that specialty and takes a subsequent comprehensive examination. Certification is more than a recognition of excellence in a specialty; it is considered an essential minimum standard of competence in the particular specialty. After certification, the candidate is known as a "diplomate," for example, Lucy C. Weng, M.D., Board-Certified Diplomate in Nuclear Medicine.

Narcotic Registration

Not all physicians prescribe medications; only those in a clinical practice do. For example, pathologists and doctors in research do not write prescriptions.

A federal permit must be obtained by a physician in clinical practice who will have occasion to prescribe or dispense narcotic drugs. A physician must register with the registration branch of the Drug Enforcement Administration (DEA). This permit must be renewed annually.

All drugs and prescription pads should be kept by the doctor in a locked area to avoid being picked up and misused by someone else. Any concerns you may have about the way in which drugs are stored or dispensed in the office should be reported to the physician.

■ MEDICAL LAW

Medical jurisprudence, or law, is the result of legislation passed by elected officials and is based on the standards of acceptable practice established by the medical profession. The standards of medical ethics are sometimes higher than the conduct called for in medical law. Thus, an illegal act by the doctor is always unethical, but an unethical act by the doctor may not be illegal. Medical law holds many responsibilities for both the doctor and the staff of a medical office. Lack of proper professional conduct on the part of the doctor or the office staff may result in a criminal offense or a civil lawsuit. Criminal law governs the rights and responsibilities of individuals within society, while civil law governs the obligations between individuals. Most lawsuits involving doctors are cases governed by civil law.

The Physician-Patient Relationship

The relationship between the doctor and the patient is entered into when the patient comes to the physician for care. Once the physician has accepted a person as a patient, the physician is obligated to provide appropriate treatment for as long as necessary or to terminate the relationship by established methods. In turn, the patient is required to pay the doctor's fee as compensation for care. Even though this agreement between the physician and the patient is rarely put in writing, it is considered a **contract**, that is, a legally binding agreement. If either party does not fulfill the obligations of the agreement, a **breach of contract**, or violation of the contract, is said to occur.

An exception to the assumed contract between patient and physician is emergency care. For example, a physician who is responsible for providing emergency care in an emergency room or a clinic cannot refuse to treat any patient who applies to that facility with an identifiable emergency. However, no legal relationship exists between the physician and the patient in such an emergency situation.

The physician-patient relationship is not always a personal one. For example, a radiologist who reads and interprets X rays or a pathologist who examines and evaluates a biological specimen may never see the patient.

The Physician's Obligations

When a **physician-patient relationship** is entered into, the physician is legally required to:

- Possess the ordinary skill and learning commonly held by a reputable physician in the same field of practice in a similar locality. (The patient has the right to believe the physician is so qualified. Accordingly, the doctor's license should be displayed in the office.)
- Use his or her learning, skill, and best judgment for the benefit of the patient.

- Preserve confidentiality.
- Act in good faith.
- Perform to the best of his or her ability.
- Advise against needless or unwise treatment.
- Inform and advise the patient when the physician knows a condition is beyond his or her scope of competency.

The physician is not legally required to:

- Accept as patients all who seek the physician's services.
- Restore a patient to the same condition that existed before illness occurred.
- Obtain recovery for every patient.
- Guarantee successful results from an operation or a treatment.
- Be familiar with the reactions of patients to various medicines.
- Make a correct diagnosis.
- Be free from errors in judgment in complex cases.
- Possess the maximum amount of education possible.
- Continue care after a patient discharges himself or herself, even if harm could come to the patient.

The family practitioner is not required to have all of the specialized knowledge that a specialist in another field would have.

The Patient's Obligations

The Patient's Bill of Rights of the American Hospital Association, shown in Figure 3-3 on page 40, states some of the patient's responsibilities. These include the willingness to follow the treatment plan and to provide the physician with complete and accurate information. The patient is also responsible for paying for the treatment received.

PROJECT 7   Obligations of the Patient and the Physician

WP 5 contains numbered items that refer to the obligations of the physician and of the patient. Mark each statement completion either "T" for *true* or "F" for *false*. Be prepared to discuss your answers in class.

■ PRIVILEGED COMMUNICATIONS

All information furnished to a physician by a patient is considered confidential and may not be divulged to any unauthorized person. The medical assistant who processes the doctor's correspondence and works with patients' medical records is considered such an authorized person. However, the assistant must not convey this information to anyone, not even the patient, without expressed **authorization** from, or permission of, the doctor. If the assistant gives out such informa-

A PATIENT'S BILL OF RIGHTS

The American Hospital Association presents a Patient's Bill of Rights with the expectation that observance of these rights will contribute to more effective patient care and greater satisfaction for the patient, his physician, and the hospital organization. Further, the Association presents these rights in the expectation that they will be supported by the hospital on behalf of its patients, as an integral part of the healing process. It is recognized that a personal relationship between the physician and the patient is essential for the provision of proper medical care. The traditional physician-patient relationship takes on a new dimension when care is rendered within an organizational structure. Legal precedent has established that the institution itself also has a responsibility to the patient. It is in recognition of these factors that these rights are affirmed.

1. The patient has the right to considerate and respectful care.

2. The patient has the right to obtain from his physician complete current information concerning his diagnosis, treatment, and prognosis in terms the patient can be reasonably expected to understand. When it is not medically advisable to give such information to the patient, the information should be made available to an appropriate person in his behalf. He has the right to know, by name, the physician responsible for coordinating his care.

3. The patient has the right to receive from his physician information necessary to give informed consent prior to the start of any procedure and/or treatment. Except in emergencies, such information for informed consent should include but not necessarily be limited to the specific procedure and/or treatment, the medically significant risks involved, and the probable duration of incapacitation. Where medically significant alternatives for care or treatment exist, or when the patient requests information concerning medical alternatives, the patient has the right to such information. The patient also has the right to know the name of the person responsible for the procedures and/or treatment.

4. The patient has the right to refuse treatment to the extent permitted by law and to be informed of the medical consequences of his action.

5. The patient has the right to every consideration of his privacy concerning his own medical care program. Case discussion, consultation, examination, and treatment are confidential and should be conducted discreetly. Those not directly involved in his care must have the permission of the patient to be present.

6. The patient has the right to expect that all communications and records pertaining to his care should be treated as confidential.

7. The patient has the right to expect that within its capacity a hospital must make reasonable response to the request of a patient for services. The hospital must provide evaluation, service, and/or referral as indicated by the urgency of the case. When medically permissible, a patient may be transferred to another facility only after he has received complete information and explanation concerning the need for and alternatives to such a transfer. The institution to which the patient is to be transferred must first have accepted the patient for transfer.

8. The patient has the right to obtain information as to any relationship of his hospital to other health care and educational institutions insofar as his care is concerned. The patient has the right to obtain information as to the existence of any professional relationships among individuals, by name, who are treating him.

9. The patient has the right to be advised if the hospital proposes to engage in or perform human experimentation affecting his care or treatment. The patient has the right to refuse to participate in such research projects.

10. The patient has the right to expect reasonable continuity of care. He has the right to know in advance what appointment times and physicians are available and where. The patient has the right to expect that the hospital will provide a mechanism whereby he is informed by his physician or a delegate of the physician of the patient's continuing health care requirements following discharge.

11. The patient has the right to examine and receive an explanation of his bill regardless of source of payment.

12. The patient has the right to know what hospital rules and regulations apply to his conduct as a patient.

No catalog of rights can guarantee for the patient the kind of treatment he has a right to expect. A hospital has many functions to perform, including the prevention and treatment of disease, the education of both health professionals and patients, and the conduct of clinical research. All these activities must be conducted with an overriding concern for the patient, and, above all, the recognition of his dignity as a human being. Success in achieving this recognition assures success in the defense of the rights of the patient.

Figure 3-3   American Hospital Association Patient's Bill of Rights

tion without proper authorization and it is later misused, the doctor may be sued for invasion of privacy.

The assistant is responsible for informing the doctor of all information given to the assistant by the patient. If the patient has questions, appears confused, or seems not to understand, the assistant should inform the physician. Likewise, any unpleasant incident that may have occurred between the patient and any member of the staff should be brought to the physician's attention. This is accomplished by a notation to the doctor and does not become part of the medical record. The doctor will then act on the assistant's observation and discuss the matter with the patient.

Statutory Reports

Exceptions to the doctor's confidentiality are **statutory reports**. The doctor is required by law to file such a report of confidential information to state departments of health or social services under certain circumstances. Mandatory reports are generally made to protect the health of the community. In the physician's office within the scope of employment, a person should file a statutory report only when delegated to do so by the physician. Agencies provide guidelines for filing complaints.

The individual states are responsible for making and enforcing these laws. Some examples of circumstances requiring statutory reports are:

- Births.
- Deaths.
- Abuse of a child, a vulnerable or elderly adult, or a battered woman. In private life, anyone may file a complaint with a protective agency. State law requires physicians, teachers, and licensed health care workers to report cases of suspected abuse.
- Injuries resulting from violence, such as gunshot or stab wounds, and, in fact, any evidence of criminal violence.
- Occupational illnesses, such as chemical poisoning.
- Communicable diseases, including acquired immune deficiency syndrome (AIDS), hepatitis, neonatal herpes, Lyme disease, rabies, and venereal disease.
- Cases of food poisoning.

Access to Health Records

Although strict confidentiality must be maintained for patients' medical records at all times, proper treatment and billing often require these records to be released to insurance companies and other medical facilities or to other physicians.

Because much of the information used in health care is stored and accessed using computers, special care must be taken to preserve the confidentiality of computerized information about patients. For example, do not leave your desk and allow a computer screen showing information about a patient to remain visible to others. Be aware of any unusual changes in patients' billing or treatment information that is stored in a computer. It is possible for people outside the medical office to gain access to this information and to alter it if the computer is part of a network. A network links several computers together so that software, hardware, and data files can be shared.

Patients also have a right to access their medical records. Preferably, this will be done with the participation of the physician so that the report can be properly interpreted for the patient. The physician should always be notified if a patient wishes to see this information; the assistant should never simply hand the patient a medical record upon request.

A doctor may choose to give a copy of the patient's record to the patient or may choose to give only copies of X ray or lab reports. This may be done when a patient is leaving on a vacation or moving out of the area. In this situation, the doctor will tell the assistant what materials to photocopy, and the assistant will make a notation in the patient's record of the materials that were sent with the patient.

When a doctor "sells" the practice, retires from the practice, or dies, patients' clinical records are not considered the same as other property and dispersed of as such; rather, patients must give permission for the transfer of the records to another physician or clinic. The records are not generally given to the patient.

Release of Information

When a medical office receives a request for information about a patient, the legal obligation of the doctor and the assistant is to keep the patient's records out of the wrong hands and get them into the right hands as promptly as possible. This can be ensured by double-checking the source and validity of the request. In addition, permission to release the information must be obtained from the patient. This permission is obtained in writing in the form of an authorization for **release of information** (sometimes called a "release").

In a doctor's office, the best rule is to refuse to give information unless instructed to do so. The assistant should become familiar with federal, state, and local laws regarding release of information. Be particularly cognizant of releasing information that pertains to minors, family members, attempted suicides, personal injuries, accidents (including industrial accidents), and mental-health problems.

Contents of a Proper Authorization

Valid authorizations must meet several legal requirements, which include the following:

- Name of the facility releasing the information.
- Name of the individual or facility receiving the information.
- Patient's full name, address, and date of birth.

RECORDS RELEASE

TO: _____ Health care provider
_____ Address

I hereby authorize the above-named health care provider to release the specified information below to

Mark Newman, M.D.
2235 South Ridgeway Avenue
Chicago, IL 60623-2240
FAX: 312-555-0025

PATIENT: _____
Address: _____
Birth Date: _____

Please include
___ Specific Records _____

Signed _____ Date _____

RELEASE OF MEDICAL RECORD

Date _____

HEALTH CARE PROVIDER _____

Address _____

I hereby authorize release of the health record(s) to
Mark Newman, M.D.
2235 South Ridgeway Avenue
Chicago, IL 60623-2240
FAX: 312-555-0025

Patient's Name _____

Address: _____

Date of Birth:: _____

Signed _____

Figure 3-4   Authorizations for Release of Information

- Specific dates of treatment.
- Description of the information to be released.
- Signature of the patient.
- Date the form was signed.

A witness to the patient's signature is sometimes used for additional validation of the authorization form. Information about patients from a third party (for example, hospital records or records from other clinics) cannot be forwarded by the doctor's office. Such information must be requested from the source that generated it. Two examples of authorization forms are shown in Figure 3-4.

Methods of Honoring an Authorization

Use the following procedures in fulfilling an authorization for release of information:

- Photocopy all information, records, and chart material to be sent out; never send out originals.
- In the event the record contains information that might be harmful to the patient, the doctor probably would make an abstract of the record containing only the information specifically requested. (For example, confidential material about marital discord should not be sent for a request involving a work-related injury.)
- Send insurance companies only the portion of the medical record specifically requested. If there is no specific request, release the dates of office visits, a list of procedures performed, the diagnosis, and the disability dates, if applicable.

Requests from insurance companies should be accompanied by a valid authorization. The doctor's office may charge the insurance company a **search-and-view-fee** and a fee to copy each page of the record. Such fees sometimes are requested in advance, and the information is not sent until the fee is paid. Figure 3-5 shows a letter requesting a search-and-view fee from an insurance company seeking information about a patient.

MARK NEWMAN, M.D.

2235 South Ridgeway Avenue
Chicago, IL 60623-2240

Board Certified in Family Medicine

312-555-6022

March 16, 19--

Ms. Tracy Anderson, Claims Examiner
State-Wide Insurance Company
4400 Kessler Boulevard
Lexington, KY 40504-8234

Dear Ms. Anderson:

PATIENT: HOWARD POWERS--GROUP NO. 3423-K
                        POLICY NO. 322-48-0933

Your letter of March 9, 19--, arrived requesting information on my patient Howard Powers.

The request for providing information to your company is not a part of the continuing medical care of this patient, and no provision has been made in my office charges to include a complete review of our records for Mr. Powers. The charge for copies of our office records is $45. Also, Mr. Powers must provide us with a signed authorization to release this information to you.

Please enclose the authorization along with your payment in full so that we may promptly provide you with the requested information.

Sincerely,

Mark Newman, M.D.

MN:lj

Figure 3-5 Letter Requesting a Search-and-View Fee

Keep the original release request in the patient's medical record. On the form, make a notation of the records that were sent and when they were sent. A photocopy of the release typically is sent along with the photocopied records to show that there was legal authorization to forward the records.

PROJECT 8   Authorization for Release of Information

WP 6 contains numbered items that refer to the release of information. Mark each statement completion either "T" for *true* or "F" for *false*. Be prepared to discuss your answers in class.

■ CONSENT

When a patient comes to a physician for treatment, the patient enters into a contractual relationship with the physician from which consent is implied rather than stated outright. However, **implied consent** applies to routine treatment only. In more complicated procedures, especially surgery, diagnostic tests, and X-ray treatments, it is important to have **expressed consent** to avoid later lawsuits or, even more serious, criminal accusations. Expressed consent may be written or oral. It is standard practice for the patient to give written consent by signing a special consent form before any special procedure is performed. An exception is the patient who is incapable of giving consent when an emergency necessitates immediate action.

A telephone conversation can be used as legal consent providing it is a three-way conversation between the patient and two office personnel. Both office employees then must sign as witnesses to the telephone conversation giving consent for treatment.

Example

A child is injured in a basketball game while the parents are away on vacation. A long-distance telephone conversation between the parents, the physician, and a medical assistant could be used to obtain consent to treat the child.

The patient's consent to treatment is of little value if the patient does not fully understand the treatment to be administered. The doctor must explain to the patient in simple, understandable terms the illness or problem to be treated, the options for treatments (with their individual benefits and risks), and the prognosis so that the patient can give **informed consent** to the treatment.

The patient must be legally competent to give consent for treatment. This means the patient must have attained legal majority (adult age by law) and be of sound mind. When a patient is not competent to give consent, the consent must come from the next of kin, the legal guardian, or a court-appointed guardian. A minor in the following situations is considered legally capable of giving consent:

- A minor in the military service.
- A minor living away from his or her parents and able to manage his or her own financial affairs.
- A college student living away from home.
- A minor who is married or divorced.

In most cases, minors may give consent to the following:

- Pregnancy tests.
- Prenatal care.
- The diagnosis and treatment of venereal disease.
- The diagnosis and treatment of alcohol or drug abuse.

No particular consent form is designated by law, but the consent should contain the following:

- The date.
- The patient's name.
- The procedure to be performed.
- The name of the doctor performing the procedure.
- The patient's signature.
- The signature of a witness (optional) testifying to the patient's signature.

Figure 3-6 shows an example of a **written consent** form. Printed form consent forms for many different purposes are readily available.

INFORMED CONSENT FOR FLEXIBLE SIGMOIDOSCOPY

1. EXPLANATION OF THE PROCEDURE

    A flexible instrument that allows your doctor to see the inside of the lower intestine will be inserted through the rectum as you lie on your side. The instrument will be advanced to the extent that you do not experience undue discomfort and that allows a thorough examination.

2. RISKS AND DISCOMFORTS

    There exists the possibility of certain changes occurring during the test. These include abdominal discomfort and, in rare instances, injury to the colon. Every effort will be made to minimize these during the examination. Emergency equipment and trained personnel are available to deal with any unusual situations that may arise.

3. BENEFITS TO BE EXPECTED

    The results obtained from the test may assist in the diagnosis of your illness or in detecting early signs of bowel cancer.

4. INQUIRIES

    Any questions about the procedures used in the test are encouraged. If you have any doubts or questions, please ask us for further explanation.

5. FREEDOM OF CONSENT

    Your permission to perform this test is voluntary. You are free to deny consent if you so desire.

THE PATIENT HEREBY STATES:
I have read this form, and I understand the test procedures that will be performed. I consent to undergo this examination.

_____   _____
Signature of Patient   Date

Figure 3-6   Informed Consent Form

CONSENT FOR VIDEOTAPING

I, _Anita Melendez_ , give my consent for the videotaping of my appointment with Mark Newman, M.D., including medical history and examination on this date.

I understand that I have a right to private, confidential medical consultation and treatment, and I voluntarily waive that right so that the videotape may be used for teaching purposes at the University Medical School.

I am in agreement that my medical history, which is related to the taped examination, may be disclosed during the described use of the videotape for <u>teaching purposes</u>.

I further understand that at any future time I may request in writing that certain parts or the entire recording may be deleted and not used.

Signature _Anita Melendez_   Date _7/10/--_

Witness _Joanne Diaz_   Date _7/10/--_

Figure 3-7   Consent for Videotaping Form

The booklet entitled *Medicolegal Forms With Legal Analysis*, published by the American Medical Association, shows many different samples. It is available upon request from the American Medical Association. Consents must be carefully worded so that they will be admissible in court, if needed.

Frequently used consent forms should be readily available. When the consent form is completed and signed by the patient, it is placed in the patient's file. Figure 3-7 shows an example of a completed consent form.

The physician may dictate a notation in the patient's chart such as the following:

Risks and benefits of the procedure were discussed and understood by the patient.

or

Side effects of the medication were discussed with the patient, and she appeared to understand. All of her questions were answered.

PROJECT 9   Consent

WP 7 contains numbered items that refer to a patient's consent for treatment in medical offices. Mark each statement completion either "T" for *true* or "F" for *false*. Be prepared to discuss your answers in class.

Medical liability is the physician's obligation to perform the duties of his profession in a responsible manner. Negligence, as applied to the medical profession, is called "**malpractice**." Malpractice is defined as the "doing of some act that a reasonable and prudent physician would not do, or the failure to do some act that such a physician would do."

In spite of vigilance on the part of the physician and office staff, accidents may occur during treatment, and patients may be dissatisfied with the care that has been given. In such cases, a patient may file a malpractice suit against the doctor. It must be emphasized, however, that the patient must prove **negligence**, or want of ordinary care or skill. Neither the failure to effect a cure nor an error in judgment is cause for a malpractice suit. Doctors can protect themselves against financial liability by purchasing medical malpractice insurance.

The number of malpractice suits increases every day and has become a major health care issue in this country. Because of the increased number of malpractice suits, doctors are practicing defensive medicine, which means they are ordering additional tests and follow-up visits to confirm a diagnosis or treatment result. This practice, however, drives up the cost of health care, which has also become a national problem. Many concerned groups, such as the AMA, are seeking a workable solution to the problem of malpractice costs.

Contributory Negligence

A patient's refusal to have tests, X rays, or vaccinations, or a patient's failure to follow the doctor's instructions might be considered **contributory negligence**. The doctor must prove contributory negligence by the use of evidence, carefully written at the time of the patient's actions. For example, notations in the chart would protect the doctor against a later claim that reasonable precautions had not been taken. Any contact by telephone or letter regarding laboratory or X-ray reports should also be indicated.

Example

Notation in a patient's medical record:
3/12/—   Patient refused to have chest
          X ray. Patient did accept
          medication.

Slander

Slander refers to oral information and **libel** refers to written information—false or true—given with intent to injure the reputation of another person. For example, if an assistant gives out oral confidential information to the wrong people, the indiscretion can lead to a lawsuit for slander. A doctor may lose such a suit even though the informa-

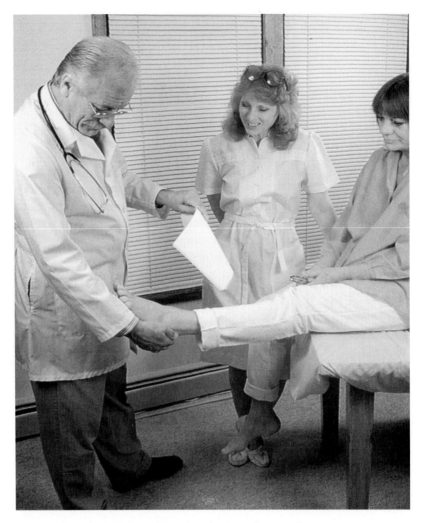

To protect against malpractice suits, doctors often require a follow-up visit to confirm treatment results.

tion was correct if invasion of privacy can be claimed. An assistant may give out incorrect information by mistake that could also lead to conviction on a slander charge. Any unfavorable criticism of another doctor or patient may be construed as defamation of character. In view of these legal considerations, the assistant must at all times be aware of the obligation to be discreet and to keep information about doctors and patients confidential.

Abandonment

Part of the contractual agreement between the patient and the physician is the doctor's responsibility to furnish care for a particular illness as long as it is required, unless the patient is discharged in an appropriate manner. A patient may file a lawsuit against a physician claiming **abandonment** if the physician fails to furnish this care. Again, good medical record keeping is essential as proof that the doctor did not abandon the patient.

Example

Notations in a patient's medical record:

4/6/—	Patient canceled appointment. Rescheduled for 4/13/—.
4/13/—	Patient did not show for follow-up appointment.

A doctor may choose to terminate the physician-patient relationship because of a patient's failure to comply with treatment instructions. In such cases, the physician is required to notify the patient of that intention and to allow the patient a reasonable length of time to obtain another doctor.

The notification should be in the form of a letter sent to the patient by registered or certified mail. It should state the reason for withdrawal, the date of severance, and the doctor's willingness to continue treatment if the patient complies with treatment instructions and needs further care. An example of such notification is shown in Figure 3-8.

After a withdrawal letter has been sent, the doctor should provide the patient's name (confidentially) to the office appointment desk. If the patient calls and requests an appointment, the assistant should transfer the call to the physician, who will then explain what needs to be done to reestablish care.

MARK NEWMAN, M.D.

2235 South Ridgeway Avenue
Chicago, IL 60623-2240

Board Certified in Family Medicine

312-555-6022

April 15, 19--

Mr. Ted Marshall
5678 Ridge Avenue
Chicago, IL 60623-5423

Dear Mr. Marshall:

I must withdraw from your further professional care. You did not follow my advice and treatment plan by not following through on your scheduled series of chemotherapy.

Your condition needs medical care; therefore, this letter is to request that you please place yourself immediately under the care of another physician.

I will be available for your medical treatment until April 20. At that time, after receiving your written permission, I will make available to the physician of your choice your medical records.

Sincerely,

Mark Newman, M.D.

MN:lj

By Registered Mail

Figure 3-8 Withdrawal of Services Letter

Assault and Battery

Strictly speaking, **assault** is when a person threatens another person with the intention to hurt; **battery** is the actual hurting. Under medical law, battery has been interpreted to include surgical and medical procedures performed without the patient's consent or extended beyond the consent given.

Example

> Removal of a badly damaged uterus during exploratory surgery when the patient had not signed a consent for a hysterectomy could be considered battery.

Battery has been claimed even in cases where the procedure was in the interest of the patient. Unless there is a severe emergency, a doctor may well lose a suit as a result of not having proper consent.

The Physician's Liability for Employees

In addition to concern for the welfare of the patients, the physician must be aware of other potential **litigations** (lawsuits) such as those in the area of employment. There are laws that cover all aspects of the hiring process, drug testing of employees, equal opportunity, sexual harassment, disability, discrimination, equal pay, fair labor, and workers' compensation. A well-trained staff minimizes the likelihood of litigation.

Each employee is responsible for his or her own behavior. Nonetheless, liability for negligence is recognized by law to include not only the physician's actions but also the actions of the physician's employees. While acting within the proper assignment and job description, the assistant is the agent of the physician. Therefore, a physician should not delegate to an assistant tasks requiring professional judgment regarding diagnosis or treatment, nor should an assistant undertake such tasks.

The physician should be aware of the assistant's job capabilities. An assistant who is unable to perform a required task should explain this situation to the physician and offer to learn the correct procedure.

It is also the physician's responsibility to define and regulate office policies, assist with the teaching of these policies, and see that they are properly implemented. It is the assistant's responsibility to know the office policies and perform them properly. If an assistant finds employment at an office where unlawful or unethical procedures are practiced, the assistant will be wise to terminate that employment. Situations that might arise include suspected fraud, health insurance scams, kickbacks, and embezzlement (an employee's taking money and using it personally).

When a physician is out of town and unable to care for a patient, another physician may be called to provide care. The absent physician typically is not liable for the negligence of a substitute physician.

Nonetheless, the primary physician should provide the patient with the name of a doctor equally qualified to provide necessary care during the primary physician's absence.

If the physician is part of a group practice, the patient most likely will be treated by another doctor in the group. Malpractice insurance costs are generally shared in group practices, so it is likely that the cost of defending a suit arising from the negligence of another physician in the group would also be shared. Appropriate notations should be entered in the patient's medical record when the physician is away.

Example

Notation in a patient's medical record:

> Dr. Mukerjee on vacation, 10/9/—. Patient telephoned with complaint of calf pain and tenderness. Patient referred to Dr. Lemaire or to emergency room at County Hospital.

Office Safety

Litigation may also result from injuries due to falls or other office accidents. The assistant must be aware of patients' safety at all times. Always alert patients to steps, stairs, and slippery floors. Be sure to assist patients who use walkers, crutches, or wheelchairs. Do not leave sharp objects or medical equipment lying around the waiting area, and take appropriate measures to repair broken furniture and equipment in the office. Always be aware of patients in the waiting area, since a patient who becomes faint may fall to the floor and sustain further injury. The waiting area must be made safe for young children.

The Occupational Safety and Health Act (OSHA) is intended to prevent injury to employees. It is used to enforce standards for providing a workplace free from recognized hazards (toxic material, malfunctioning equipment, bad air quality, high noise levels). It was the originator of the "right-to-know laws" specifically addressing hazardous chemical materials, regulation of blood-borne pathogens (particularly HIV and hepatitis B) and infectious body fluids, and disposal of medical wastes (human tissues, specimens, dressings, needles, and medical equipment).

Liability Insurance

The cost of professional liability insurance, or malpractice insurance, has risen dramatically in the past 20 years as a result of the increasing number of malpractice suits and the large monetary damages awarded in some cases. This insurance is a necessity for all medical professionals since it also helps cover legal expenses even if a **settlement**, or agreement on the suit, is reached out of court.

Although the actions of the physician's staff are covered by the physician's insurance, liability insurance for medical assistants is available.

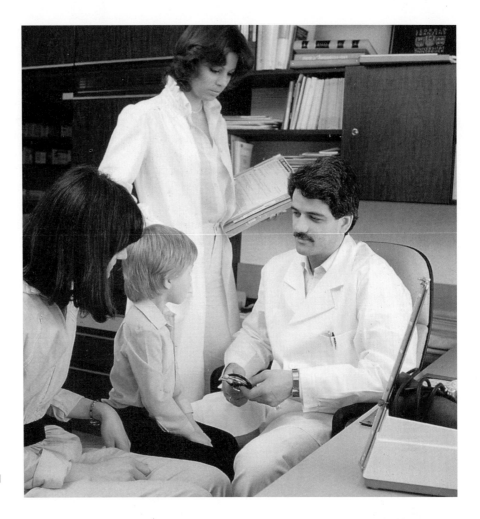

Maintaining good interpersonal relationships with patients and staff helps reduce the likelihood of litigation.

Safeguards Against Litigation

The conscientious assistant plays an important role in the prevention of malpractice cases. Remember that it is easier to prevent a malpractice claim than to defend one. Maintaining good interpersonal relationships with patients and staff helps reduce the likelihood of litigation. In particular, remember the following:

- Keep everything you hear, see, and read about patients completely confidential.
- Never criticize a doctor to a patient.
- Do not discuss a patient's condition, diagnosis, or treatment with the patient or with other patients. Remember, what the doctor tells the assistant about a patient is to be kept confidential, even from the patient.
- Do not diagnose or prescribe, even though you feel sure you know what the doctor will prescribe. (There may be other circumstances in the case of which you are unaware. Prescribing constitutes the practice of medicine and is unlawful unless you are licensed to practice.)
- Notify the doctor if you learn that a patient is under treatment by another physician for the same condition.

- Notify the doctor if the patient mentions that he or she has no intention of returning to the office or complying with the treatment plan.
- Be available to assist the patient and the doctor.
- Obtain proper authorizations for release of information and consents. File these with the patient's records.
- Keep complete and accurate records, including notations about a patient's failure to show for an appointment, cancellation of an appointment, or failure to follow treatment instructions.
- Be selective in giving information over the telephone.
- Keep prescription pads and medications in a secure place.
- Be safety conscious. See that all equipment is in safe working condition, and be alert for potential hazards.

PROJECT 10 Malpractice and the Assistant's Responsibility

In WP 8, the numbered items relate to the assistant's responsibility in preventing malpractice claims. Mark each statement completion "T" for *true* or "F" for *false*.

■ THE PHYSICIAN AND THE COURT

A doctor may be called to appear in court to testify either as an expert witness or as a defendant in a lawsuit. Credibility of the record may be challenged for the following reasons: delayed filing of lab reports, illegible record data, altered record, loss of information, or forged signatures.

The Physician as Defendant

Today, people do not form the same bond and close relationship with their doctors as in the past. A patient will receive care from at least three to five physicians during a lifetime. Because people are more health conscious and knowledgeable, they also are more likely to question the doctor's treatment and to sue when they feel they have been harmed.

A patient, as a **plaintiff**, may file a malpractice lawsuit at any time. Filing does not imply a claim has any merit; the patient must prove negligence. When a claim is filed, the patient's attorney will immediately **subpoena** all relevant medical records of that patient. To subpoena means that all named documents are ordered to be brought to court. In many cases, a settlement between the physician's malpractice insurance company and the patient can be reached, and the case may not go to court.

The doctor may be able to make a statement, or **deposition**, under oath in the lawyer's office, or the doctor may have to appear in court.

If a plaintiff who is a patient claims the doctor was negligent, the physician may have to appear in court as the **defendant**, to defend the care given to the patient. Even when such claims are not substantiated, there is financial loss and stress on the physician's reputation. It is easier to prevent a claim than to defend one.

Statute of Limitations

A **statute of limitations** is a law that sets a time limit for initiating litigation. This time limit varies from state to state, not only in its length but also as to the event from which it dates. That is, the span of time during which a lawsuit for malpractice may be brought may begin when the negligence first occurred, when the negligence was first discovered, or when the physician-patient relationship was ended. In pediatric cases, the statute of limitations may begin after the patient reaches majority, so doctors treating children should keep records beyond this time.

Good Samaritan Act

The purpose of a **good samaritan act** is to protect the physician from liability for civil damages that may occur as a result of providing emergency care. Because there are minor variations in this law from state to state, the assistant's role in emergency situations is defined by the state in which the assistant works.

The Physician as Witness

Physicians may be called as witnesses in the course of their practices for a great variety of reasons, depending, of course, on their specialties.

A doctor who gives testimony regarding the case of a patient is permitted to consult the patient's records during the trial to refresh his

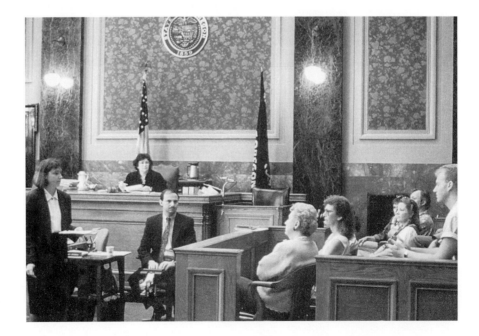

Medical records must be complete, up-to-date, and in order since they may be subpoenaed as evidence in the courtroom.

or her memory. The doctor must, therefore, take to court all papers on the case: the medical history, an account of the first examination and of the diagnosis, treatment and prognosis reports, the number and dates of office visits, and the charges billed and collected. All X-ray and laboratory reports also must be included. The assistant must compile these records so that they are complete, up to date, and in order.

Damage Suits

One of the most frequent occasions for a doctor to appear as a witness is in damage suits after accidents or in cases of negligence by another person where there is a claim for monetary compensation. The claimant's physician will testify to the court about the following information:

- The type of injury.
- The patient's condition when first seen by the doctor.
- The length, type, and progress of the patient's treatment.
- How much the patient has suffered.
- Whether there is permanent or partial disability.
- The extent to which earning capacity has been damaged.

A Patient's Competency

When a will is contested in court, the court is asked to determine whether the person who made the will was in a condition to use the judgment necessary to do so. The testimony of that person's physician will be an important factor in the ruling of the court.

Expert Testimony

Physicians also may be asked to give testimony as experts in their respective fields. In criminal trials, for example, if the defendant's lawyers bring a plea of insanity, psychiatrists specializing in legal cases are called in by both sides for their expert opinions. If there is an accusation or suspicion of homicide, doctors may be required to testify as to the cause and time of death. Physicians are entitled to monetary compensation for expert testimony.

PROJECT 11 Legal Terms

On WP 9, match each legal term in Column 2 with the proper definition in Column 1. Be prepared to discuss your answers in class.

Key Terms

The following terms appear in **boldface** type in this chapter. Do you recall what they mean? Refer to the chapter for definitions you need to review.

abandonment
assault
authorization
battery
breach of contract
contract
contributory negligence
defendant
deposition
ethics
etiquette
expressed consent
good samaritan act
implied consent
informed consent
libel

litigation
malpractice
negligence
physician-patient
  relationship
plaintiff
reciprocity
release of information
search-and-view fee
settlement
slander
statute of limitations
statutory reports
subpoena
written consent

Topics for Discussion

1. Debate current bioethical topics such as how a limited supply of health care services should be alloted, genetic research, prolonging life via respirators and other artificial means, and so forth.
2. Discuss your duty as a medical assistant regarding confidential information in the following situations:

a. Parents requesting medical information about their child.
b. A phone call from a person who says he is a police officer and needs some information about a patient.
c. A local newspaper reporter requesting information about the condition of an accident victim.
d. An employer calling to check on the condition of a worker injured in a fall on the job.
e. A wife requesting information about her husband's examination.
f. A parent requesting laboratory results for a 23-year-old son.

Role-Playing

1. Mr. Pierce, a lawyer, phones to ask you whether a Mrs. Sundquist is a patient of Dr. Newman, your employer.
2. Mr. Jamison, a patient, calls the office to say he does not think his medication is working so he has stopped taking it. He also says he is thinking about consulting another physician.
3. Sara Matthews telephones the office and asks you for the results of her throat culture, which you know to be positive.

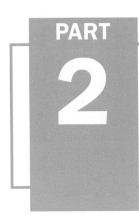

PART

2

Administrative Responsibilities

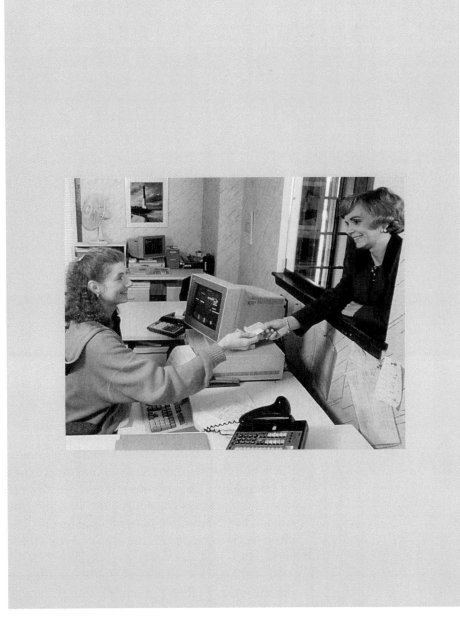

Telephone Procedures

OBJECTIVES

Upon completion of this chapter, you should be able to:

■ List at least five principles of good telephone etiquette.

■ Discuss the following telephone skills:
   Answering
   Identifying
   Handling emergency calls
   Putting callers on hold

■ Appropriately screen the following incoming calls:
   Appointments
   Prescription refills
   Personal calls
   Calls from another doctor
   Questions from patients
   Emergency calls
   Hospital reports

   Laboratory reports
   Nonmedical calls

■ Discuss the procedures for taking complete and accurate messages and for following through on incoming calls.

■ Discuss the procedures for placing outgoing telephone calls, including planning and following through on calls.

■ Explain the use of telephone directories as reference sources.

■ Explain how to place a long-distance call.

■ Discuss the importance of a telephone log.

■ List and discuss special features of telephone systems.

■ THE IMPORTANCE OF THE TELEPHONE

The main channel of communication between the patient and the doctor is the telephone. Almost all patients make their first contact with the doctor by telephone; urgent and emergency cases are also reported by telephone. The assistant must handle telephone calls in such a way as to reassure the caller but not interrupt the doctor, who may be engaged with another patient's problems. The medical assistant also must learn to recognize the situation in each type of call and handle it correctly.

Attitudes are contagious. Patients judge the care they receive by the attitude of office personnel (reflected by voice in telephone situations) as well as by the actual medical service provided by the doctor. Unhappiness with the quality of personal attention can affect the patient's perception of care. A patient may listen more to the tone of the assistant's voice than to what the assistant says. The caller should be paid the same attention given a person in a face-to-face conversation.

■ TELEPHONE SKILLS

Telephone calls may be incoming, outgoing, or interoffice. The telephone on the assistant's desk may have several call buttons, which, when pressed, connect the telephone to the doctor's private office or to other staff offices in the building. This feature makes it possible for the assistant to ask a question and relay the answer to the caller. Medical assistants typically handle all incoming calls to the medical office and should use the opportunity to present a positive image for the physician and the practice.

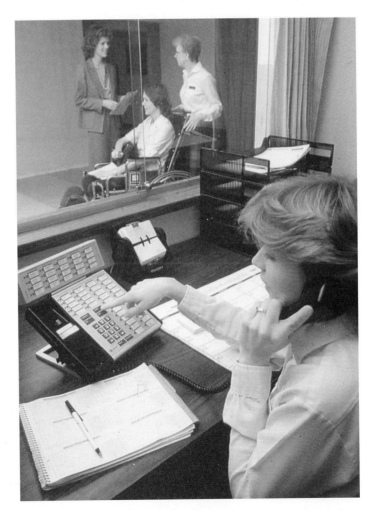

When answering the telephone, use the opportunity to present a positive image for the physician and the practice.

Telephone Etiquette

When answering the telephone, try to visualize the person with whom you are talking. Think about who the caller is, what the caller is asking, how the caller feels, and whether he or she is a patient. By doing this, your voice will sound alert, interested, and concerned during the conversation.

Use a pleasant tone that conveys self-assurance to the caller along with a genuine desire to be understanding and helpful. This is what is meant by the phrase *using a* **"voice with a smile."**

Use variations in pitch and phrasing to avoid sounding monotonous, and never indicate impatience or annoyance through the sound of your voice. The caller may sense this mood and react accordingly, making communication more difficult.

When speaking into the telephone, hold the mouthpiece about an inch from your mouth to avoid distortion or faintness of voice. Speak clearly and distinctly; do not run words together or mumble. Even if you answer the phone with the same greeting many times a day, say the words slowly enough for the caller to understand. Always speak at a moderate pace throughout the conversation, giving the caller time to think about and understand what was said.

When concluding a conversation, say "Good-bye" and use the caller's name. This will leave the caller with a pleasant impression. Finally, replace the receiver gently when you hang up.

Following are some tips to remember in using proper **telephone etiquette**:

- Use proper identification.
- Identify the nature of the call.
- Use courteous phrases such as *please* and *thank you.*
- Listen carefully.
- Use words appropriate to the situation, but avoid using technical words.
- Offer assistance as necessary.
- Avoid unnecessarily long conversations.
- Avoid using colloquial or slang expressions such as *you know, bye-bye, ain't,* and *uh-huh.*
- Conclude calls properly by saying "Good-bye" and using the caller's name.

Promptness

Courtesy begins with promptness in answering the call. The ideal time to answer a call is on the second ring. Answering on the second ring does not make the caller wait and yet allows the caller a moment of preparation time to begin the conversation (the caller will expect to hear at least one ring before there is an answer). If there is a delay, even a brief one, the caller may hang up or become irritated.

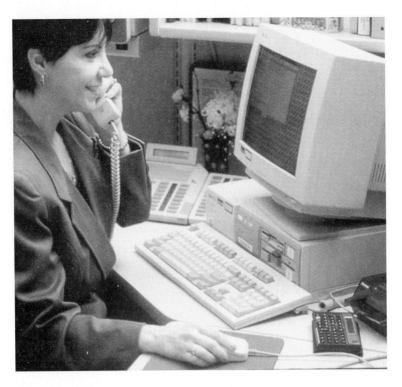

By visualizing the person calling on the telephone, the assistant's voice will sound alert, interested, and concerned during the conversation.

Greeting and Identifying

There are many ways to answer the phone, but the preferred method is to answer with the name of the physician or clinic followed by the assistant's name. Answering with "Good morning" or "Good afternoon" adds a personal touch but may be inefficient in a busy office. It may be more important to take the time to say the name of the office slowly and distinctly. If the doctor has a common surname, the doctor's full name may be used to avoid confusion.

Example

ASSISTANT: Dr. Mark Newman's office, Linda speaking.

In large clinics, an assistant who acts as a receptionist may answer the call by identifying the name of the clinic. After a call has been transferred, employees in individual departments will then identify themselves.

Example

ASSISTANT: Northeast Clinic. May I direct your call?
PATIENT: I'd like to make an appointment with Dr. Nasser.
ASSISTANT: I will transfer you to Sharon at the appointment desk.
SECOND ASSISTANT: Appointment desk. This is Sharon. How may I help you?

A group practice made up of only two or three physicians might be identified with all of the doctors' names.

Example

ASSISTANT: Doctors Newman, Berg, and Martin, Linda speaking.

Saying only "Doctors' office" is likely to be confusing to the caller, whose response may be, "Is this Dr. Newman's office?"

■ SCREENING CALLS

Most incoming calls concern matters that can be handled by a well-trained assistant guided by the individual preferences of the doctor. Some doctors may prefer to speak to patients no matter what the circumstances. However, this is likely to be inefficient because it can cause interruptions to the patients being seen at the time by the doctor. Also, medical records are probably not available for the doctor's reference at the time of the call. In some offices, a nurse is available to answer patients' questions.

Screening calls is often a difficult problem for the beginner, who may be afraid to assume the responsibility of making decisions. It is important to discuss this aspect of the job with the doctor at the very beginning and to ascertain to what extent the assistant will handle calls alone, what information should be given out, when messages should be taken, and when to tell the patient that the doctor will return the call. A call screening sheet, such as the one shown in Figure 4-1 can be used to assist you in screening and transferring calls.

The assistant must be guided by the doctor's wishes in deciding whether to handle a call or to transfer it to the doctor. The first priority is to determine the nature of the call. You will then have a good idea of how to handle the call.

Screening Situations

Many calls can be handled by taking a message. Some examples of such calls include the following:

- An ill new patient wants to talk with the doctor.
- A patient already under treatment who wants to talk with the doctor.
- A relative of a patient who requests information about the patient.
- A relative or personal friend of the doctor who calls for the doctor.
- Business calls from attorneys, accountants, or hospital personnel.
- Satisfactory and unsatisfactory progress reports given by a patient (for example, a patient who was told at time of appoint-

CALL SCREENING SHEET

PURPOSE OF INCOMING CALL	Doctor	Nurse	Message	Other
MEDICAL				
Emergency: Dr. in				Come in
Emergency: Dr. out of office				Send to ER
Seriously ill		✓		
Test results from lab			✓	
Information; advice; test results			✓	
Rx renewal			✓	
Doctor	✓			
Hospital: ER, ICU			✓	
Other				
NONMEDICAL				
Appointment				Appt. desk
Medical records				Arlene
Insurance				Tina
Billing/charges				Tina
Personnel				Gary

Figure 4-1   Call Screening Sheet

ment to call back with how a medication or treatment is working).
- Results from a lab or X ray department.
- Prescription refills.

The following calls are usually put through to the doctor:

- Calls from another doctor.
- Urgent calls from the hospital, such as from the intensive care unit or the emergency room.
- Calls from patients who have been specifically identified by the doctor. (For example, this might include out-of-town patients, the family of a seriously ill patient calling to check on the patient's condition, or a patient in labor.)
- Calls from a patient with an acute illness, such as a severe reaction to a medication.

If there is a nurse in the office, many of these calls can be routed to the nurse, who will then decide whether to interrupt the doctor in an examination room.

Some examples of various screening situations follow:

Example: Call to Schedule an Appointment

ASSISTANT: Dr. Newman's office, Linda speaking.
CALLER: I would like to speak to Dr. Newman.
ASSISTANT: Dr. Newman is with a patient. May I help you?

CALLER: Well, I need to make an appointment for next week.

ASSISTANT: Mary, at the appointment desk, will be able to help you. Let me transfer your call to her.

or

I can schedule an appointment for you. Are you a patient of Dr. Newman's?

The assistant can then proceed to schedule an appointment for the patient.

Example: Call to Discuss a Medical Question

ASSISTANT: Dr. Newman's office, Linda speaking.

CALLER: I need to talk to Dr. Newman.

ASSISTANT: Dr. Newman is with a patient. May I help you?

CALLER: I'm a patient of Dr. Newman's, and I have some questions about my medications.

ASSISTANT: May I ask who is calling?

CALLER: This is Wendy Chen.

ASSISTANT: I will transfer you to the nurse, Ms. Chen. She should be able to help you.

or

The nurse should be able to help you with those questions, but she will need to pull your medical records. Let me take a message and ask her to return your call.

Example: Personal Call for the Doctor

ASSISTANT: Dr. Newman's office, Linda speaking.

CALLER: I'd like to talk to Dr. Newman.

ASSISTANT: Dr. Newman is with a patient. May I help you?

CALLER: I'm a friend of Dr. Newman's, and I need to speak with him. This is a personal call.

ASSISTANT: Dr. Newman usually returns phone calls right after lunch. If you give me your name and number, I will ask him to get back to you.

CALLER: My name is Chris Floyd. He can reach me at 555-6789 before 2 p.m.

ASSISTANT: I will give the message to Dr. Newman as soon as he is available.

Transferring Calls

Most telephone systems give you the ability to transfer calls to another line by pressing a button that corresponds to that line or by pressing a combination of numbers to reach the proper extension. When calls are transferred, most systems allow private consultation between the two office lines while the outside caller is on hold. This makes it possible for the assistant to ask a question and relay the answer to the caller without putting the doctor or nurse on the line. When transferring a call to another line, always announce the caller. For example: "Susan, Ms. Chen is on Line 2 with a question about her medications."

If an **intercom** system (paging system) is used in the office or clinic, the assistant presses the appropriate intercom button and says "Nurse, call on Line 2" into the receiver in order to notify the nurse of a call.

Some doctors carry a **pager** (or beeper) so they can be easily located. A pager is a small, portable device that allows doctors to be alerted (typically by dialing a special telephone number) when they are needed and are away from the office. Once alerted, the doctor can call the office for the message. Just as when the doctor is in the office, it is important to use good judgment in determining whether a situation warrants paging the doctor.

Emergency Calls

An emergency call may come at any time, and the assistant must be able to handle any situation. The person who telephones will probably be upset, and people who are excited often forget to give the most important information. It is imperative that the assistant remain calm and handle the call efficiently, reassuring the caller that help will come as quickly as possible. The importance of obtaining the name, address, and telephone number of the patient cannot be emphasized too strongly. The more information you can obtain, the better.

If the doctor is in the office when an emergency call comes through, he or she will speak with the patient. However, it is recommended that the assistant screen the call to determine whether or not it really is an emergency. Great tact and excellent judgment are needed to do this.

Nonmedical Screening Situations

One of the most difficult people to deal with over the telephone is the person who refuses to state the purpose of the call, saying that it is a "personal call" or a "personal matter." A personal friend does not hesitate to state that fact. If the caller is mysterious about the reason for calling, it is a pretty safe assumption that the matter is of more importance to the caller than to the doctor. If the doctor has given such instructions, the assistant should explain that the doctor will not return the call unless the nature of the call is known.

If the caller absolutely refuses to give information, it is permissible to suggest that a letter be written so that the doctor can become acquainted with the matter and give a response. A legitimate caller will give a name and state the reason for the call. A confident, pleasant voice will help you make the doctor's position clear while avoiding needless disputes.

Handling a Complaint

At times it may be necessary for you to handle a call from a patient who has a complaint. Following are procedures for handling a caller with a complaint:

- Listen attentively.
- Determine the key points of the complaint.
- Speak in a soft, calm voice.
- Try not to interrupt the caller.
- Avoid putting the caller on hold; being on hold may increase the caller's anger.
- Express regret that the caller has a complaint, but do not necessarily admit an error or apologize for an error.
- Avoid blaming another staff member or a computer for an error.
- Explain the action to be taken regarding the complaint, but be careful of commitments. It is better to tell the caller that you will investigate the problem and then call back.
- Do not allow an angry caller to become abusive. If this happens, speak up at once by saying, "I know that you are upset, but raising your voice won't help the situation."

Example

ASSISTANT: Dr. Newman's office, Linda speaking.
CALLER: I have to talk to Dr. Newman.
ASSISTANT: Dr. Newman is with a patient. May I help you?
CALLER: I have a complaint about this bill I received from him. I did not have an appointment last month, and I will not pay this bill!
ASSISTANT: I understand that you are upset. If you will tell me your name, I will pull your records so that we can clear up the misunderstanding.

PROJECT 12 Screening Calls

Dr. Newman is in the office seeing patients. Complete WP 10 on screening telephone calls by choosing which action in Column 2 should be taken for each situation in Column 1. Be prepared to discuss your answers in class.

■ PUTTING CALLERS ON HOLD

Most office telephone systems allow the person receiving an incoming call to put the caller on hold. The hold function allows the assistant to keep one or more callers waiting while handling another call or retrieving information such as a patient's file. When a call comes into the office, it is better to answer the call and put the caller on hold than to allow the line to continue ringing with no answer.

If you must break away from a call to retrieve information, ask the caller whether he or she would prefer to have you call back or to be placed on hold. (If it will take more than a few minutes to find the information, it is better to call back.) When you return to the line with the caller on hold, politely reestablish the call.

Example

ASSISTANT: Thank you for holding, Mr. Erickson. I have that information now.

If only two lines are ringing, the assistant should answer one line, "Dr. Newman's office. Could you please hold?" and wait for the caller to say yes or no. If the response is no, follow through on the call. If the answer is yes, the second line should be answered and the second call completed. Most telephone systems have **automatic call distribution** by which the calls are taken in the order received. An efficient method for remembering each call is to make a notation on a piece of paper about the nature of each call.

Line 1	Line 2	Line 3	Line 4
Appointment	Insurance	Doctor	Nurse

Updating Callers on Hold

Remember that the hold function of the telephone can be abused. Callers will not want to be kept waiting longer than 1 minute. If the person the caller is holding for cannot be located within that amount of time, do not keep the caller on hold. Instead, offer to take a message.

Keep the caller who is on hold informed about the status of the call once every 30 seconds.

Example

ASSISTANT: The appointment desk is still busy. Will you continue to hold?

After returning to a caller on hold several times, offer again to take a message.

Example

ASSISTANT: Gary in insurance is still unavailable. Could I take a message and ask him to return your call?

It is important to be polite when placing people on hold, since keeping them waiting in this manner can be annoying to the caller.

Because most calls cannot be taken immediately by the doctor or nurse, the assistant must take clear messages so that the telephone calls can be returned later.

Remember the following procedures for taking efficient, informative telephone messages:

- Always have pencil and paper at hand.
- Make notes as information is being given.
- Ask politely to have important information repeated.
- Verify information such as names, spellings, numbers, and dates for accuracy. You might ask "Would you spell your name, please?" or "Let me repeat that to be sure I have noted it correctly."
- Make inquiries tactfully. A tactful question might be, "Will Gary know what this is about?" or "Could I tell Sue what this is about?" or "Is this a medical matter? If so, the doctor will need your medical record."

The more information you include in the message, the better. Be brief, yet thorough. The doctor will have a much better understanding of the conversation if he or she is given a clear, concise report. Certain statements by a patient may convey a very significant piece of information to the doctor, such as complaints of pain or discomfort, a chance remark regarding an inability to work, or a reference to illness in the family. The assistant's impression of the conversation is also important to the doctor. The assistant might note, for example, "The patient seemed depressed."

When taking a phone message, do not say, "I will have the doctor call you." This makes a commitment on behalf of the doctor. It is better to say "I will give the message to the doctor" or "I will ask the doctor to call you."

After taking a message regarding a patient's care, the assistant should obtain the patient's chart. The telephone message should be attached to the chart with a paper clip and placed in the message center for the nurse or the doctor.

The doctor may wish to have all telephone messages entered into the patient's medical record. In such cases, the message can be filed inside the chart after it has been acted on. Some offices may have a page in the patient's record specifically for messages. In other cases, the doctor may dictate a note to be entered into the patient's medical record instead of entering the actual message form. Figure 4-2 (a) shows an example of a chart note that might be entered in the patient's record from a telephone message taken by the assistant. Figure 4-2 (b) shows a telephone message to be taped directly into a patient's chart.

Verifying Information

When you are not sure what a caller has said or you have difficulty understanding the caller, you should say something like, "I want to get your name correctly. Will you spell it for me, please?" Many names

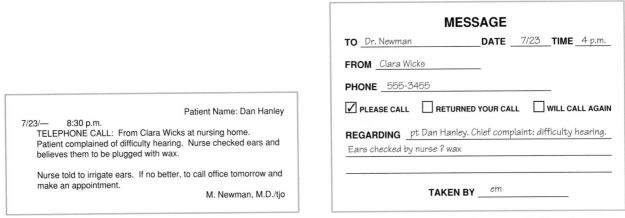

Patient Name: Dan Hanley

7/23/—   8:30 p.m.
   TELEPHONE CALL: From Clara Wicks at nursing home.
Patient complained of difficulty hearing. Nurse checked ears and
believes them to be plugged with wax.

   Nurse told to irrigate ears. If no better, to call office tomorrow and
make an appointment.

                                             M. Newman, M.D./tjo

Figure 4-2 *(a)*   Telephone Message Keyed and Placed in Patient's Chart

MESSAGE

TO Dr. Newman   DATE   7/23   TIME 4 p.m.

FROM   Clara Wicks

PHONE   555-3455

☑ PLEASE CALL   ☐ RETURNED YOUR CALL   ☐ WILL CALL AGAIN

REGARDING   pt Dan Hanley. Chief complaint: difficulty hearing.
Ears checked by nurse ? wax

TAKEN BY   em

Figure 4-2 *(b)*   Telephone Message to be Taped Directly Into Patient's Chart

sound alike over the telephone—for instance, *Wood* and *Woods*, *Romanoff* and *Romanov*, *Johnson* and *Janson*. The doctor may also have several patients with the same last name, and, in such cases, it is imperative to know the first name of the person. It is a good idea to repeat the date and time of an appointment if it is made over the phone.

Writing Down the Message

Printed telephone message forms are available from stationers. All printed message forms have blanks for noting basic information about the phone call. See Figure 4-3 for an example of a printed message form.

Some doctors design their own telephone message forms and have them printed. Such a customized form may contain some of the questions most frequently asked of a patient. For example, the message form used in a pediatrician's office might include a blank for the child's temperature or for the time of the last meal eaten by the child. Each doctor in a group practice would include several standard questions on a personalized office message form such as the one shown in Figure 4-4.

MESSAGE

TO Dr. Newman   DATE 10/6   TIME   9:00

FROM   Alma Jackson

PHONE   555-1102

☒ PLEASE CALL   ☐ RETURNED YOUR CALL   ☐ WILL CALL AGAIN

REGARDING   Test results from 10/1

TAKEN BY   tjo

Figure 4-3   Telephone Message Slip

TELEPHONE MESSAGE

DATE	TIME	PHYSICIAN
10/8/--	1:30	Ellis
PATIENT	**AGE**	**PHONE**
Patricia Strand	18 months	555-7643
		Mother—Betty

___ Abdominal pain	___ Earache	___ Sore throat
___ Cough	___ Headache	___ Swollen glands
___ Cramps	___ Nasal congestion	✓ Temperature 100 R
✓ Diarrhea	___ Rash	___ Urinary
___ Dizziness	___ Runny nose	✓ Vomiting

REGARDING: Patricia sick x 24 hours. Keeps some clear
liquids down. Just finished 10 days of Septra DS.
        tjo

Figure 4-4   Telephone Message Slip Designed by Physician

Responding to Calls for Prescription Refills

One common message the assistant may take by telephone is for a prescription (Rx) refill. To handle this situation, the assistant needs to know common abbreviations used in recording medications. A few of the more common abbreviations and their meanings are listed here:

Dosage Times		Dosage Amounts	
a.m.	Morning	g	Gram
b.i.d.	Twice a day	gr	Grain
p.m.	Afternoon	ml	Milliliter
hs	Bedtime	mcg	Microgram
qd	Every day	mEq	Milliequivalent
qh	Every hour	mg	Milligram
q.i.d.	Four times a day		
t.i.d.	Three times a day		

The usual procedure is for the patient to return the empty bottle to the pharmacist, asking for a refill. The pharmacist calls the physician for an authorization to refill, if one does not already exist. This telephone call is handled by the assistant, who takes a message.

Example

ASSISTANT: Dr. Newman's office, Linda speaking.
CALLER: This is Consumer Pharmacy with a refill for Dr. Newman. Carla Sanchez needs Digoxin 0.25 milligram, one every day, number 100. This was last refilled on June 10.
ASSISTANT: May I have your telephone number there, please?
CALLER: The telephone number here is 555-1252.
ASSISTANT: Let me repeat that prescription to make sure I have it correctly.

Specially designed forms can be made for **prescription refill** messages. See Figure 4-5 for an example of the completed refill form for this call.

PRESCRIPTION REFILLS

NAME _Carla Sanchez_

RX	DOSE	AMT.	LAST REFILL
Digoxin	0.25 mg	100	6/10
	one q.d.		

PHARMACY _Consumer Pharmacy_   TEL. _555-1252_

Figure 4-5   Prescription Refill Slip

PROJECT 13 Taking Messages

While Dr. Newman is busy with a patient, Mr. Kramer calls about his son Jeffrey, who is complaining of a sore throat and an earache. The patient is unable to come to the office for an appointment, and the telephone number is 555-1913. Today's date is October 8, and the time is 11:10 a.m. Write out a telephone message for Dr. Newman using one of the message forms on WPs 11 through 18. What other information, if any, will you need to obtain from Mr. Kramer? Write your questions on the back of the message form. Place the completed message in the Miscellaneous folder for future use.

Remove the remaining telephone message forms from the working papers and place them in your Supplies folder for future use.

PROJECT 14 Telephone Skills

Circle the best answer in each of the telephone situations described on WP 19. Be prepared to discuss your answers in class.

Using Electronic Mail (e-mail)

Messages can be transmitted in digital form from computer to computer through an **electronic mail** system, commonly known as **e-mail**. The message is keyed by the sender at a computer terminal, and it is then transmitted electronically to the receiver's computer. If the receiver is not available, the message is stored until the receiver retrieves it. Both the sender and the receiver may print the message or forward it to another electronic mailbox. Electronic mail saves time, conveys messages rapidly, and promotes flexibility. Users may access the system through outside telecommunications sources enabling users to access the system from home or other locations to send or receive messages. Electronic voice mail operates in the same manner, storing voice messages.

■ OUTGOING CALLS

A medical assistant will make many local and long-distance telephone calls for the employer. As a medical assistant, you will probably place calls to patients, hospitals, clinics, and laboratories. You will also make a variety of other business and professional calls for the doctor.

Planning the Call

Plan the conversation before making a call by obtaining necessary information and outlining questions to ask. Know the specifics of the call before you dial. Ask yourself who, what, where, when, and why, and make appropriate notations. Be aware of the following:

- Whom to call and ask for once the phone is answered.
- What information to give or obtain.

- Questions to ask.
- When to call.
- Possible situations that might arise during the call (what-if situations).

Example

> DR. NEWMAN: Linda, please call Dr. Martin and ask him to see Lucy Barlow.

To successfully complete the call requested in the example above, Linda will need to ask Dr. Newman the following:

- What is Lucy's diagnosis (if applicable)?
- When should Lucy be seen by Dr. Martin?
- What are the contingency plans (what-ifs)? For example, what is the alternative if Lucy is to be seen today but Dr. Martin is not in the office today?

Always obtain necessary information and have it at hand before scheduling services (such as referrals, laboratory and X-ray procedures, surgery, and hospital admissions) for patients.

Placing the Call

When you have the proper information and are prepared to place a call, use the following procedures:

- Identify yourself and the doctor's office. If you are calling for the doctor, identify the doctor.
- State the reason for the call.
- Provide the necessary information.
- Ask tactfully for information.
- Listen carefully and make notes as needed.
- Verify information.
- If the person you are trying to reach is unavailable, leave a message for that person to call you back.

Example

> PATIENT: Hello?
> ASSISTANT: Hello, this is Linda at Dr. Newman's office. Is this Mr. Long?
> PATIENT: Yes, this is Mr. Long.
> ASSISTANT: Mr. Long, we have scheduled your stomach X ray for Wednesday, June 2, at 9 a.m. The X ray will be taken at the Metro Radiology Clinic on Fourth and Greenview.
> PATIENT: Good.
> ASSISTANT: Please remember, Mr. Long, that you can't have anything to eat or drink after midnight on Tuesday. Also, don't smoke or chew gum Wednesday morning. Did you get those instructions written down?

PATIENT: Yes, Wednesday at 9 a.m. Metro Radiology Clinic. No food or drink after midnight on Tuesday.
ASSISTANT: Good. Do you have any questions?
PATIENT: No. Thanks for calling.

Example

The assistant places a call to Dr. Martin for Dr. Newman. Dr. Newman may need to be paged or called out of a patient's examination room when Dr. Martin comes on the line.

ASSISTANT: This is Linda at Dr. Newman's office. Dr. Newman would like to talk with Dr. Martin. Is Dr. Martin available now?
ASSISTANT (WHEN DR. MARTIN ANSWERS): Just a moment, Dr. Martin. I will get Dr. Newman for you.
(*Then, paging*): Dr. Newman, Dr. Martin is on Line 2.

In a busy office, Dr. Newman can use the waiting time to examine patients while an assistant locates Dr. Martin. It is true that Dr. Martin will be placed briefly on hold, waiting for Dr. Newman. However, in most cases, to use this example, the waiting time for Dr. Martin would not be as long as it would have been for Dr. Newman had the assistant not set up the call. If Dr. Martin is not in the office, the assistant needs to know whether Dr. Newman wants Dr. Martin located and if the answer is yes, how urgently this needs to be done.

PROJECT 15   Outgoing Calls

Dr. Newman has been asked to speak at the in-service education meeting at University Hospital. He asks you to get specific details about the meeting when Mrs. Yates calls from the hospital. Today's date is October 8, and the time is 10:25 a.m. On plain paper, write a list of questions to ask Mrs. Yates.

Place this message in the Miscellaneous folder for future use.

Faxing Information

A facsimile (fax) machine is now used to send or receive information about patients immediately. The doctor must develop and follow guidelines for faxing information about patients.

A patient's confidentiality must be protected—the fax machine must be in a secured location where only authorized personnel have access to it. Federal and state laws must be followed for maintaining medical records. Send a release of information with a cover letter (see the example shown in Figure 4-6 on page 76). Contact the receiver before transmitting the information. File the original cover letter in the chart. Request a signed return receipt of the faxed information. Transmitted documents received on thermal fax paper must be photocopied before

MARK NEWMAN, M.D.

Board Certified in Family Medicine

2235 South Ridgeway Avenue
Chicago, IL 60623-2240
312-555-6022
FAX: 312-555-0025

FACSIMILE COVER LETTER

DATE: ____________ **TIME:** ________ a.m./p.m.

TO: ______________________
(name)
____
(facility)
____
(address)

FAX NUMBER: ______________________

RE: ______________________

FROM: ______________________
(name/department)
MARK NEWMAN, M.D.

Number of pages including cover letter: ____________

NOTICE OF CONFIDENTIALITY: The faxed document or documents contain confidential information. The information is only for use by the above-named receiver. Use of the information in any form is strictly prohibited if you are not the intended receiver. Please notify our office immediately if you received this fax in error. Contact our office by telephone to arrange for the return of the original fax document.

RETURN RECEIPT: Please complete the following statement and return it to the above-stated fax number.

I, ______________________, verify that I have received ___ pages
Authorized Receiver

from ______________________.
Sending Facility

Figure 4-6 Facsimile Cover Letter With Return Receipt

being placed in a patient's chart because thermal fax paper deteriorates over time.

Cellular Telephones

The physician may have a **cellular phone** (mobile service). The cellular phone may be installed in an automobile or may be a portable type with a battery pack. With the advance of cellular phones, the doctor may be contacted at all times.

Follow Through

Proper handling of telephone calls does not end after the phone is hung up. The medical assistant must follow through on all requests made and instructions provided in the conversation. See Figures 4-7 through 4-10 for examples of **follow-through** methods.

A record of incoming telephone calls can also be made using a journal with columns for the date and time of the call, the name of the

MESSAGE

TO _Nurse_   DATE _10/6_   TIME _10:20_

FROM _Laura Paulson_   *11:00 Told to come for cultures*
                                         for all family members.

PHONE _555-7261_   *Sue, R.N.*

☑ PLEASE CALL   ☐ RETURNED YOUR CALL   ☐ WILL CALL AGAIN

REGARDING _Jason has strep. Andy + Eric now have sore_
throats. Should family come in for cultures?

TAKEN BY _tjo_

Figure 4-7 Follow-Through Notation Made Directly on a Telephone Message Skip

---

MEMO TO: Mark Newman, M.D.

FROM: University Hospital

DATE: September 25

SUBJECT: Dr. Dean Ashcroft's seminars

The University Hospital telephoned at 4 p.m. today about a series of four seminars titled "Educating Caregivers."

1. Early Care: Prenatal
2. Prevention of Accidents Involving Household Poisons
3. Early Abusive Behaviors
4. Addictive Caregivers

Dr. Ashcroft is the sponsor of the series. Please let me know if you would like to register for any of these seminars.

TJO

Figure 4-8 Follow-Through Memo Summarizing a Telephone Call

TO DO
DATE _7/23_

RUSH	ITEMS	DONE
	~~Send records to Dr. Peters re: Jill Sommers.~~	7/26
	~~Reserve conference room 7/31 at 8 a.m.~~	7/26
	Remind Dr. Newman to get slides for 7/31.	
*	Call Brent Ashwood 7/23 re: disability form	
	at 555-7287.	

Figure 4-9 Follow-Through Notation on a To-Do List

IN-HOUSE WORK SHEET

NAME _Marlene Goodin_   DATE _8/6/--_

PROBLEM _Difficulty breathing_

INJECTIONS:

LAB: Theophylline level next week—pt
       to call us to schedule.

X RAYS: Sinus films 8/6
          Chest PA 8/6

SPECIAL PROCEDURES: EKG 8/6

INSTRUCTIONS:

RTC: 6 weeks

OLD RECORDS: Eastside Clinic
                 requested 8/8

Figure 4-10 Follow-Through Notation About Telephone Calls on a Medical Work Sheet

---

caller, and a brief notation regarding the purpose of a call. Figure 4-11 shows an example of a **telephone log** for incoming calls. Notice that a follow-through notation can be made in such a log.

TELEPHONE LOG
DATE _10/6_

TIME	CALLER	TELEPHONE	REASON	DONE
9:00	Alma Jackson	555-1102	Test results	
10:10	Hank Baxter	555-3721	Schedule GI + GB appt.	✓ 2:30
10:15	Matt Colburn		Appt.	✓
10:20	Laura Paulson	555-7261	Andy + Eric, sore throats, TC?	✓ 11:00

Figure 4-11 Follow-Through Notation on a Telephone Log

■ TELEPHONE STANDARDS

Many clinics and businesses monitor their employees' performance in handling telephone calls. This enables the employer to maintain a high standard of customer service, which helps to keep patients satisfied with the care they receive. An example of a checklist for evaluating telephone performance is shown in Figure 4-12.

<table>
<tr><td>**PROJECT 16**</td><td>**Telephone Situations**</td></tr>
</table>

Circle the best answer in each of the telephone situations on WP 20. Be prepared to discuss your answers in class.

■ TELEPHONE DIRECTORIES

Telephone directories are a valuable resource for the medical assistant. A variety of information is contained in the directories, including crisis numbers, area codes, local ZIP Codes, a time zone map, and a list of services provided by the telephone company.

TELEPHONE PERFORMANCE

Name of Employee: _____ Date: _____

Beginning and Closing of Call

____ Answered promptly (2 or 3 rings).

____ Gave proper identification (clinic or office name, department, and name).

____ Left a pleasing impression at close of call.

Development of Call

____ Ready to offer assistance to caller.

  Made inquiries tactfully regarding:

  ____ Reason for call.

  ____ Caller's regular physician.

  ____ Other pertinent information.

____ Verified information.

____ Gave effective explanations.

____ Used good judgment.

  If caller was put on hold:

  ____ Waited for caller's OK to be put on hold.

  ____ Updated caller on status of call.

  ____ Offered to take a message.

____ Recorded an accurate message.

Voice Personality

____ Spoke pleasantly.

____ Spoke courteously.

____ Spoke distinctly.

____ Used correct grammar.

____ Used caller's name.

  Rated by: _____

Figure 4-12   Telephone-Performance Checklist

Alphabetic Directory

An **alphabetic directory**, or white pages, lists telephone customers by name in alphabetic order. As an aid in looking up numbers, the directory lists cross-references to the various spellings of similar-sounding names. The white pages usually contain other information such as directory-assistance numbers, billing information, long-distance calling procedures, and area code maps. In large cities, information concerning government agencies, including phone numbers, is often listed in the blue pages section of the alphabetic directory.

Classified Directory

A **classified directory**, or yellow pages, lists telephone subscribers under headings for types of businesses such as "Office Supplies or Laboratories—Medical." Classified directories also contain advertising for subscribing businesses and sometimes contain local street maps and ZIP Code listings.

After looking up a telephone number, jot it down for future reference. If a number cannot be found in the directory, call directory assistance to ask an operator for help.

Personal Directory

A personal directory is used for phone numbers that are frequently called by the office staff. The personal directory should be kept near the phone for easy access and would probably include a list of the following phone numbers:

- Hospitals
- Insurance companies
- Laboratories
- Medical supply companies
- Pharmacies
- Hospital emergency room
- Specialists for referrals made to patients

Long-Distance Calls

Information about placing special long-distance calls such as operator-assisted calls and conference calls is provided in telephone directories. Long-distance calls can be dialed direct almost anywhere in the world, and this is usually the most cost-effective way to place a long-distance call. To dial direct, dial the prefix number *1*, the area code, and then the regular seven-digit phone number (for example, 1-212-555-6022). If you know the area code but not the telephone number, you can obtain the phone number from long-distance information by dialing *1*-(area code)-555-1212 if the area code is in the United States. Many directories include a list of area codes for major United States cities.

Check the difference in time zones before placing a long-distance call so that the call will arrive at a place of business between 9 a.m. and 5 p.m.

Calling Cards

A **calling card**, which may be obtained from the telephone company, enables local and long-distance calls to be charged directly to a physician's monthly bill. The doctor may use the calling card as needed when away from the office. This card is used in place of coins and is as easy to use as a credit card.

■ TELEPHONE EQUIPMENT

There is a wide variety of telephone equipment available for the medical office. The type of system you use will depend on the size of the office in which you work. Most office telephone systems use sophisticated computer technology. The right system will improve office efficiency, reduce pressure on the office staff, and help provide better service to patients. A number of different features are commonly found in phone systems used in medical offices.

Switchboard

A call board or central switchboard monitors and directs all incoming calls. A receptionist or switchboard operator may field incoming calls and then direct them to appropriate extensions, but most systems also allow incoming calls to go directly to lines in the office.

Such a phone system uses computer software to record data pertaining to calls. The system can be programmed to provide a printout of all calls received, including the time and date of each call; how long it took to answer each call; how long the call lasted; and, for outgoing calls, the number dialed. Such programs are especially useful in providing records of long-distance calls for billing purposes and for tracking calls if a legal issue arises. See Figure 4-13 for an example of such a computerized call printout.

Desk Phones

Smaller medical practices may need only three to five phone lines to handle day-to-day business. In such offices, a basic desk phone will

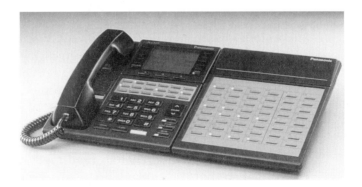

Most office telephone systems use computer technology to improve office efficiency.

DAILY PROFILE REPORT

GROUP 3
DATE: 10/16/—   17:10:01

TIME	STF	#RCVD	#ANS
8:00	6	35	27
8:30	6	22	22
9:00	6	25	25
9:30	5	21	21
10:00	4	23	22
10:30	4	18	18
11:00	6	14	14
11:30	6	22	22
12:00	2	11	11
12:30	2	16	15
13:00	4	19	19
13:30	4	13	13
14:00	6	17	17
14:30	5	8	8
15:00	3	10	10
15:30	3	12	12
16:00	3	13	12
16:30	2	8	6
		307	295

Figure 4-13 Computer Printout From a Telephone System. (*STF* is the staff phone. *#RCVD* means the number. *#ANS* means the number answered.)

be used. It is likely to have an intercom, but it will also have fewer lines available for incoming calls. Basic features for desk-phone systems include the following:

- **Call pickup**: You can answer calls from another extension on your phone by pushing specific buttons. For example, suppose the buttons to be pushed for call pickup are "#" and "7" on your telephone. If a call comes into the insurance person's line when he or she is away from the desk, you can intercept the call on your phone by picking up your receiver, pushing # and then 7 on your phone, and saying "Insurance. This is Leslie."

- **Call forwarding**: You can temporarily forward calls to another number. For example, the accounting staff could have their calls forwarded to the insurance extension during their lunchtime.

- **Call transfer**: You can put a caller on hold and then, by pushing specific buttons on your telephone, transfer the call to another extension in the office. For example, suppose a patient calls to request an urgent appointment that day, but the schedule is full. You can put the caller on hold, discuss the situation with the nurse out of the patient's hearing, and then transfer the call to the nurse's line by pushing the appropriate buttons. The nurse can then talk with the patient in order to evaluate the urgency of the medical situation.

- **Automatic hold recall**: The telephone system periodically (at 30-second intervals) reminds you that a caller is on hold.

- **Automatic call distribution**: This feature allows you to take calls in the order in which they are received. It is especially useful at the appointment desk.

■ ANSWERING SERVICES

Doctors use commercial answering services; answering machines; and, in some specialties, pagers to provide 24-hour service to their patients.

Commercial Answering Services

Commercial answering services can be hired by the doctor's office on a monthly basis to answer the office's calls from a remote location. All unanswered calls are forwarded to an operator during nonoffice hours. This operator takes messages for routine calls or pages the doctor if the call is an emergency. The doctor or the assistant checks in with the answering service for any messages after returning to the office.

Answering Machines

An answering machine consists of a tape recorder that is connected to the telephone line and is triggered by an incoming call. A message that has been prerecorded by the doctor or assistant is played to the caller. It tells the caller what to do if the call is urgent or routine. The message can be changed according to circumstances.

Example

> TAPE MESSAGE: Dr. Newman's office is closed until 1 p.m. If this is an emergency, please call University Hospital at 555-2500.

Upon returning to the office at 1 p.m., the assistant plays back the messages and follows through as needed. Then the assistant turns off the answering machine and begins taking calls again.

PROJECT 17 Recording a Message

Write a message (less than 1 minute long) to be recorded on an answering machine. Explain that Dr. Newman's office is closed for the weekend and give information for routine and emergency calls. Dr. Newman's office opens Monday at 8 a.m. The phone number of University Hospital is 555–2500. Use plain paper. Place the message in the Miscellaneous folder.

If possible, use a tape recorder to record and listen to your message.

Key Terms

The following terms appear in **boldface** type in this chapter. Do you recall what they mean? Refer to the chapter for definitions you need to review.

alphabetic directory
automatic call
  distribution
automatic hold recall
call forwarding
call pickup
call transfer
calling card
cellular phone
classified directory

e-mail (electronic mail)
follow-through
intercom
pager
prescription refill
screening calls
telephone etiquette
telephone log
"voice with a smile"

Topics for Discussion

1. You work for two doctors. A patient new to the area calls and wants to schedule a complete physical exam. The patient asks you about the qualifications of both doctors and about which doctor you would recommend. How would you answer?

2. What would you tell a person who wants to talk with the doctor when the doctor is not in the office?

Role-Playing

1. Your instructor will dictate a series of prescription refills to you. Practice completing messages for these prescription refills.

2. You receive the following calls while Dr. Newman is with patients. How would you handle each of them?

   a. A friend of Dr. Newman's calls to ask whether he is free for lunch today.

   b. Mr. Nagata is new in town and was told by his previous doctor to call Dr. Newman.

   c. A research analyst from Allied Insurance Group calls asking for Dr. Newman.

   d. A patient calls to ask what laboratory work is required for a complete physical exam.

   e. Joe Rutherford, a 73-year-old patient of Dr. Newman's, calls and sounds as if he just wants to talk with someone.

Appointments

Upon completion of this chapter, you should be able to:

- Give four guidelines for scheduling appointments.

- Discuss the following situations:
  Procedures for setting up an appointment book.
  Time allotments for various types of appointments.
  Screening (triage).
  Obtaining information from a patient when scheduling.
  Explaining office policies to new patients.
  Procedures for canceling and rescheduling appointments.
  Appointment delays by the patient and by the doctor.
  Emergencies.
  Interruptions.
  House calls.
  Failure to show for appointments.

- Provide appropriate responses to the following situations:

The schedule is full; the patient's problem is not urgent.
The schedule is full; the patient's problem is urgent.
Only a certain appointment time is available.
The doctor is not available at the time requested by the patient.
Another doctor in the clinic is available at the requested time.
The patient refuses to give a reason for an appointment.
The doctor no longer sees patients for a certain problem (for example, obstetrics or pediatrics).

- Apply the guidelines of scheduling.

- Identify measures to help protect the physician legally when there is a cancellation or no-show.

Scheduling appointments is one of the principal duties of the assistant, and being able to do so efficiently and intelligently is one of the assistant's most important skills. Appointments must be entered into an appointment book or computer scheduling software. Canceled appointments must be indicated and the time slot used for another patient whenever possible. The doctor's outside appointments should be listed and, if necessary, the doctor must be reminded of them in advance.

■ SETTING UP THE SCHEDULE

Before appointments can be made in an appointment book, you must know the basic schedule of the doctor's office. The doctor probably will have to make the rounds of patients at one or more hospitals on certain days and at certain hours. Office hours, therefore, may vary on different days. Some doctors have office hours in the evenings and on weekends. If there are several doctors in one office, the hours of each doctor may be different. Each doctor's hours should be entered into the appointment book to show at a glance the hours when each doctor is in and where each doctor can be reached at other times.

Once the basic schedule of the office is set, specific guidelines are used to schedule appointments for patients.

Following the Doctor's Policy

Policy may be affected by the doctor's specialty, the office hours, how quickly the doctor works, the treatment or procedure to be performed, the available office personnel, and the type of facility.

Screening Patients' Illnesses

When scheduling an appointment, the assistant must use good judgment to determine how soon a patient needs to be seen. This process is called **screening**, or **triage**. Some patients must come to the office immediately, some may be scheduled for later the same day or the following day, and others may be scheduled at a later time that is convenient for both the doctor and the patient.

Considering Patients' Preferences

Some patients prefer to be seen at a certain time or on a certain day of the week. Try to schedule appointments according to patients' preferences if the schedule allows it.

Consulting the Schedule

If the schedule is full, provide the patient with an alternate time.

■ APPOINTMENT BOOK

All appointments are entered into an appointment book or computer scheduling software so that an accurate record of the day's schedule is always available. A copy of the day's appointments may be given to the doctor each morning to keep the doctor informed of the schedule.

Time Allotment

Appointment books vary in size, content, and format, as do computer scheduling software programs. Each page of an appointment book divides the working day into 10-, 15-, or 30-minute intervals. In this way the assistant can control **time allotment** in scheduling each exam or procedure. Most office visits are considered routine or brief, and the patient is allotted 10 to 15 minutes in the appointment book. Problems requiring more time include minor surgery, consultations, cast applications, and some adult physicals. For example, a complete physical examination will take longer than a routine blood pressure checkup. An example of a schedule showing appointments of varying lengths is given in Figure 5-1.

In general, try not to schedule too many similar appointments together (for example, two complete physical exams or two first visits for obstetrics). The doctor may request that lengthy appointments such as complete physicals be scheduled only at certain times. For example, the doctor may ask you to schedule complete physicals as the first appointment available in the morning or the first appointment available in the afternoon or not to schedule them on Mondays or after 3 p.m.

Monday, September 29

8:00	Hospital Rounds	
8:15		
8:30		
8:45		
9:00	Jolene Sanborn - rash	555-9107
9:15	Donnette Chambers - re. ✔ BP	555-6274
9:30	Robert Crenshaw - diet	555-9771
9:45	Marilyn Skelly - re. ✔ cast	555-5732
10:00	Break	
10:15	Arnold Friske - CPE	555-1127
10:30		
10:45		
11:00		
11:15	Lynette Babbatte - renew meds	555-7241
11:30	Wade Benjamin - nausea	555-9275
11:45	Tina Gonzalez - tired	555-3057
12:00		
12:15		
12:30	Lunch	
12:45		

Figure 5-1 Schedule Noting Lengths of Appointments

Page Arrangement

Appointment books may have a single sheet for each day and a separate page for each doctor, or they may show an entire week on two facing pages. The more information required for scheduling, the larger each individual sheet will be.

■ TYPES OF SCHEDULING

Patients complain twice as much about waiting in the doctor's office as they do about any other cause, including doctor's fees and treatment results. When an appointment has been made for a specific time, it is frustrating for the patient to be kept waiting for a long period of time. An efficient scheduling system will help eliminate the waiting period for most patients.

Hospital Rounds

A primary consideration in scheduling is allotting time for the doctor's **hospital rounds**. Hospital visits at set hours should be noted in the appointment book.

The assistant may be responsible for recording daily hospital visits. Methods vary for recording this information and may include the following:

■ Index cards showing information on each patient.
■ Computer printouts from the hospital with information about each patient.
■ Telephone calls from the doctor to the assistant in which the information about each patient is written down by the assistant.

Scheduled Appointments

Most doctor's offices and clinics prefer to use a scheduling system in which each patient is given a set appointment time, which means an approximate time the patient will be seen by the doctor. This method usually decreases the waiting time for the patient and gives the office staff more control over the flow of patients in the office. Also, because the reason for each patient's visit is known in advance, the staff can make the best use of the office facilities and equipment.

Fixed Office Hours

Clinics have **fixed office hours** during which the doctor is in the office and available to see patients—from 10 a.m. to noon, for example. Patients sign in with the receptionist and are seen in the order in which they arrive. This system allows patients the freedom to come to the clinic when they wish, but it also has several drawbacks:

■ The reason for the patient's visit is not known until the patient arrives at the office.

- It is difficult to control the flow of patients. Thus, many patients may arrive at the same time, causing crowding and long waits. At other times, there may be no patients, causing the doctor's and the staff's time to be used inefficiently.
- Equipment and office facilities may be used inefficiently.

Wave Scheduling

One way to get around these problems is to combine fixed office hours with scheduled appointments. This is called **wave scheduling**. In an office using wave scheduling, the assistant tells about six patients to come between 9 a.m. and 10 a.m., then tells the next six patients who call to arrive between 10 a.m. and 11 a.m., and so on throughout the day. Wave scheduling gives patients the flexibility of open office hours while allowing the assistant more control over the flow of patients. This method works well in practices such as dermatology and endocrinology because the doctor does not have to wait for laboratory and X ray results before suggesting a treatment to the patient.

Another version of wave scheduling is to schedule a patient with a complex problem on the hour (for example, 10:00 a.m.) and short routine exams for the remainder of the hour.

Double-Column Scheduling

Double-column scheduling may be used on an emergency basis or if a patient is very sick and needs to see the doctor immediately. Some offices use double-column scheduling when the schedule is full and more patients need to be seen. When double-column scheduling is used, the extra appointments are entered in a second column beside the regularly scheduled appointments.

See Figure 5-2 for examples of appointment books using these various scheduling methods.

Computer Scheduling

A variety of computer scheduling software is used in medical offices. Most scheduling software allows the assistant to search for the next available slot for the amount of time needed. For example, if a complete physical is to be scheduled, the computer would search for the next available 1-hour appointment. After this has been located, the assistant can confirm that the date and time are acceptable to the patient and then enter the appropriate information to fill the slot.

In addition to a printout of the daily schedule, most scheduling software can generate reports of cancellations and no shows, patient's registration information, and chart labels for patient's records. Figure 5-3 on page 90 shows a scheduling program on a computer screen.

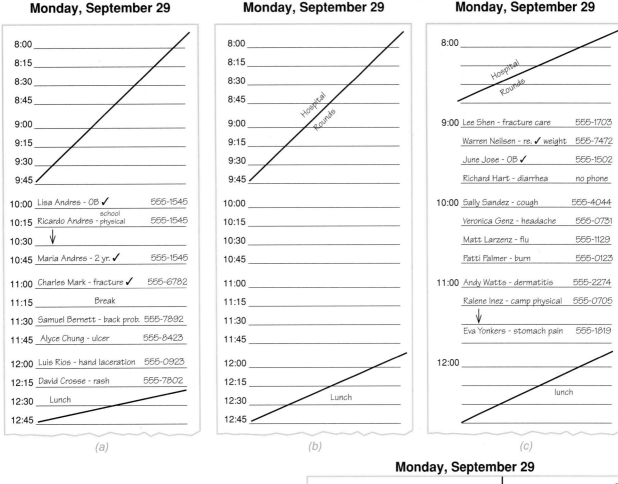

Monday, September 29 *(a)*

8:00		
8:15		
8:30		
8:45		
9:00		
9:15		
9:30		
9:45		
10:00	Lisa Andres - OB ✓	555-1545
10:15	Ricardo Andres - physical (school)	555-1545
10:30	↓	
10:45	Maria Andres - 2 yr. ✓	555-1545
11:00	Charles Mark - fracture ✓	555-6782
11:15	Break	
11:30	Samuel Bernett - back prob.	555-7892
11:45	Alyce Chung - ulcer	555-8423
12:00	Luis Rios - hand laceration	555-0923
12:15	David Crosse - rash	555-7802
12:30	Lunch	
12:45		

Monday, September 29 *(b)*

8:00	
8:15	
8:30	
8:45	Hospital Rounds
9:00	
9:15	
9:30	
9:45	
10:00	
10:15	
10:30	
10:45	
11:00	
11:15	
11:30	
11:45	
12:00	
12:15	
12:30	Lunch
12:45	

Monday, September 29 *(c)*

Time	Appointment	Phone
8:00	Hospital Rounds	
9:00	Lee Shen - fracture care	555-1703
	Warren Neilsen - re. ✓ weight	555-7472
	June Jose - OB ✓	555-1502
	Richard Hart - diarrhea	no phone
10:00	Sally Sandez - cough	555-4044
	Veronica Genz - headache	555-0731
	Matt Larzenz - flu	555-1129
	Patti Palmer - burn	555-0123
11:00	Andy Watts - dermatitis	555-2274
	Ralene Inez - camp physical	555-0705
	↓	
	Eva Yonkers - stomach pain	555-1819
12:00	lunch	

Monday, September 29 *(d)*

8:00	Hospital Rounds			
8:15				
8:30				
8:45				
9:00	Alex Marshall - CPE	555-1492	Marvin Gomez - burn	555-2010
9:15				
9:30	↓		Tom Chenz - re. ✓ wt	555-0709
9:45				
10:00	Carmen Hovik - NP OB	555-3839	Deiter Reye - flu	555-0527
10:15	Larry Reis - nosebleeds	555-1118		
10:30	Frank Skein - head injury	555-0027		
10:45	Harris Hemez - cast repair	555-9483	Elaine Roe - croup	555-1172
11:00	Bart Carmen - preop. physical	555-3001	Gayle Reamer - abd. pain	555-1523
11:15			James Reid - diabetic re. ✓	555-7229
11:30	Jeremy Lentil - 1-yr. ✓	555-8492		
11:45	Lorna Chan - earache	555-0095		
12:00				
12:15				
12:30	Lunch			
12:45				

Figure 5-2 Appointment Books Showing *(a)* Scheduled Appointments, *(b)* Fixed Office Hours, *(c)* Wave Schedule, and *(d)* Double-Column Schedule

```
┌─O F F I C E─┐ ┌─Appointment List─────────────────────────────────┐
│   H O U R S │ │ 6:00a                          1:30              │
├─────────────┤ │ 6:15                          1:45              │
│September 1997│ │ 6:30                          2:00p             │
│Su Mo Tu We Th Fr Sa│ │ 6:45                     2:15              │
│    1  2  3  4  5  6│ │ 7:00a                    2:30              │
│ 7  8  9 10 11 12 13│ │ 7:15                     2:45              │
│14 15 16 17 18 19 20│ │ 7:30                     3:00p             │
│21 22 23 24 25 26 27│ │ 7:45                     3:15              │
│28 29 30            │ │ 8:00a                    3:30              │
│                    │ │ 8:15                     3:45              │
│                    │ │ 8:30                     4:00p             │
├─Staff──────────────┤ │ 8:45                     4:15              │
│Dr. Katherine Van   │ │ 9:00a                    4:30              │
│Dr. John Rudner     │ │ 9:15                     4:45              │
│Dr. Jessica Rudner  │ │ 9:30                     5:00p             │
│                    │ │ 9:45                     5:15              │
│                    │ │10:00a                    5:30              │
│                    │ │10:15                     5:45              │
│                    │ │10:30                     6:00p             │
│                    │ │10:45                     6:15              │
│                    │ │11:00a                    6:30              │
│                    │ │11:15                     6:45              │
└─────────────┘ └─────────────────────────────────────────────────┘
F1-Help F2-Print F4-Purge F5-Staff F6-Find SPACE-Goto PgDn/Up-Next/Prev ESC-Exit
```

Figure 5-3   Computer Schedule Screen

■ GUIDELINES FOR SCHEDULING

Before scheduling a patient, find out the reason for the appointment. Once the reason for the appointment is known, you will be able to decide how much time is needed for the appointment and when the appointment should be made. You may have to ask the patient several questions before deciding how much time is needed to handle a certain appointment and how soon the patient should come to the office. When in doubt, the nurse or the physician may have to be consulted.

The following list might be used as a guideline for deciding how soon a patient needs to be seen. The term *stat* is used in health care to mean "immediately." Patients with serious or life-threatening illnesses need to be seen "stat." Some complaints are not life-threatening but should be evaluated "today." Less serious illnesses can wait until "tomorrow." Routine examinations, tests, and procedures can be scheduled "when available."

Stat	Today	Tomorrow	When Available
Breathing difficulty	Abdominal pain	Blood in stools	Mole removal
Burn	Nausea and vomiting	Cast repair	Physicals
Chest pain	Possible fracture	Dermatitis	Rechecks
Laceration	Severe headache	Flu	OB checks
Nosebleed	Visual difficulty	Rash	Vague complaints
Head injury		Vaginitis	Well-baby check

Physical exams and follow-up visits are considered routine and do not take precedence over other procedures in scheduling.

Keep in mind the flow of patients in the office when scheduling appointments. The doctor can see a patient in one room while another

WP 21 lists 40 situations an assistant may have to screen for scheduling. Determine whether the patient should be seen (a) stat, (b) today, (c) tomorrow, or (d) when available. Use an asterisk (*) to mark those situations requiring more than one time slot (10 or 15 minutes) in the appointment book. Be prepared to discuss the situations in class.

patient is in the X-ray room and a third patient is being prepared by the nurse for an examination. Schedule appointments consecutively in solid blocks of time. If there are only a few appointments on one day, schedule the appointments early in the day to allow for emergencies or changes that may occur. Such scheduling also gives the doctor a block of time in the afternoon to catch up on medical reports, correspondence, and other professional matters without being interrupted.

When a patient asks for a **routine appointment** without specifying the time, the patient should be asked, "Do you prefer a morning or an afternoon appointment?" or "There is a 2 o'clock appointment available tomorrow."

If the patient wants to make an appointment on a specific day and only a certain time is available, the patient could be told, "The only time Dr. Newman has open that day is 4 p.m. Can you come in at that time?" If the patient requests an appointment for a time when the doctor is not in, it is not necessary to say where the doctor will be at that time. You might suggest an alternate time by saying, "I am sorry, but Dr. Newman is not available at that time. He does have a morning appointment on Thursday, however."

In a busy office, there may be no appointment time available for a week or more. A patient could then be told, "Dr. Newman's schedule is filled for several weeks. The earliest appointment time is Friday, June 2, at 10:30 a.m., unless it is an emergency." This reply indicates that the doctor is available for emergencies. Most patients will cooperate and accept the first appointment available, unless there really is an emergency. The assistant may mention that an earlier appointment may become available if a cancellation occurs.

Should the assistant determine that the patient needs to be seen that day, the patient could be told, "The schedule is full today, but if you can come to the office at 2 p.m., we will work you into the schedule between other patients." Remember, the patient must be made to feel that the doctor is available when really needed.

Reason for the Appointment

Should the patient refuse to give a reason for the appointment, ask whether the appointment is for a medical problem. If the visit is for personal or business reasons, it should be noted as such in the appointment book.

Some patients may be embarrassed to talk about their medical condition, but the doctor still will expect the assistant to find out the reason for the appointment. Asking simple questions about the medical problem will encourage the patient to state the reason for the visit. Such questions include: "Have you seen the doctor about this condition before?" and "Is this a condition that requires urgent treatment?" The privacy of the patient is important, so be polite and tactful when acquiring information.

Necessary Data

The appointment book or scheduling software should provide space for recording all necessary data. In general, this includes the following information:

- Patient's first and last names.
- Account number.
- Insurance provider.
- Telephone number.
- Referring physician.
- Reason for the appointment.
- Notations regarding any laboratory tests or X rays required before the examination.
- A notation if the appointment is for a new patient.

Always verify the patient's name and its spelling and repeat telephone numbers. Confirm the appointment time by repeating it to the patient. For example, "Sara, your appointment with Dr. Newman is for Wednesday, July 16, at 2:15."

When the patient arrives in the office, the information in the appointment book should verified. Because the information required for scheduling is confidential, the appointment book should not be left where any patients can see and read it.

PROJECT 19   Setting Up Dr. Newman's Practice

Information about Dr. Newman's practice and common abbreviations used in the appointment book are found on WP 22. Remove this sheet from the back of the book, and attach it to the cover of the binder or file folder you will be using for your appointment calendar.

You will find the calendar pages dated October 13 to December 3 on WPs 23 through 37. Remove these pages, and place them in your binder or folder. You will work with these pages throughout most of the course, entering, canceling, and rescheduling appointments, as well as watching for events that must be brought to Dr. Newman's attention. For example, whenever Dr. Newman states he will be attending a meeting or scheduling surgery, make the appropriate entry.

Check the calendar for the week of October 13 against Dr. Newman's schedule listed on WP 22. The calendar pages have been prepared for you with the exception of the week of October 20. On those calendar pages, cross out the hours that Dr. Newman is making hospital rounds, teaching at the University Medical School, and so forth.

On the appropriate pages, enter the following commitments:

October 16, 3:00 p.m., Dr. Newman's physical exam with Dr. Hugh Arnold.

October 29, 4:00 p.m., lecture by Dr. Margo Matthews at University Hospital.

Second Tuesday of every month at 8 p.m., Chicago Medical Society Meeting.

* is an icon indicating that all or part of the exercises may be done using MediSoft and the Student Data Disk. Read Appendix A at the end of this textbook before proceeding.

Occasionally a patient will walk in without an appointment. If the doctor is busy and it is judged that the **walk-in patient** should be seen at that time, you may explain that the doctor will see the patient for a few minutes when the patient can be worked into the schedule.

A patient with a true emergency should be seen upon arrival. The assistant should notify the nurse or doctor of the emergency and escort the patient to the examination room. The assistant must tactfully explain the presence of walk-in and emergency patients to other waiting patients who have made appointments that will now be delayed. If a physician outside the office calls to request that a patient be seen that day by one of the doctors in your office, that patient must also be worked into or added to the day's schedule.

On days when the schedule is full, the office nurse may be used to help determine whether a patient is truly an emergency case and to ask the doctor for further instructions. In some cases, the doctor may request that emergency patients who telephone be referred to the emergency room. A number of emergency scheduling situations might occur in a group practice.

Example: Emergency Patients Referred to the Hospital

ASSISTANT: Dr. Newman's schedule is extremely busy today, so he has asked me to refer emergency patients to the University Hospital Emergency Room.

Example: Scheduling the Appointment With Another In-House Physician

ASSISTANT: Dr. Werner does not have an appointment available today, but Dr. Long could see you at 1:45. Would you like to schedule an appointment with Dr. Long?

Example: New In-House Physician Handling a Patient

ASSISTANT: I am sorry to inform you that Dr. Howard is no longer seeing pediatric patients. Our new physician, Dr. Arenson, is a pediatrician. Dr. Arenson has an appointment available tomorrow at 8:30 a.m. Would you like me to schedule you for that appointment?

Do not refer the patient to another doctor or clinic unless you are directed to do so by your doctor or employer.

In addition to appointments for patients, the doctor will have hospital commitments, seminars, lectures, meetings, and personal appointments. All of these must be marked in the appointment calendar so that there is no conflict. In addition, it is often helpful to give the doctor a reminder of such commitments that do not involve patients ahead of time. Figure 5-4 on page 94 shows an example of such a reminder with a corresponding entry in the appointment book.

Friday, October 3

8:00	
8:15	
8:30	
8:45	Hospital
9:00	Rounds
9:15	
9:30	
9:45	

10:00	Alicia Lopez - postpartum ✓	555-2407
10:15	Julie Anderson - dressing change	555-0224
10:30	Rex Duncan - re. ✓ cast	555-9870
10:45	Karen Tomas annual physical	555-6422
11:00		

3:00	Staff meeting Conference Room A
3:15	
3:30	
3:45	
4:00	Meeting with Infection Control Comm.
4:15	Room 620
4:30	Whitman Hall
4:45	
5:00	
5:15	
5:30	
5:45	
6:30	Charity Ball Sunburst Hotel

MESSAGE

TO Dr. Newman   **DATE** 10/2   **TIME** _____

FROM _____

PHONE _____

☐ **PLEASE CALL**   ☐ **RETURNED YOUR CALL**   ☐ **WILL CALL AGAIN**

REGARDING Reminder! Infection Control Committee
meeting — 4 p.m., Friday, October 3, Room 620, Whitman Hall.

TAKEN BY 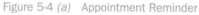 tjo

Figure 5-4 *(a)* Appointment Reminder

Figure 5-4 *(b)* Corresponding Schedule Entry

■ REGISTERING ARRIVALS

Patients are asked to **register**, or **sign in**, upon arrival at a doctor's office or clinic. It is the assistant's duty to verify the patient's name, address, and other information with the patient's record. Verify the spelling of each patient's name. This daily register provides a record of who came first and prevents the awkward mistake of ushering a late-comer into the examination room ahead of an earlier arrival.

When making an appointment for a new patient, he or she may be asked to arrive a few minutes early to complete registration forms and visit with the assistant or manager for new patients. At this time, the practice's policy regarding payment can be explained to the patient, especially if the policy is to have patients pay for the first appointment at the time of the visit.

Example

> ASSISTANT: Your appointment with Dr. Newman is Wednesday, April 3, at 2 p.m. Please try to arrive about 15 minutes early to complete our new-patient registration form. You will also need your insurance policy numbers.
> *or, if the patient does not have health insurance:*
> It is our office policy to request that new patients pay for their visit at the time of the first appointment to establish credit.

When the patient has signed in, the assistant should leave the medical file for the nurse, indicating that the patient is ready to be seen. A check mark is entered in the appointment book to show that the patient has arrived. It may be the assistant's responsibility to see that the patient's chart is in order and that all forms are completed before the patient is seen by the physician.

The registration record can be periodically checked against the appointment schedule to make sure that a patient who has arrived has not forgotten to sign in.

PROJECT 20 **Scheduling Appointments**

Dr. Newman's policy for scheduling is to enter the first and last name of the patient (correctly spelled), the reason for the visit, and the telephone number. The amount of time needed for the appointment is blocked out with arrows. Today's date is October 13. On your calendar pages, enter the following appointments:

October 13, 11:00 a.m., Thomas Baab, CPE, 555-3478

October 14, 10:45 a.m., Erin Mitchell, new patient, OB check, 555-8153

October 14, 11:00 a.m., Gary Robertson, urinary problem, 555-9565

October 14, 11:15 a.m., Laura Lund, cramps, 555-4106

October 14, 11:45 a.m., Charles Jonathan III, knee pain, 555-3097

October 15, 10:30 a.m., Ardis Matthews, nausea, 555-3178

October 20, 11:45 a.m., Doris Casagranda, rash, 555-1200

October 21, 11:00 a.m., Sara Babcock, CPE, 555-5441

October 22, 11:15 a.m., Ana Mendez, neck pain, 555-3606

■ KEEPING TO THE SCHEDULE

Late Patients

The entire schedule may be thrown out of balance because a patient is late. Patients who are late for appointments may have to be asked to wait until the doctor has seen the next patient or until a treatment room is available. It is not the assistant's place to criticize a patient for tardiness, but most doctors wish to be notified of a patient who is habitually late since it is an inconvenience to other patients. Sometimes, the patient who is late may have to be asked to reschedule.

Extended Appointments

Schedules also fall behind when either the doctor or the patient loses track of the time during an examination, causing the appointment to go past the allotted period. The assistant may have to remind the doctor if the visit runs over the scheduled time. The assistant can use the intercom or knock on the examination room door and hand the doctor a written reminder when the doctor comes to the door. The doctor can then decide whether or not to conclude the visit with the patient.

Out-of-Office Emergencies

The schedule may also be disrupted when the doctor is called out of the office for an emergency. The assistant should explain the situation to waiting patients and ask patients whether they wish to wait for the doctor or to reschedule their appointments.

Example

> ASSISTANT: Dr. Newman has been called out on an emergency. He is not likely to be back for at least an hour. Would you like to wait for him to return, or shall I reschedule your appointment?

As a courtesy, patients should also be informed if the doctor is running late as a result of unforeseen interruptions. The assistant might say, "Dr. Newman is running behind schedule by about 30 minutes. Would you like to wait, or shall I reschedule your appointment?" Do not offer to reschedule if the schedule is behind by only a few minutes.

Open Slots

No matter how carefully appointments are scheduled, crowding is sometimes unavoidable and appointments fall behind schedule. Leaving a 15- or 20-minute interval free in the late morning and again in the middle of the afternoon will help you to straighten out a delayed schedule. If no delays occur, these open slots can be used to catch up with other work. Open slots also allow time for emergency patients and unscheduled patients.

■ CANCELING APPOINTMENTS

Almost every patient will cancel an appointment at one time or another; some patients make a habit of doing so. When a patient calls to cancel an appointment, a new appointment time should be suggested.

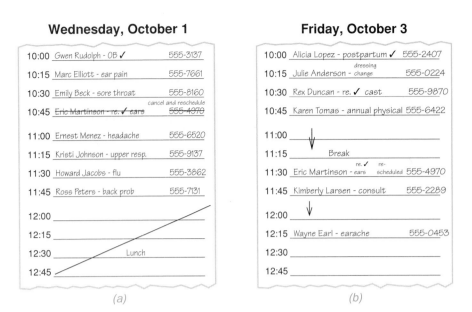

Wednesday, October 1

10:00	Gwen Rudolph - OB ✓	555-3137
10:15	Marc Elliott - ear pain	555-7661
10:30	Emily Beck - sore throat	555-8160
10:45	~~Eric Martinson - re. ✓ ears~~ *cancel and reschedule*	~~555-4970~~
11:00	Ernest Menez - headache	555-6520
11:15	Kristi Johnson - upper resp.	555-9137
11:30	Howard Jacobs - flu	555-3862
11:45	Ross Peters - back prob	555-7131
12:00		
12:15		
12:30	Lunch	
12:45		

(a)

Friday, October 3

10:00	Alicia Lopez - postpartum ✓	555-2407
10:15	Julie Anderson - *dressing* change	555-0224
10:30	Rex Duncan - re. ✓ cast	555-9870
10:45	Karen Tomas - annual physical	555-6422
11:00		
11:15	Break	
11:30	Eric Martinson - ears *re. ✓ re-scheduled*	555-4970
11:45	Kimberly Larsen - consult	555-2289
12:00		
12:15	Wayne Earl - earache	555-0453
12:30		
12:45		

(b)

Figure 5-5 *(a)* Canceled Appointment; *(b)* Rescheduled Appointment

If an appointment book is being used, make the appropriate **cancellation** entry by drawing a line through the appointment or erasing the appointment. If computerized scheduling is being used, choose the appropriate cancellation directive from the menu; the time will now be available for another appointment. The policy of the practice may be to identify the rescheduled appointment in a distinctive way that shows it is the result of a cancellation. Figure 5-5 shows an example of (a) a canceled appointment and (b) the rescheduling of the appointment on another day.

A notation regarding the cancellation may also be entered into the patient's medical record (especially if the cancellation is made on the same day as or the day before the scheduled appointment).

Also make a notation in the patient's medical record if the patient fails to keep an appointment and does not call to cancel. Figure 5-6 shows an example of a chart note recording a no-show appointment.

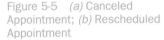

Name	Dan Hanley	**Telephone**	555-1875
Date of Birth	7/27/36	**Age**	59

7/23/--, 8:30 p.m.	TELEPHONE CALL: From Clara Wicks at nursing home.
	Patient complained of difficulty hearing. Nurse checked ears and believes them to be plugged with wax.
	Nurse told to irrigate ears. If no better, to call office tomorrow and make an appointment.
	M. Newman, M.D
8/14/--	Failed to show for appointment.
	tjo

Figure 5-6 Chart Notation for a No-Show Appointment

The doctor will decide what action to take if a patient repeatedly makes appointments and does not keep them. Specialty practices sometimes charge patients for canceled appointments when notification is not made 24 hours in advance.

There are times when the doctor will have to cancel an appointment. The patient should be notified by phone of a cancellation as early as possible to avoid an unnecessary trip to the office. In an emergency, it may not be possible to notify the patient of a cancellation in time. If that is the case, explain the circumstances tactfully when the patient arrives and schedule a new appointment.

As changes in the appointment book are made throughout the day, remember also to make the changes on the work station schedule used by the doctor and nurse.

Next Appointment

Before a patient leaves the examination room, the doctor will tell the patient when to return. When the patient stops at the check-out area, the assistant should inquire whether another appointment is needed.

In most cases, the doctor will tell the patient when to return to the office for follow-up with instructions such as "return in 10 days" or "return in three weeks." The assistant should schedule the patient's next appointment for a convenient time as close as possible to the suggested return date.

Get into the habit of entering the appointment information into the appointment book or computer and then writing an **appointment card**, which will serve as a reminder for the patient of the next visit. Never trust an appointment time to memory with the intention of entering it later, no matter how hectic the office is. See Figure 5-7 for an example of an appointment card.

Many offices use a system of follow-up telephone calls to remind a patient of an appointment for the next day. If the follow-up appointment is several months in the future, the patient may be asked to complete a postcard with the patient's address before leaving the office so the card can be sent as a reminder to the patient. If the office uses a computerized scheduling system, the computer can print reminders to be sent to patients scheduled for follow-up visits.

Bill Fleming

YOUR APPOINTMENT IS:

July 1   AT 10:30

SPECIAL INSTRUCTIONS:

MARK NEWMAN, M.D.
2235 South Ridgeway Avenue
Chicago, IL 60623-2240
312-555-6022

PLEASE CALL IF YOU CANNOT KEEP THIS APPOINTMENT.

Figure 5-7   Appointment Card

PROJECT 21 · Rescheduling Appointments and Preparing Appointment Cards

Today's date is October 13. Reschedule each of the following patients according to instructions given below. Dr. Newman's policy is to draw a single line through canceled appointments.

1. Thomas Baab telephones to say that he has to cancel his appointment on October 13 at 11:00 a.m. and would like to reschedule for the same time on October 15. Make the appropriate changes in the appointment book.

2. Charles Jonathan III stops at your desk to change his appointment for October 14. You reschedule him for October 21 at 10:45 a.m. Complete an appointment card using the form on WP 38, and file the card in the Miscellaneous folder. Make the correct entries in the appointment calendar. Place the unused appointment cards in your Supplies folder for future use.

■ OUT-OF-OFFICE APPOINTMENTS

House Calls

Some doctors make **house calls,** and these visits should be entered in the appointment book with a notation indicating that the appointment is a house call. In scheduling a house call, the assistant needs to obtain the following information:

- ■ The patient's name.
- ■ The patient's address, with directions to the house if it is in an unfamiliar area.
- ■ Home telephone number, in case the assistant needs to contact the doctor during the house call.
- ■ The reason for the visit.

Because procedures such as laboratory tests and X rays cannot be performed in the home, most doctors prefer that patients come to the office or hospital emergency room for treatment.

PROJECT 22 · Completing a House-Call Slip

Dr. Newman hands you some handwritten notes that he made at a house call for Raymond Murray on October 12. He asks you to key the notes on a house-call slip, since he did not have any forms with him at the time. The notes and the house-call slip are on WP 39. Place the completed house-call form into your Miscellaneous folder. Put the blank form in your Supplies folder.

Other Appointments

Other appointments that may be scheduled outside the office include laboratory tests, X rays, surgery, special procedures, and hospital admissions. Follow basic scheduling procedures for such appointments, adding any pertinent information such as:

- Possible diagnosis.
- The patient's age (for surgery or hospital admission) or date of birth.
- Special instructions from the doctor (for example, asking the pathologist to call after a procedure is completed).

These appointments should not be scheduled in your office appointment book if the doctor will not be performing the procedure.

Patient Referrals

A patient sent to a **consultant** (specialist) for **referral** may be introduced by a letter of introduction sent by the **attending physician**, who is sometimes called the **primary physician**. This correspondence will be kept at the consultant's office marked "Future Appointments."

The assistant in the consultant's office should indicate the name of the referring physician in the appointment book. A medical record will not be started until the patient arrives for the scheduled appointment. If the consultant needs the patient's past records, such as test results or X-ray reports, the patient will be asked to complete a release of information form. See Figure 5-8 for an example of appointments scheduled for referred patients.

Tuesday, September 30

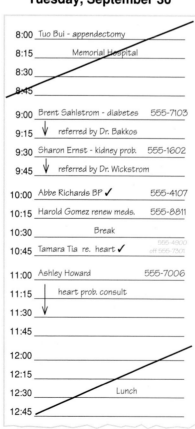

8:00	Tuo Bui - appendectomy
8:15	Memorial Hospital
8:30	
8:45	
9:00	Brent Sahlstrom - diabetes 555-7103
9:15	↓ referred by Dr. Bakkos
9:30	Sharon Ernst - kidney prob. 555-1602
9:45	↓ referred by Dr. Wickstrom
10:00	Abbe Richards BP ✓ 555-4107
10:15	Harold Gomez renew meds. 555-8811
10:30	Break
10:45	Tamara Tia re. heart ✓ 555-4900 off 555-7301
11:00	Ashley Howard 555-7006
11:15	heart prob. consult
11:30	↓
11:45	
12:00	
12:15	
12:30	Lunch
12:45	

Figure 5-8   Schedule Showing Referrals

Key Terms

The following terms appear in **boldface** type in this chapter. Do you recall what they mean? Refer to the chapter for definitions you need to review.

appointment card
attending physician
cancellation
consultant
double-column scheduling
fixed office hours
hospital rounds
house calls
primary physician

referral
register (sign in)
routine appointment
screening
stat
time allotment
triage
walk-in patient
wave scheduling

Medical Vocabulary

The following medical terms were used in one of the projects for this chapter. Review each term and its meaning.

bronchitis: inflammation of air pathways leading to the lungs.
COPD: chronic obstructive pulmonary (lung) disease.
cor: cardiac or heart.
crackles: abnormal breathing sounds.
dyspneic: having trouble breathing.
edema: swelling caused by excess fluid in the tissues.
end-stage: terminal, nearing completion.
erythromycin: an antibiotic medication.
exacerbation: the return of or worsening of an illness.
O$_2$: oxygen.
pedal: pertaining to the foot or ankle.
sputum: material coughed up from the airways.
wheezing: abnormal breathing sounds in the chest.

Topics for Discussion

1. Dr. Newman requires a 1-hour appointment for a complete physical. The patient requests a physical next week, and there is no opening for 1 hour until 3 weeks from now. Discuss how this situation should be handled.

2. A patient calls complaining of chest discomfort. Dr. Newman has a full schedule, and you have already added four emergencies to today's schedule. Dr. Newman told you to send any other urgent problems to the hospital emergency room. What should you tell this patient?

Role-Playing

You are the assistant with telephone duty at the appointment desk.

1. With a classmate, role-play the following telephone situations:
   a. PATIENT: I fell off a ladder and bruised my knee. Could I get an appointment with Dr. Newman today?
   b. PATIENT: My child needs an appointment for an athletic physical.
   c. PATIENT: Is the doctor in? *(Pause here to allow the assistant to respond.)* My two-year-old son has been in the medicine chest, and the aspirin bottle is open. He may have eaten some pills.
   d. PATIENT: I have a wart on the palm of my hand. Could I make an appointment to have it removed?
   e. PATIENT: I'd like to speak with Dr. Newman about the results of my gallbladder X rays.

2. Call a patient to handle the following situations:
   a. Reschedule a patient's appointment because the doctor is ill.
   b. Reschedule a patient's appointment because the doctor has an emergency case.
   c. Reschedule a patient's appointment because you discovered that you had not allowed enough time for the patient's complete physical.
   d. Reschedule a patient's appointment for later the same day because the doctor will be running two hours late in seeing patients with scheduled appointments.
   e. Reschedule a patient's appointment because the doctor decided to take a vacation day.

Records Management

Upon completion of this chapter, you should be able to:

- Compare the different filing methods—alphabetic, geographic, subject, numeric, and phonetic.

- Demonstrate the correct use of an alphabetic filing system.

- Perform the steps in the filing process.

- Describe the uses of a tickler file.

- Prepare patient's files in alphabetic order.

- Discuss the use of electronic files.

- Apply subject filing techniques.

- Identify the types of filing equipment and supplies.

- Review techniques to locate misfiled or lost records.

Efficient records management is essential in any medical office. **Records management** is the systematic control of the steps involved in the life of a record, or file, from creation through maintenance to disposition. The organization of an office is evident in its files.

An office may have **centralized** files where items such as patients' medical records are stored in one location for the entire office to access them, or it may have **decentralized** files where information such as a doctor's correspondence is easily accessible to an individual user.

The assistant can learn how the office operates by observing its records management program. Therefore, an assistant must recognize the types of records, know the organization of the office files, apply filing procedures, and assist the employer in choosing suitable equipment and supplies.

A resource for the assistant is ARMA (Association of Records Managers and Administrators, Inc.). ARMA is a well-known authority on filing rules, guidelines, and procedures.

■ TYPES OF RECORDS

The various records in an office should be classified into categories according to office operations. In a medical office, records would be

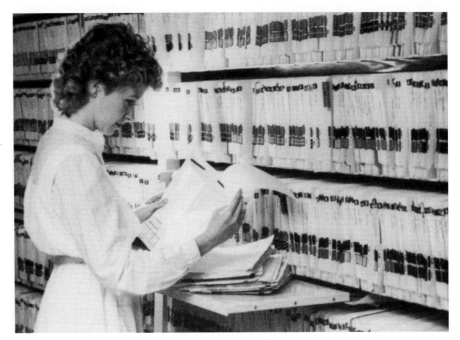

The medical assistant must recognize the types of records, know the organization of the office files, and apply filing procedures.

classified primarily into patients' files (which include patients' charts and ledgers), medical and general correspondence, and business and financial records.

Patients' Files

A **patient'' file** includes the clinical data sheet, the medical reports, and the correspondence pertaining to each individual patient. These records are filed alphabetically or numerically with an alphabetic cross-index file.

Patients' ledgers (statements) need to be easily accessible and should be arranged alphabetically.

General and Medical Correspondence

General correspondence pertaining to the operation of the office and medical correspondence unrelated to individual patients should be filed by subject separately from patients' records. Medical correspondence may include items such as articles from journals and research reports, materials from professional organizations, and so forth.

Business and Financial Records

These records pertain to management of the office. Examples include insurance policies (both professional and personal), income and expense records, financial statements, and tax records. These records should be filed **chronologically** (by date, with the most recent date in front) within the subject area.

■ SUPPLIES AND EQUIPMENT

An assistant must be familiar with the kinds of filing supplies and equipment available in order to aid the employer in selecting suitable filing essentials for the office.

Card Files

Patients' ledgers, patients' index cards, telephone numbers, and various other records may be kept in a **card file**. Card files are usually kept in a conventional file box or cabinet.

The **rotary card file** is the most space-saving system. The rotary card file is a small, desktop file designed to rotate, which permits the use of both sides of each card. Addresses and phone numbers of associates are easily accessible in a rotary card file.

File Cabinets

A common type of file cabinet is the **vertical file**. Vertical files can differ in drawer size, in number of drawers in a unit, in color, and in construction material.

Drawers or shelves open horizontally in **lateral file** cabinets to provide easy access to records. In lateral file cabinets, files are arranged sideways from left to right instead of front to back.

Open-shelf files are popular in offices with limited space. These shelves can extend to the ceiling and require less floor and aisle space than do file cabinets. (The picture on page 103 shows open-shelf files in the background.) The folders are placed in the file sideways with the tabs protruding. Many clinics use open shelves for patients' charts.

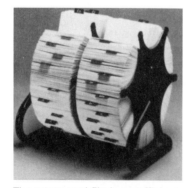

The rotary card file is an efficient way to store addresses and telephone numbers of business associates.

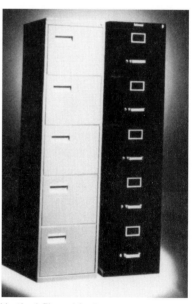

Vertical file cabinets are commonly used to store business documents and files.

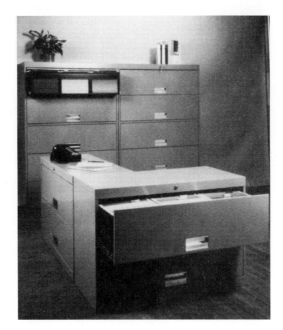

Drawers open horizontally in lateral file cabinets to provide easy access to files.

Other files that save space and are easily accessible include **mobile-aisle files**. These files are considered compacted open-shelf files and are mounted on tracks on the floor. Mobile-aisle files hold a large volume of records and can be accessed electronically.

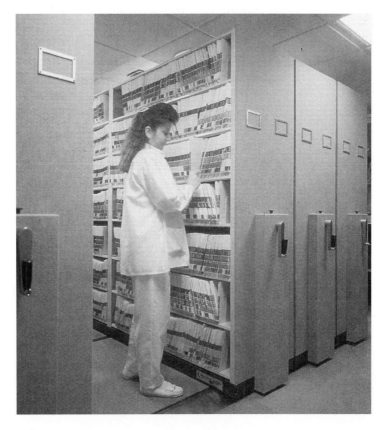

Mobile-aisle files save space and are easily accessible.

Electronic Files

The files in a medical office can also be stored on electronic media such as hard disks, floppy disks, or compact discs (CD-ROM). On a personal computer or a word processing system using either a hard disk or floppy disks, files such as patients' information, patients' ledgers, or even patients' medical records can be stored.

Patients' confidentiality can be maintained in **electronic files** by using **passwords** (individual security entrance codes) to the files. Care must be taken in labeling disks and in storing them in protective containers. On computer systems with hard disks, careful attention should be paid to naming (labeling) items, using passwords, and deleting nonessential files. Compact discs have the largest capacity for storage and need the same care as hard disks and floppy disks.

Micrographics

The process of storing records in miniaturized images to reduce filing space requirements is called **micrographics**. Thousands of paper records can be stored on microfiche or ultrafiche; the paper records then can be destroyed or put in dead storage, and only the micrographic media has to be filed.

Microfiche reproduces information onto a sheet of film (a card) which can hold up to 90 frames. **Ultrafiche** holds even more compacted information and can contain up to 1000 frames. The types of microfiche and ultrafiche readers (machines used to enlarge images for viewing or reproduction) also vary. The microfiche and ultrafiche can be filed in a card file or in a book-type binder.

Folders

File folders can be purchased in various styles, weights, colors, and tab cuts. A **tab** is a portion of the file folder that extends beyond the rest of the folder so that it can be labeled and easily viewed. Folders should be filed so that the tab cuts are read in an orderly fashion from left to right. Color-coded folders can be purchased for patients' files to help identify filing categories visually. For example, the first two letters of patients' last names might be designated by colored tabs or markings on the folder.

Labels

Labels, which vary in color and width, are used to identify files. They are available in perforated rolls, on self-adhesive strips, or as computer forms designed for use with dot-matrix or laser printers.

Guides

Guides are rigid dividers placed between sections of files to indicate where a new section or category of files begins.

Out Guides

An **out guide** is a card that substitutes for a file that has been temporarily removed. The name of the person who has the file, the date it was removed, and the material the file contained are recorded on the front of the out guide so that others can locate the file. When the file is returned, these notations are crossed out, and the out guide can be reused.

Cross-Reference Sheets

A **cross-reference sheet** is used to indicate that material may also be filed elsewhere and to note where the original material is filed. This sheet can be a different color so that it can be recognized quickly.

■ FILING PROCEDURES

Following systematic steps for preparing materials for filing enables the assistant to file accurately and effectively and to use filing space efficiently.

Releasing

Before an item can be filed, it must bear a release mark showing that the material has been inspected, acted on, and is now ready for filing. The mark used for **releasing** varies from office to office; the material can be stamped, initialed, or coded.

Indexing

Indexing is the process of selecting the name or words under which an item will be filed and putting the units of that name or the words in proper order. For example, a patient named Jose Gomez would be filed under G, for *Gomez*.

Coding

Coding involves putting a code (a number, a letter, or an underscore beneath a word) on a document to indicate where it should be filed. For example, in correspondence regarding Jose Gomez, *Gomez* would be underscored (or coded in some way).

Cross-Referencing

Any material that could be coded and filed under more than one heading requires **cross-referencing**. A cross-reference sheet or card (illustrated in Figure 6-1 on page 108), which indicates other places the document may be filed, should be prepared and filed for the item.

Figure 6-1   Cross-Reference Card

Sorting

Papers should be arranged in filing sequence before they are actually placed in the folders. This process is called **sorting**.

Storing

Storing is the actual placement of items in a folder or on a computer disk. If the item is to be placed in a folder, the top of the item should be to the left.

Ensuring Follow-Up

So many patients need follow-up visits that a special file, commonly called a **tickler file**, or follow-up file, is useful. Patients who want a regular checkup once or twice a year appreciate reminders. A patient may also need to be reminded of a series of injections or a course of treatments.

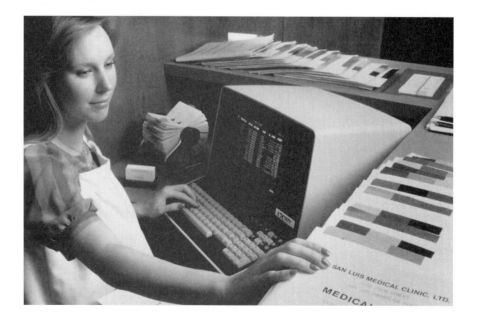

Many modern offices use computer files to store information on patients.

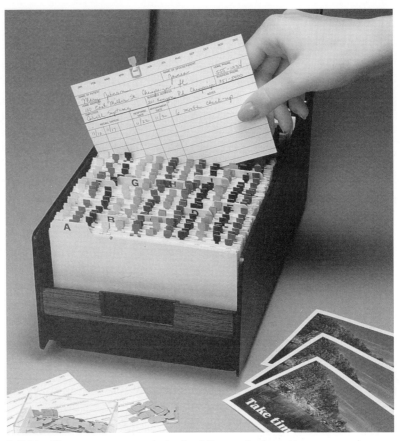

A tickler file serves as a reminder for follow-up tasks and appointments.

A practical tickler file system involves a monthly, chronological arrangement of index cards. Notations of actions to be taken are placed behind specific dates of the month. At the end of the month, cards are distributed behind the specific dates of the next month, and so on. A tickler file must be used daily in order to be effective.

Another reminder method is to use a colored index tab clipped to a patient's record. The colored tab indicates that the patient needs some type of follow-up. Different colors may be designated for different purposes.

Transferring of Files

Every office needs a system for the regular transfer of files. The three classifications commonly used in a medical office are *active, inactive,* and *closed.* Active files include current patients; inactive, patients who have not been seen by the doctor in six months or more; closed, patients who have died, moved away, or have terminated their relationship with the doctor. Each office must establish guidelines for transferring, or moving, files from one classification to another.

■ FILING METHODS

Records are filed according to how information is sought; the critical factor is that they must be readily accessible. Therefore, several filing systems have been developed: alphabetic, geographic, subject, numeric, and phonetic. Each system has certain advantages.

Alphabetic Filing

Alphabetic filing, the most popular system, is arranging names in alphabetic order. The advantages of alphabetic filing include a direct reference (there is no need for another type of file), an order that is easy to understand, simple storage (just follow the standard procedures), ease in finding misfiled items, a system that is inexpensive to operate and to maintain, and the need for only one sorting. A disadvantage is the risk of misfiling if operators do not follow the rules, transpose letters, select wrong file names, or file items under similar names or spellings. Some other disadvantages are that alphabetic filing is neither confidential nor secure in open files and there is limited space for expansion of files.

Before accurately filing and retrieving records in an alphabetic system, an assistant must thoroughly understand the following basic rules for alphabetizing and indexing.

Each part of a name is considered an **indexing unit**. Alphabetizing is done unit by unit. In comparing two words, alphabetic order is determined by the first letter that is different. Also remember, "Nothing comes before something." Thus *Mane* is filed before *Manes*. Ignore the punctuation or space within the name.

Rule 1. Names of individuals should be indexed in the following order: surname (last name), given name (first name), and then middle name or initial.

Names	Indexing Units		
	1	2	3
Wade R. Benjamin	Benjamin	Wade	R
Wayne M. Benjamin	Benjamin	Wayne	M
Juan Benje	Benje	Juan	

Rule 2. Prefixes such as *d', D', de, De, Del, De la, Di, Du, El, Fitz, La, Le, Los, M, Mac, Mc, O', Saint, San, St., Van, Van de, Van der, Von,* and *Von der* are considered part of the surname, not separate units.

Names	Indexing Units		
	1	2	3
Lorne Fitz Gerald	FitzGerald	Lorne	
Esther Ann O'Reilly	OReilly	Esther	Ann
David R. Von der Wan	VonderWan	David	R

Rule 3. A hyphenated name is considered one indexing unit. (For example, *Ann Ames-Batte* is filed as *AmesBatte, Ann*.

Rule 4. Abbreviated and shortened forms of personal names are not spelled out. Use the abbreviation or the shortened form unless you are certain that the spelled out name is the patient's legal name. When in doubt, ask the patient.

Names	Indexing Units		
	1	2	3
Carol A. St. James	StJames	Carol	A
Bill J. Wicks	Wicks	Bill	J
W. Ray Wicks	Wicks	W	Ray
Geo. Lester Wilson	Wilson	Geo.	Lester

Rule 5. Professional or personal titles and seniority designations are the last indexing unit if needed to distinguish between two or more identical names. If you only have a title and one name, index the name as it is written.

Names	Indexing Units		
	1	2	3
Alan Berg, M.D.	Berg	Alan	M.D.
Charles Jonathan III	Jonathan	Charles	III
Charles Jonathan, Jr.	Jonathan	Charles	Junior
Sister Mary-Margaret	Sister	MaryMargaret	

Rule 6. When names are identical, index the names by address in the following order: city, state (spelled in full), street name, quadrant (NE, NW, SE, SW), and house or building number in numeric order (lowest number first).

Names

Emily Beck
1055 Maple Lane
Chicago, IL 60623-9623

Emily Beck
8275 Maple Lane
Chicago, IL 60623-9623

Indexing Units

1	2	3	4	5	6	7
Beck	Emily	Chicago	Illinois	Maple	Lane	1055
Beck	Emily	Chicago	Illinois	Maple	Lane	8275

Rule 7. Index business and organizational names in the order in which they are written. When *The* is the first word of the name, it is indexed as the last unit. If a business name contains a word that is written as two words but is normally one word, index it as a single unit. Single

letters in a business name are indexed as separate units. Index each part of a geographic name as a separate unit.

Names	Indexing Units			
	1	2	3	4
Air Port Clinic	AirPort	Clinic		
The Children's Hospital	Childrens	Hospital	The	
Dason's & Weiss' Supplies	Dasons	and	Weiss	Supplies
JD Consultants	J	D	Consultants	
Jan Dupont Consultants	Jan	Dupont	Consultants	
Los Mosa Clinic	Los	Mosa	Clinic	
U.S. Medical Ltd.	U	S	Medical	Ltd

Rule 8. Arabic numerals (1, 2, 3) and roman numerals (I, II, III) are considered a single unit and are filed in numeric order before alphabetic characters. Arabic numerals precede roman numerals. Hyphenated numbers are indexed according to the number before the hyphen. Ignore the number after the hyphen, and index the number as a single unit. Ignore the letters *st, d,* and *th* after an arabic numeral. Spelled out numbers are filed alphabetically as they are written.

Names	Indexing Units		
	1	2	3
5th Avenue Clinic	5	Avenue	Clinic
Sixty-third Street Pharmacy	Sixtythird	Street	Pharmacy

Rule 9. Hotels, motels, churches, hospitals, and universities are indexed as written unless the name starts with hotel, motel, university, and so forth. Treat each indexing word as a separate unit.

Names	Indexing Units		
	1	2	3
Alexander Hotel	Alexander	Hotel	
Motel Atler	Atler	Motel	
University of Illinois Hospital	Illinois	Hospital	University
St. Paul's Clinic	St Pauls	Clinic	

Rule 10. Index government names as follows:

Federal Government	Indexing Units		
	1	2	3
U.S. Department of Health,	United	States	Government
Education, & Welfare	4	5	6
(After *United State Government,*	Health	Education	Welfare
index department name and then	7		
lower divisions.)	Department		

State and Local Government	**Indexing Units**			
	1	2	3	4
Bellville County Health Council	Bellville	County	Health	Council
Illinois Bureau of	1	2	3	4
Health	Illinois	State	Health	Bureau

Foreign Government	**Indexing Units**		
Republic of Sweden	1	2	3
Finance Division	Sweden	Republic	Finance
	4		
	Division		

PROJECT 23 Preparing Index Cards and Patients' Files

Dr. Newman maintains an index card and a file folder for each patient. The index card contains pertinent information about the patient for easy reference. Information from the indexes is on WPs 40 and 41. Compute the year of birth for each patient by subtracting the patient's age from the current year, and insert it on the card.

In addition, label a file folder for each patient, "(last name), (first name)." Duplicate the clinical data sheet on WP 42, and prepare one for each patient.

Each patient will now have an individual chart, or file. Except for the index card, material pertaining to each patient should be filed chronologically in its respective folder. File additional material on a patient accordingly.

Prepare an index card, clinical data sheet, and file folder whenever a new patient arrives for an appointment.

Dr. Newman's policy for updating addresses and telephone numbers on index cards and charts is to draw a line through the old information and re-write the new information.

Place the completed, alphabetized index cards in your Supplies folder, and put the alphabetized patient file folders in your expanding portfolio.

Geographic Filing

Geographic filing classifies the records filed by particular regions. Divisions in this system involve a sequence such as nations, states, cities, and so forth. Within each file, records are arranged alphabetically. Research statistics, medical sales records, and medical suppliers are examples of files that might be arranged geographically.

Subject Filing

Correspondence and other kinds of records that pertain to the same subject should be filed alphabetically by subject categories. **Subject filing** is often used for a doctor's research. It enables a doctor to classify material by disease or condition, for example.

The subject headings will depend on the specific needs of the doctor and on the amount of material that has accumulated under each heading. Manuscripts are filed alphabetically under the title of the article

RELATIVE SUBJECT INDEX

Advertisements
Drugs
Medical
Office
Automobile
Insurance
Maintenance
Clinic Property
Building
Inventory
Maintenance
Medical Equipment
Office Equipment
Collections
Accounts Receivable
Agency Contracts
Form Letters
Education
Doctor's Continuing
Employee
Patient
Entertainment
Financial
Annual Financial
Banking
Monthly Financial
Forms
Applications
Consent

Release From
Work
Release of
Information
Hospital
Policy
Reports
Staff Meetings
Insurance
Clinic
Fire
Liability—Doctor's
Patients
Index Control File
Patient Billing List
Personnel
Applications—
Inactive
Benefits and
Policies
Current
Employees
Doctor's Personal
File—
Diplomas,
Licenses
Referral Information
Society Information
American Medical
Association

Seminars
State Medical
Society
**Subscriptions and
Publications**
Drug Companies
Lobby Magazines
Medical
Magazines
Newspapers
Professional
Library
Supplies
Inventory
Medical
Office
Order Forms
Taxes
Payroll
Personal (Doctor's)
Property
Travel
Expenses
Pending
Utilities
Electricity
Gas
Telephone
Water

Figure 6-2   Relative Subject Index

or book. Abstracts, excerpts, and reviews may be clipped from journals or newspapers. Whether to file clippings by the author's name or the subject depends on how the doctor plans to use the items. All reviews of and references to the doctor's own writing should be filed together under the title of the article or the book.

Figure 6-2 shows an example of a relative subject index with a sample of captions (headings) that may be used in subject filing.

Subject filing saves time because all items pertaining to a subject are kept in one location; therefore, statistics and information are easily accessible. The relative subject index is easy to expand. Some disadvantages of subject filing are that subjects may overlap, extensive cross-referencing might be required, and it is time-consuming even for experienced filers to file and to retrieve material.

Numeric Filing

Offices with a large volume of patients' records may use a **numeric filing** system. Each new patient is assigned a number from an **accession book** (a book of consecutive numbers indicating the next available number to be assigned), and a cross-index is prepared to identify the number with the name.

Straight-numeric filing is a system that uses consecutive numbers in ascending order. For example, File 125203 would be filed after 125202 and before 125204.

Terminal-digit filing uses the last digit or set of digits as the primary indexing unit. The folder numbered *33-52-12* would be filed in Section 12, behind Guide 52, and the 33d item in sequence.

Numeric filing is considered the most accurate system; it is harder to lose files or to misfile them than with other systems. Expansion in numeric filing is unlimited, and both storage and retrieval can be quickly accomplished. However, a numeric filing system is costly—more guides are needed, extensive training must be given to all users, and an alphabetic cross-index must be maintained.

PROJECT 24 | **Using Subject Filing**

As Dr. Newman's assistant, you must retain and file the following items. On a plain sheet of paper, write the subject heading under which each would be filed. Use Figure 6-2 as a guideline and be prepared to discuss your answers in class.

1. A copy of a medical article that Dr. Newman wrote to be submitted to the local newspaper.
2. A pending new contract from a collection agency.
3. A bulletin about an educational seminar next month for the nursing staff.
4. A summary of monthly long-distance telephone calls.
5. A maintenance contract for the office.
6. An itinerary for a seminar next month sponsored by the state medical society.
7. The minutes from October's staff meeting at University Hospital.
8. An inventory of laboratory supplies.
9. A statement showing a paid fire insurance premium.
10. A notice of change in medical insurance coverage for office employees.

Phonetic Filing

When the exact spelling of a name is not known, a **phonetic filing** system, such as Soundex, can be used. This phonetic system groups all names that are pronounced alike under a simple code, reducing each name to a letter and a three-digit code number. When applying the Soundex system, observe the following rules:

1. The first letter of the name remains unchanged and is not coded.
2. Vowels and the letters *h, w,* and *y* are not coded.
3. Double consonants are treated as one consonant.
4. If two or more letters of one code number are next to each other or are separated by *h* or *w*, only one of the letter equivalents is coded. If these letters are separated by a vowel or *y*, each is coded separately.
5. If there are not enough code consonants for a three-digit code, zeros are added as needed to complete the code.
6. The following consonants are coded by these letter equivalents.

Key Letters	Code Numbers
b, f, p, v	1
c, g, j, k, q, s, x, z	2

Key Letters	Code Numbers
d, t	3
l	4
m, n	5
r	6

After the coding of the surname, like codes would necessitate using the next unit to determine alphabetic order.

Example: Phonetic Code for *Anderson*

A, not coded (initial letter)
n, 5
d, 3
e, not coded (vowel)
r, 6
son, not coded (maximum three digits already coded)
Anderson = A-536

Example: Phonetic code for *Schmidt*

S, not coded (initial letter)
c, not coded (same category as S)
h, not coded
m, 5
i, not coded (vowel)
d, 3
t, not coded (same category as d)
0, added as third digit
Schmidt = S-530

◼ COMPUTERIZED FILING

Computer filing software is available to file office documents such as patients' records, research records, and business and financial records. This software can use all of the standard filing methods, including alphabetic, geographic, numeric, and subject. Data can be entered into the computer, indexed, stored, and retrieved for specific purposes such as scheduling, reviewing patients' ledgers, or processing insurance forms.

◼ RETENTION

Every office should establish a system of record **retention**, or storage, including the replacement of outdated documents.

Case Histories

Case histories are kept permanently. Micrographic systems can solve the space problem of storing old records.

Insurance Policies

Current polices are kept in safe storage. Professional liability policies are kept permanently.

Tax Records

Tax records are kept permanently. Keep three current years where they are readily accessible; keep the remaining records in dead storage. Records in dead storage are not thrown away but are stored in an area away from current files.

Receipts for Equipment

Receipts for both medical and office equipment are kept until they are fully **depreciated** (until the value of the equipment is completely diminished).

Personal Records

Professional certificates and licenses are kept permanently in safe storage. Banking items such as statements and deposit receipts are kept in the files for three years and then transferred to dead storage. Some other personal items that should be kept permanently are old partnership agreements, other old business agreements, and old major property records.

■ LOCATING MISSING FILES

Even a well-organized office will at some time misfile or lose a document. Some procedures to locate a missing file include:

- Looking directly in front of or behind where it should be filed.
- Looking between other files in the area.
- Looking under the files, if possible.
- Checking for transposition of first and last names (for example, *Wheng, Hart* instead of *Hart Wheng*).
- Checking alternate spellings of the name (for example, *Thomasen* for *Thomason*).
- In a numeric filing system, checking for transposed numbers (for example, *19-63-01* instead of *19-01-63*).
- In a subject filing system, checking related subject files or the Miscellaneous file.
- Searching the desk or work area of previous users of the missing file.
- Checking with other personnel in the office.

Key Terms

The following terms appear in **boldface** type in this chapter. Do you recall what they mean? Refer to the chapter for definitions you need to review.

accession book	numeric filing
alphabetic filing	open–shelf files
card file	out guide
centralized	passwords
chronologically	patient files
coding	phonetic filing
cross-reference sheet	records management
cross-referencing	releasing
decentralized	retention
depreciated	rotary card file
electronic files	sorting
geographic filing	storing
guides	straight-numeric filing
indexing	subject filing
indexing unit	tab
labels	terminal-digit filing
lateral file	tickler file
microfiche	ultrafiche
micrographics	vertical file
mobile-aisle files	

Topics for Discussion

1. Display the various types of filing supplies.
2. Examine filing supplies in catalogs.
3. Using the Soundex system, assign the correct file number to your name.

Role-Playing

1. The file clerk has asked you to help file patient records. As you file, you note that quite a few records are misfiled. How would you handle the situation?
2. After you have been working in the file room for several weeks, you believe you have a more efficient method for filing reports. Discuss your procedure with the supervisor.

Written Communications

OBJECTIVES

Upon completion of this chapter, you should be able to:

- Process incoming mail.

- Describe mail classifications.

- Contrast the various methods of mail delivery offered by the postal service.

- Prepare outgoing mail.

- Discuss the use of electronic mail.

- Compose written communications for a variety of situations.

- Apply correct letter formatting and letter styles.

- Discuss the steps involved in word processing.

- Discuss the procedures involved in machine transcription.

Processing the mail and writing correspondence are a major part of each day's work for a medical assistant. A physician receives an enormous amount of mail every day, so the assistant's handling of correspondence is vital to an efficient office.

■ PROCESSING INCOMING MAIL

Sound judgment in sorting and processing incoming mail will save the doctor a great deal of time each day.

The assistant must learn to distinguish quickly between the different types of mail most frequently received. Mail must be sorted according to importance and then placed on each doctor's desk, generally into the following categories:

- Important items, such as those sent special delivery, Express Mail, registered mail, and certified mail.
- Regular first-class mail.
- The doctor's personal mail.
- Periodicals and newspapers.

- Advertising materials.
- Samples.

Processing Guidelines

Use the following guidelines to process incoming mail, sorting it by category of importance:

1. Open all letters except those marked "Personal" (unless you are authorized to open all mail).
2. Check the envelope's contents carefully.
3. Attach the envelope to the correspondence if there is no sender's address on the correspondence.
4. Stamp the date on each item to show when it was received.
5. Attach enclosures to each item.
6. Carefully put patients' checks aside to be recorded and deposited later.
7. Check to be sure that the envelope is not needed and is empty before discarding it.
8. Write a reminder on the calendar or in the follow-up file for material that is being sent separately.
9. Attach the patient's chart to correspondence regarding the patient. Such correspondence should be placed in a high-priority area on the physician's desk.
10. If a business letter responds to a request, pull the relevant file and attach the letter to it.
11. Set aside the correspondence—such as payments requiring receipts, insurance forms or questions, bills, and other routine business matters—that can be answered without the doctor.

The dates of medical meetings or seminars must be noted on the appointment calendar if the doctor plans to attend. Requests for contributions may be reviewed by the doctor, unless the assistant knows the charities and other causes to which the doctor contributes regularly. Any advertising matter that pertains to the doctor's specialty or interests should be placed in the designated area on the doctor's desk. General-interest magazines should replace outdated magazines in the reception area.

Medical journals should be placed on the doctor's desk. Reprints of journals can be obtained by contacting the publisher.

Medical samples should be unpacked and placed in the doctor's supply cabinet if they can be used. If they cannot be used, follow office policy, which may include saving them for a charity. They should not be thrown into the trash.

In some offices, the assistant is required to **annotate** communications. That is, the assistant scans the item and writes any necessary or helpful notes in the margin or on an attached adhesive note.

The assistant is responsible for processing all the mail when the physician is absent from the office. Decisions must be made about each piece of mail—whether to telephone the doctor about it; forward it to the doctor; answer it immediately; or just acknowledge receipt of the mail, explaining that the doctor is out of the office.

An assistant should keep a record of mail that arrives during a doctor's absence, noting when it arrived, what action was taken concerning the item, and if it was forwarded to the doctor. If an item is to be forwarded, a copy of the item should be sent, not the original.

PROJECT 25 | **Processing Incoming Mail**

The following items arrive in the morning mail. On a plain sheet of paper, explain how each item should be processed. Be prepared to discuss your answers in class.

1. A letter from a consultant about one of the doctor's patients.
2. An announcement of a medical society meeting.
3. A drug sample that the doctor can use.
4. A check from a patient.
5. A letter from a current patient complaining about being overcharged by the doctor.
6. The *Journal of the American Medical Association*.
7. An open house announcement for a local specialty clinic.

■ PREPARING OUTGOING MAIL

Outgoing mail consists of professional, business, and personal correspondence. Professional correspondence concerns patients, clinical matters, and research. Business letters are necessary to the management of the office and may concern insurance companies, lawyers, supply houses, and bills to the patients. If the doctor publishes an article, reprints are sent to interested persons. Personal correspondence pertains to the doctor's personal rather than professional life; examples are letters sent to friends and to the doctor's personal business interests.

Supplies

Stationery supplies should be stored in a special cabinet or on shelves reserved for such materials. These supplies should include such items as letterhead stationery, copy paper, manuscript paper, prescription blanks, patients' chart forms, and patients' ledger cards.

The following is a list of other supplies every office should have on hand:

- Envelopes
- Business (calling) cards
- Appointment cards
- Manila envelopes in assorted sizes
- Memorandum pads
- Notebooks
- Index cards
- File folders
- Labels for file folders
- Printed labels for postal packages

- Pencils
- Pens
- Large and small paper clips
- Rubber bands
- Erasers

A postage scale is essential in a busy office. Ordering stationery and other office supplies may be the assistant's responsibility. Check storage cabinets regularly so that new stationery and supplies can be ordered before existing supplies run out.

Mail Classifications

In order for mail to be dispatched efficiently, the assistant must know the various classifications of mail.

First Class. First-class mail includes letters of any form (handwritten or typewritten), postal cards, postcards, business reply cards, bills, and statements of accounts. First-class mail is sealed against postal inspection.

Priority Service. Priority service provides first-class handling for items that weigh more than 12 ounces but less than 70 pounds. Priority service provides the fastest way to send heavier mail to its destination. The rate is determined by weight and by distance sent.

Second Class. A special second-class rate may be used for mailing newspapers and periodicals. Publishers and news agencies must obtain second-class privileges from the post office in order to use the special rate. Clinic newsletters can be sent by second-class mail if they are unsealed.

Third Class. Mail that cannot be classified as first or second class and that weighs less than 16 ounces is classified as third class. Such an item might be a brochure the doctor wants to send to a patient or to another physician.

Fourth Class. Books, printed matter, merchandise, and other items weighing at least 16 ounces and not exceeding 70 pounds are sent fourth class. The rate depends on the weight of the item and on the distance it is to be transported.

Mail Delivery by the Postal Services

Every post office has leaflets available or a special number to call to provide the latest information about domestic and international postage rates and fees. The assistant must continually be aware of current postal rates, requirements, and available services.

The following services are available through the post office:

Express Mail. The post office offers **Express Mail** service, which guarantees next-day delivery (within a specified time limit) between certain designated locations in the United States. If Express Mail does not reach its destination by the required time, the sender is entitled to a refund. (Private shipping companies, such as Federal Express and United Parcel Service, also offer next-day delivery service.)

Special Delivery. Any class of mail can be sent **special delivery**. An item sent special delivery will immediately be delivered to the addressee as soon as it arrives at the designated post office.

Registered Mail. Additional protection can be provided for valuable first-class mail if it is registered with the post office. The fee for **registered mail** varies according to the declared actual value of the registered item. The post office keeps a record of the mailing.

Certified Mail. For items that have no intrinsic value, certified mail may be used. **Certified mail** provides a mailing receipt, and the post office keeps a record of delivery. Items that should be sent by certified mail because they are hard to replace include insurance policies, birth certificates, passports, contracts, deeds, and bank books.

Special Handling. For third- or fourth-class mail, **special handling** provides the fastest handling and transportation available. This service is often used for sending X rays. The service is not applicable to special delivery.

Insured Mail. Mail may be insured against damage or loss. The post office will reimburse the sender for a lost or damaged item sent by **insured mail** according to the amount of insurance purchased.

Return Receipts. For a small fee, a signed receipt from the addressee may be obtained on registered, certified, and most insured mail. A signed **return receipt** provides legal evidence that the addressee received the item.

Combination Mailing. Any **combination mailing** must be declared. For example, if a letter accompanies an X ray, the letter (with the proper postage) could be attached to the outside of the envelope containing the X ray. Alternatively, the letter could be placed inside the envelope containing the X ray with the outside marked *letter enclosed*.

Electronic Mail

Electronic mail, as discussed on page 73, is the use of telecommunication devices to send or receive messages. These devices include computers, computer-based message systems, and facsimile (fax) equipment.

Information can be exchanged with compatible computers through telephone links using a **modem**. Computer-based message systems are computers that are directly connected with each other (**on-line**) and exchange information generally within an organization or business.

Exchanging information by fax is increasing in popularity because of its speed. A fax machine can be used to transmit laboratory reports, insurance claims, medical reports, and so forth. Techniques to ensure confidentially are discussed in Chapters 3 and 4.

■ COMPOSING CORRESPONDENCE

The assistant is responsible for composing correspondence regarding a variety of office matters. The letters an assistant composes must be pleasing in appearance and written in a professional style. Correspondence represents the office and the doctor and should look as professional as it sounds.

Equipment

In order to complete tasks connected with outgoing mail, the assistant needs a computer with **word processing** (**information processing**) capabilities. Word processing software improves the efficiency of processing text, eliminates rekeying during editing or revising, and improves **turnaround time** (the time between creating the document and obtaining the final copy).

A wide variety of computer word processing software is available, and each package has its own commands. The software and commands to use it can be learned using training manuals or tutorial programs. Information processing involves the following steps:

- **Input**: To key the text of correspondence.
- **Revision**: To edit the text of the document.
- **Output**: To print the final copy.
- **Reproduce**: To duplicate or photocopy the document.
- **Distribute**: To send copies of the document to designated persons.
- **Store**: To save the document on disk.

The **monitor** enables you to view what you have inputted. A **mouse** (a manual device that controls the movement of the cursor) can be used to access commands or different software programs quickly. The computer system may be connected to a **network** where the files are shared by many **users** (operators). Information may be stored on a **hard disk** or on a **floppy disk** (a separate storage media). The system may also have various databases that can be accessed and used within the office. A **database** file usually contains a set of records, each with the same group of fields (for example, patients' names, addresses, telephone numbers, account numbers, and so forth).

To protect against loss or damage of computer files, the assistant should frequently make **backup** copies of files onto disks or tapes. Also, the assistant must **archive**, or collect, documents from a hard disk by transferring documents onto a floppy disk or tape to be stored in a separate location. The assistant must carefully label disks and maintain disk libraries so that any information is readily available.

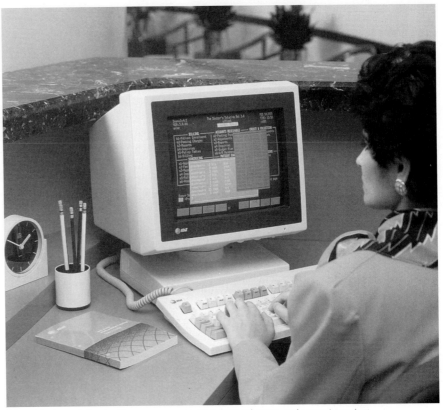

A medical assistant often composes correspondence and reports using word processing software.

Formatting

Proper spacing is necessary to produce a well-balanced and attractive letter. Use single spacing. Double-space between paragraphs. Use top and bottom margins appropriate for the length of the correspondence. If the letter is longer than one page, use blank sheets (not letterhead) of the same quality paper for additional pages and add an appropriate second-page heading.

Figure 7-1 on page 126 shows examples of two common letter formats: *(a)* block style and *(b)* modified block style. Consult *The Gregg Reference Manual*, Seventh Edition (by William A. Sabin, Glencoe/ McGraw-Hill, Westerville, Ohio, 1992) for detailed formatting instructions. A two-page letter with a second–page heading is shown in Figure 7-1 *(c)* and *(d)*.

Style

Good writing style demands accuracy, clarity, simplicity, and courtesy. Keep sentences short and vary sentence structure. Use limited technical language and be sure the material is understandable to the reader. Letters should be personalized, have a positive tone, and focus on the viewpoint of the reader. If possible, avoid starting paragraphs with the word *I*.

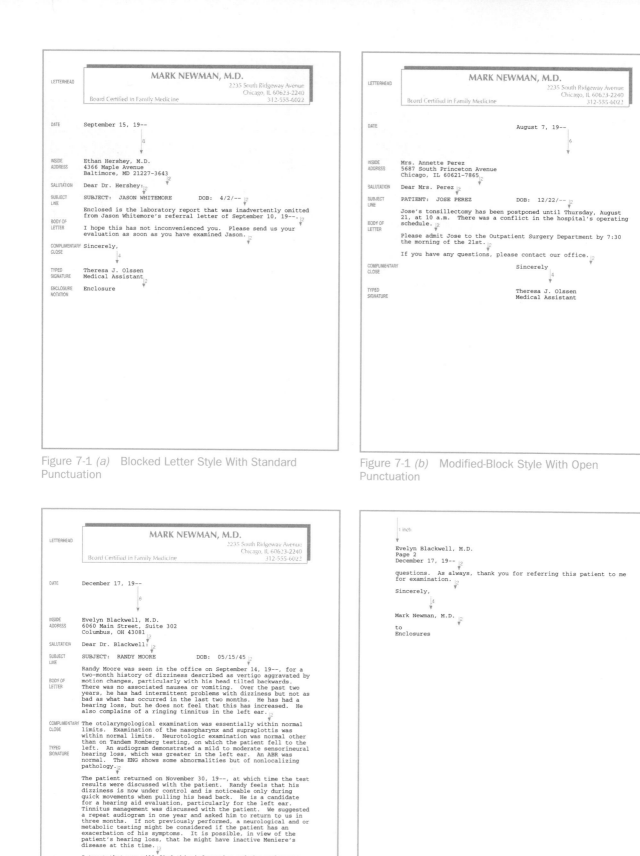

Figure 7-1 (a)   Blocked Letter Style With Standard Punctuation

Figure 7-1 (b)   Modified-Block Style With Open Punctuation

Figure 7-1 (c)   First Page of a Two-Page Letter

Figure 7-1 (d)   Continuation Page

On some occasions, you may compose letters for the doctor's signature. Information may have to be abstracted from the patient's chart. This will take a certain amount of experience and familiarity with the doctor's directions and writing style.

Use the abbreviation *Dr.* before the doctor's name in writing—for example, *Dr. Mark Newman.* However, after the doctor's name in the closing and on professional stationery, use initials indicating the type of degree—for example, *Mark Newman, M.D.* The title *Dr.* and the initials indicating the degree are never used together.

When there is no professional title, the courtesy title *Mr., Mrs., Miss,* or *Ms.* may be used. The salutation for a physician consists of the professional title plus last name—for example, *Dear Dr. Newman.* Consult *The Gregg Reference Manual* to find commonly used forms of salutations for other professions.

Commonly used complimentary closings are *Sincerely, Sincerely yours, Cordially,* and *Cordially yours.*

Even though an assistant must have well-rounded language arts skills, reference books should always be available for use when necessary. Before a letter is given to the doctor for signature, the assistant should proofread it carefully. Consult a dictionary, and use the spell-check feature available with most word processing software to search for spelling errors. Also, proofread carefully to be sure the copy makes sense. A good general dictionary, a medical dictionary, and writing reference manuals should be accessible.

Make a copy—either a photocopy or an additional computer printout—of any correspondence before mailing it. If a letter is answered by telephone or by fax machine, a notation giving the main idea and date of the reply, should be made on the original letter.

After correspondence has been composed and an envelope has been properly prepared, the physician should read and sign or initial the correspondence.

Next, the assistant should fold each item to fit the size of the envelope. Check the enclosures that are listed on the correspondence to make sure the correct item is in the appropriate envelope. Seal each envelope securely, and weigh the letter if necessary so that the proper postage can be attached. See Figure 7-2 on page 128 for an example of a properly addressed envelope and for addressing guidelines.

Referral Letters

If a patient has been referred (sent to your office) by another doctor, a note of thanks must be sent to the referring physician, giving a brief referral report of the medical examination after the patient is seen. Also, when one doctor refers a patient to another doctor, a letter should be sent or a telephone call should be made to the other physician stating the reason for the referral along with the results of any tests and examinations that have been performed. Thus, the other doctor knows that a patient is to be expected and has a brief history of the patient's problem. A release form must be signed by the patient before any records are sent to the consulting physician.

MARK NEWMAN, M.D.
2235 South Ridgeway Avenue
Chicago, IL 60623-2240

JOSHUA COLLINS MD
GREENWAY MEDICAL CENTER
340 CHESTNUT ST
SAN FRANCISCO CA 94133-1043

1. Use a return address.
2. Use all capital letters and no punctuation, except for the hyphen between the ZIP Code and the four-number extension.
3. Use proper postal abbreviations:

APT	- Apartment	RD	- Road
AVE	- Avenue	RM	- Room
CIR	- Circle	S	- South
E	- East	ST	- Street
N	- North	STE	- Suite
PL	- Place	W	- West

4. Place the ZIP Code on the last line next to the city and the two-letter state abbreviation.

Figure 7-2 Envelope, With Postal Guidelines

Figure 7-3 *(a)* shows a sample letter referring a patient to another physician and Figure 7-3 *(b)* shows a sample letter thanking a doctor for referring a patient. These samples may serve as guides in drafting such letters for the doctor's signature.

Sometimes a referral letter has been received, but the patient neither makes an appointment nor comes into the office. After a reasonable period of time, a letter should be sent to the referring doctor explaining that the patient did not appear for treatment.

PROJECT 26 **Composing Referral Letters**

WP 43 contains the names of all doctors and businesses that Dr. Newman contacts. Dr. Newman requests that you key index cards for each of the contacts on the list and for all contacts in the future.

After you complete the index cards, Dr. Newman asks you to compose two referral letters for his signature. Photocopy the letterhead on WP 44 to use as stationery, and address envelopes for each of the letters. Date the letters October 13.

Florence Sherman is being referred to an ophthalmologist, Richard Diangelis, M.D. Enclose a copy of Florence's clinical data sheet (WP 45). This referral letter is to confirm a telephone conversation on October 8.

Dr. Newman is also referring Ardis Matthews to Elizabeth Miller-Young, M.D. Enclose a copy of the clinical data sheet (WP 46) with this letter.

File the referral letters and the clinical data sheets in the patients' files. Keep the business index cards together alphabetically in the front of your Miscellaneous folder.

MARK NEWMAN, M.D.

2235 South Ridgeway Avenue
Chicago, IL 60623-2240
312-555-6022

Board Certified in Family Medicine

September 16, 19--

Lynn Corbett, M.D.
Professional Building, Suite 300
8672 South Ridgeway Avenue
Chicago, IL 60623-2240

Dear Dr. Corbett:

RE: JANET SCHMIDT   DOB: 09/30/--

Janet Schmidt, a four-year-old female, has had a heart murmur
since birth and recently has had extreme pressure on her chest.
I am referring Janet to you for examination.

Enclosed is Janet's complete medical history, along with the
results of the latest tests.

Janet's mother is to call you for an appointment within the next
two weeks.

I would appreciate receiving your evaluation.

Sincerely,

Mark Newman, M.D.

tjo
Enclosures

Figure 7-3   *(a)* Letter Informing
Physician of Referral of a Patient

MARK NEWMAN, M.D.

Chicago, IL 60623-2240
312-555-6022

Board Certified in Family Medicine

August 14, 19--

Hugh Arnolds, M.D.
Suite 440
2785 South Ridgeway Avenue
Chicago, IL 60647-2700

Dear Dr. Arnold:

RE: FRANZ GUEHN   DOB: 08/05/--

Thank you for referring Franz Guehn to me. I have just completed
his examination. Mr. Guehn was first examined by me on June 4.
His diagnosis at that time was otitis externa, bilaterally;
defective hearing, mixed type, bilaterally. The results of the
audiogram are enclosed.

In July, Mr. Guehn had another audiogram (results are also
enclosed). At that time, a considerable loss of high tones
indicated a beginning degeneration of the auditory nerve,
associated with severe tinnitus.

Thank you for referring this patient to me.

Sincerely,

Mark Newman, M.D.

tjo
Enclosures

Figure 7-3   *(b)* Letter Thanking
Physician for Referral of a Patient

Letters From the Assistant

There are many letters that may be written and signed by the assistant. Examples are routine letters about appointments or test reports, requests for information, routine business letters, and, even more important, letters sent in the doctor's absence. It is also one of the assistant's duties to remind an employer to answer letters.

Follow-up letters may be required in a variety of instances. For example, if a letter sent by the assistant has not been answered within a reasonable time, a follow-up letter should be sent. An example of a follow-up letter is shown in Figure 7-4.

Interoffice Memorandums

Informal messages exchanged within an organization may be written as interoffice memorandums on stationery with printed guide words. Memorandums do not contain an inside address or a complimentary closing. An example is shown in Figure 7-5.

Using Transcription Equipment

Equipment for dictation and transcription makes it possible for the doctor to dictate letters, reports, or articles while the assistant is busy elsewhere. Dictation machines come in various sizes, including mini, micro, and standard. Recording time varies with the recording device and its size.

MARK NEWMAN, M.D.

2235 South Ridgeway Avenue
Chicago, IL 60623-2240
Board Certified in Family Medicine   312-555-6022

September 8, 19--

Ms. Tanya Sissell
Standard Medical Supplies
883 Cardinal Avenue
Norfolk, VA 23508-3969

Dear Tanya:

Thank you for your informative presentation regarding your new *Cancerous Agents* patient information program. We received the cassette tapes we ordered last week.

We would also like to receive further information concerning your upcoming seminar on breast cancer research. This seminar was mentioned in your presentation, but you did not give informatiom concerning where the seminar will be held. Will this seminar be coming to Chicago soon? Also, will there be a fee for attending? Please send us additional information.

Sincerely,

Theresa J. Olssen

Theresa J. Olssen
Medical Assistant

Figure 7-4   Follow-Up Letter

```
                        INTEROFFICE MEMORANDUM


    MEMO TO:  Gary Libinksi, Laboratory Manager

    FROM:     Mark Newman, M.D.

    DATE:     September 15, 19--

    SUBJECT:  Outside Laboratory Usage

    After careful study, I have decided that Penway Laboratory will
    be our outside resource laboratory for the next three months.
    They have contracted to provide us with fast, reliable service.
    They are certified by Medicare to provide all necessary lab test
    results.

    Our contact person at Penway will be Gina McPherson.  She will
    bill us directly for any outside services we use with Penway.
    Also, she will send us monthly reports on our usage of their
    facility.  Gary, I also want you keep an accurate report of
    turnaround results and other problems encountered with the lab
    tests we send to Penway.

    During the week of December 20, we will have a meeting to discuss
    our usage of Penway.  You and Gina will meet with me to discuss
    the continued usage of Penway Laboratory.

    to
```

Figure 7-5 Interoffice Memorandum

Some machines are used for both recording and transcribing; in others, these functions are separate. Instruction booklets, usually provided with each instrument, explain how to place recorded material on the machine and how to operate it. You can learn to operate such machines in a few minutes, but a certain amount of practice is necessary to become proficient in transcribing.

Principles of transcription are the same regardless of the equipment. Tone, volume, and rate of speed can be regulated for the assistant's own comfort and rate of transcription. A foot pedal is used for starting the machine and for reversing it. Another helpful item is a counter, which makes it possible to locate a specific reference speedily and to judge the length of a document.

It is most important that the transcriber listen carefully for instructions and corrections. Skill in spelling, knowledge of punctuation and capitalization, and familiarity with medical terminology will determine the assistant's efficiency in transcribing a doctor's dictation. On almost all machines, dictation can be erased and the recording medium can be used over and over again.

PROJECT 27 Composing a Letter

Dr. Newman asks you to write a letter to Martinez Transcription Service requesting information about obtaining telephone transcription online service. Using letterhead stationery, inquire about the turnaround time for transcription using this service and its cost. Date the letter October 13, and address an envelope for it.

File the letter in your Miscellaneous folder.

Reprographics

It is sometimes necessary to make copies of certain office documents—letters, bills, memorandums, announcements, or patients' histories. *Reprographics* describes any process used to duplicate printed material.

Photocopiers are most commonly used to make copies in medical offices. If a large number of copies is needed, such as of a newsletter or report, the assistant may decide to have the copying done by an outside commercial copier or printer. Purchasing a high-speed copier may be the most cost-effective reprographic method if large volumes of documents are routinely produced by the medical office. The assistant should be familiar with the reprographics needs of the employer and should weigh the following factors in choosing the method of copying each document:

- Quantity of copies needed.
- Quality of copy appearance.
- Turnaround time required.
- Cost of duplication.

Key Terms

The following terms appear in **boldface** type in this chapter. Do you recall what they mean? Refer to the chapter for definitions you need to review.

annotate
archive
backup
certified mail
combination mailing
database
distribute
electronic mail
Express Mail
floppy disk
hard disk
input
insured mail
modem
monitor
mouse
network

on–line
output
priority service
registered mail
reproduce
reprographics
return receipt
revision
special delivery
special handling
store
turnaround time
users
word processing
    (information
    processing)

Medical Vocabulary

The following medical terms were used in the projects for this chapter. Review each term and its meaning.

ablation: detachment, separation, or removal.
colposcopy: visualization of the vagina using a special magnifying instrument.
condyloma acuminata: a wartlike growth of the external genitalia.
consort: sexual partner.
detachment: separation or pulling away.
dysplastic: pertaining to abnormal development.
excrescence: an abnormal growth.
exophytic: growing outward on the exterior surface of an organ.
HIV: human immunodeficiency virus.
introitus: entrance to the vagina.
migraine: a condition characterized by headaches, nausea, vomiting, and sensory disturbances.

nulligravida: a female who has never been pregnant.
perineum: the area between the anus and the genital organs.
podophyllum: a type of medication.
retina: the innermost layer of the eyeball, which transmits visual impulses to the brain.
vaginal vault: root of the vagina.
vulva: the external female genitalia.

Topics for Discussion

1. Dr. Newman is away on vacation. The following items arrive in the mail. Decide what must be done with each item.
    a. A letter marked "Personal."
    b. Another doctor's request for a consultation on a patient.
    c. An electric bill.
    d. A check from a patient.
2. Decide how to send the following items in the mail:
    a. A copy of an article Dr. Newman wrote that needs to be sent to the publisher as soon as possible.
    b. A passport belonging to Dr. Newman's son in New York City.
    c. A sales contract for a new X–ray machine. The contract has some errors that Dr. Newman has noted on it.
    d. A letter to Dr. Ethan Hershey in Baltimore. Dr. Newman needs to know that Dr. Hershey received the letter.

Role-Playing

1. A coworker has asked you to photocopy correspondence from a doctor to a referring physician. You notice a gross error in the letter.
2. You have learned the procedure for sorting, opening, and processing mail. The person presently doing this task does not follow the procedure and thus spends twice the time to complete the task.

SIMULATION 1

Simulation 1 is the first of four simulations. These simulations provide an opportunity for you to experience what it is like to work in a doctor's office. You will discover how various tasks relate to each other. Your work will include making and canceling appointments, preparing medical forms, handling telephone communications, and following through on work left over from the previous day.

GENERAL PROCEDURES

The following suggestions apply to all four simulations:

1. Review the content of the appropriate chapters to be sure that you are familiar with the procedures. You may refer to the text at any time during a simulation, just as you would use any available reference sources in an office setting.
2. Prepare three file folders—one labeled "Day 1," one labeled "Day 2," and one labeled "To Do." Assemble the materials you will need; these are indicated in the specific directions for each simulation.
3. Set priorities each day—that is, organize your work in order of importance, and complete it accordingly. Any work left over from the first day should be carried over to the second day and taken into account when new priorities are set for the second day. It is quite possible that you may have work left over at the end of the second day as well. The important thing is to make sure that all the major tasks have been taken care of each day.
4. Be prepared for interruptions. These will occur frequently during the simulation, just as they do in a doctor's office. No matter how carefully you plan your work, interruptions will disrupt your schedule. Do not let interruptions upset you, but rearrange your priorities accordingly.
5. Remember that on the job you will develop shortcuts, easier procedures, and better ways of doing certain things. Try to develop such improvements now.

SPECIFIC PROCEDURES

Day 1: Tuesday, October 14

1. Check the appointments that are scheduled to refresh your memory of the day's events. Pull chart folders for those patients with appointments today, and place them in the To-Do folder.
2. Assemble any other materials you will need. Arrange them on your desk in such a way that you still have room to work. Keep only what you are working with in front of you. Go to your Supplies folder to obtain necessary supplies just as you would go to a shelf, drawer, or file in an office.
3. Use your To-Do list, checking off tasks as you complete them.
4. Using brief notations, log calls reported by the answering service and all incoming telephone calls.
5. The simulation begins when the tape is started with the call to the answering service. You will hear telephone conversations between the medical assistant and the answering service, the patients, and other callers. (You are taking the place of Linda Jenson, administrative medical assistant for Dr. Mark Newman.) You will hear the voice of Dr. Newman giving you directions and dictation; you will hear the voices of patients as they enter the office, make appointments, and so forth; and you will hear the conversations of the assistant as calls are placed. (You will not hear the voices of all patients, only those who ask you to do something.)
6. The doctor may give new directions, and there may be additional telephone calls. Listen to the tape continuously, stopping it as necessary to obtain information; to have information repeated; and to obtain the appointment calendar, appointment cards, message blanks, and other items. Make appropriate notes as you listen.
7. As you complete tasks, place them in the Day 1 folder. At the end of the simulation, submit the folder to your instructor. Place any incomplete work in the To-Do folder, and make notations on the To-Do list as well.

Day 2: Wednesday, October 15

1. Follow the same procedure in planning your work as you used for Day 1. Remember that some of the new things that occur may be more important than work left over from Day 1. Again, listen to the tape continuously, stopping it as necessary.

2. At the end of Day 2, put all of your completed work in the Day 2 folder and turn it in to your instructor. Again, leave any incomplete work in the To-Do folder.

MATERIALS

You will need the following materials to complete the assignments in Simulation 1. If these materials are not already in the proper folders, obtain them from the sources indicated.

Materials	Source
Appointment calendar	
Supplies folder	
Appointment cards	WP 38
Clinical data sheets	*WP 42
Index cards	You provide.
Letterhead	*WP 44
Notepad	You provide.
Plain paper	You provide.
Patients' registration forms	WPs 47 and 48
Records release forms	WP 49
Telephone log	*WP 50
Telephone message blanks	WPs 11 through 18
To-Do list	*WP 51

*Photocopy from the working paper indicated.

To-Do folder
Remove the following completed projects from your Miscellaneous folder, and place them in the To-Do folder.

Message for Mrs. Yates	Project 15
Patients' charts for October 14	
Patients' charts for October 15	

Day 1 folder

Day 2 folder

Patients' folders

The following patients' folders (charts) should contain the clinical data sheet and any other items listed:

Armstrong, Monica
Baab, Thomas
Babcock, Sara
Burton, Randy
Casagranda, Doris
Castro, Joseph
Dayton, Theresa

Grant, Todd
Jonathan, Charles, III
Kramer, Jeffrey
Lund, Laura
Matthews, Ardis

Letter and envelope	
Clinical data sheet	Project 26

Mendez, Ana
Morton, Sarah
Murrary, Raymond

House-call slip	Project 22

Phan, Marc
Richards, Warren
Roberts, Suzanne
Robertson, Gary
Rogers, Clarence
Sherman, Florence

Letter and envelope	
Clinical data sheet	Project 26

Sinclair, Eugene
Sun, Cheng
Villano, Stephen

Miscellaneous folder

Martinez Transcription Service	
Letter and envelope	Project 27
Professional index cards	

If you have not completed all the projects and do not have all these records set up in advance, talk with your instructor.

EVALUATION

You will be evaluated as follows:

1. In terms of the work you completed each day and the work you did not have time to do, did you use good judgment? Did you at least get the most important things accomplished?
2. Is the work you completed of good quality? Is it accurate and neat?
3. Does all the work you completed represent a reasonable amount of work? Would a doctor be satisfied with your rate of accomplishment?

Remember: It is not likely that you will complete all the work that comes in on both days. What counts most is:

1. Good judgment in establishing priorities.
2. Good quality in the work you actually do.
3. A reasonable quantity of work produced.

Patient Records

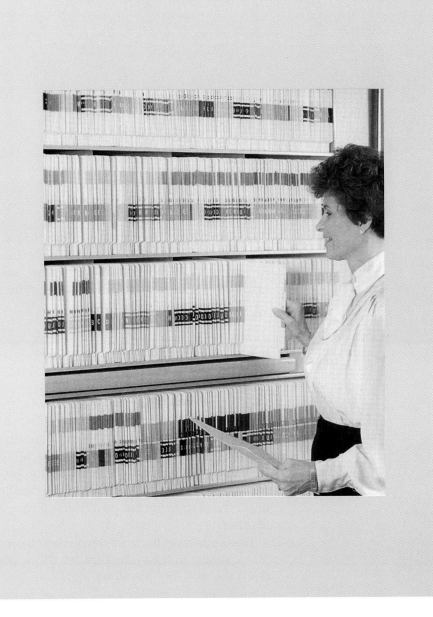

Preparing Medical Records

Upon completion of this chapter, you should be able to:

■ List six reasons for maintaining a patient's record.

■ Discuss the components of the medical record format referred to as SOAP.

■ Transcribe dictation and enter reports into a patient's chart.

■ Give the meanings of common medical abbreviations found throughout the reading material and the chart notes.

■ Explain the method for correcting an error made in a patient's chart.

There are two main categories of records in the medical facility: medical records of the patient's state of health and business papers that consist of financial records and other documents necessary to the management of the doctor's practice. The patient's medical record is the topic of this chapter.

■ THE MEDICAL RECORD

Medical records have been found among the earliest writings in Egypt and India, but they are simple compared to the medical records of today. A systematic method of maintaining medical data enables the assistant to compile accurate statistical, financial, and legal records; to record the results of research; and to provide a record of the quality of care provided to patients. Accurate medical records are also of great importance in ensuring continuity of care from one medical facility to another.

Hospitals have libraries devoted exclusively to patients' records with an extensive index system under the supervision of a records librarian. Likewise, the physician may use any of a variety of systems to record and file the medical data of patients efficiently. A patient's chart is the accumulation of all data pertaining to that patient and may include any of the following documents:

- History and physical examination.
- Notes made by the doctor or nurse.
- Laboratory and X-ray reports.
- Special procedure reports.
- Correspondence.
- Hospitalization summaries.

Medical records provide the doctor with complete information regarding the patient and the patient's illness. Thus, they are used by the doctor in the following ways:

- As a basis for planning the care of the patient.
- As evidence of the course of the illness.
- As a record of the treatment being used.
- As an evaluation of the medical care provided.
- As statistical value in evaluating a certain type of treatment.
- As proof of the incidence of a particular disease.

Medical records are used in processing insurance claims, and they may also be used by medical personnel as background material for preparing a lecture, an article, or a book. On occasion, patients' records may have to be produced in court, either to uphold the rights of the doctor if the doctor is involved in litigation or to substantiate the claim of the patient if the doctor is called as a witness.

■ OBTAINING CLINICAL DATA

When a doctor sees a patient for the first time, the doctor obtains necessary information for diagnosing the condition, prescribing treatment, and forming an opinion as to the chances of recovery. On subsequent visits, the progress of the patient's condition is noted, and when the patient has recovered from the illness, the doctor discharges the patient from treatment for that condition. At the time of discharge, a final statement about the patient's health is included in the chart. This complete documentation of the patient's case is called the patient's "medical record," "chart," or "file."

■ CLINICAL DATA SHEETS

Whether the doctor writes directly onto the chart or the notes are transcribed from the doctor's dictation, the arrangement of the information should be clear and readable. Headings are displayed and set off from the rest of the text.

There is an entry or notation in the chart each time the patient visits the office—whether the patient is seen by a doctor or a nurse, is seen for a blood pressure check or a special procedure, or is seen on a return visit for a medication. Entries must be typewritten or handwritten in ink. All entries must include the date of the patient's visit. Entries are signed with the name of the dictator, followed by the initials of the transcriptionist. A space may be left on the record for the dictator's handwritten signature. The dates of dictation and transcription may follow the signature line or be a double space below the signature line at the left margin.

Example:

Mark Newman, M.D./tjo   D & T: 3/12/xx

or

Mark Newman, M.D./tjo
D: 3/12/xx
T: 3/14/xx

Figure 8-1 shows an example of a clinical data sheet with both typewritten and handwritten notations.

Medical records are legal documents. Since it is not permissible to use an eraser on legal documents, use the following procedure if you make an error while recording an entry on a medical record:

- .Draw a line through the incorrect statements in the medical record.
- Write the word *error* next to the deleted statement.
- Write your initials next to the correction.
- Enter the correct information into the medical record.

Great care must be taken when entering data to ensure that it is inserted onto the correct chart. If an error or discrepancy is discovered on the medical record at a much later date, the doctor may dictate an addendum to the record to correct the discrepancy. The use of word processing software should help eliminate spelling and keyboarding errors. See Figure 8-2 for an example of a clinical data sheet with an error notation.

Name Alma Jackson	Telephone 555-1102
Date of Birth 8/6/--	Age 47

2/6/--	CHIEF COMPLAINT: Sensation of plugged ears x3 days. Denies earache,sore throat,or cold symptoms.
	EXAM: Oropharynx, negative. Cerumen bilaterally.
2/6/--	DIAGNOSIS: Cerumen impaction.
2/6/--	TREATMENT: Ear irrigations. TMs appear normal after washing.
	Mark Newman, M.D./tjo
4/6/--	BP, 132/86. K.B., R.N.

Figure 8-1   Clinical Data Sheet With Typewritten and Handwritten Notations

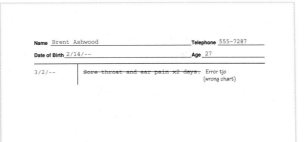

Figure 8-2   Clinical Data Sheet
With Error Notation

When using a word processing system, revisions are easily made without major rekeying of text. Blocks of text can be quickly moved to improve how a document reads. Paragraphs or statements, such as signature lines, special format codes, or standardized paragraphs, can be stored on disk to recall and to use with a minimum of keystrokes. Many medical specialties, such as pathology, can use standardized paragraphs for repetitive technical language. However, even documents prepared on word processing equipment must be carefully proofread for accuracy; spelling and grammar checkers would not locate an error such as "tot he" instead of "to the."

■ NARRATIVE NOTES

A medical record usually begins with a statement about why the patient is seeking the physician's advice. This reason is sometimes stated as a symptom and is known as the **"chief complaint (CC),"** or problem. The details of each record will depend upon the nature of the patient's problem. The record for a self-limiting problem such as a simple laceration will not be as detailed as the record for a patient with a continuing problem such as high blood pressure or diabetes.

Taking the History

Frequently, the medical assistant is given the task of obtaining the patient's present complaint. Care must be taken to avoid asking personal questions in the presence of other patients, relatives, or friends accompanying the patient; therefore, this history is obtained after the patient has been escorted to the examination room. The doctor may ask the assistant to elicit specific information from the patient; the assistant will gradually learn what pertinent questions to ask the patient.

Subjective Information

Information given by the patient is sometimes recorded under the heading **"subjective"** and may include any or all of the following subheadings.

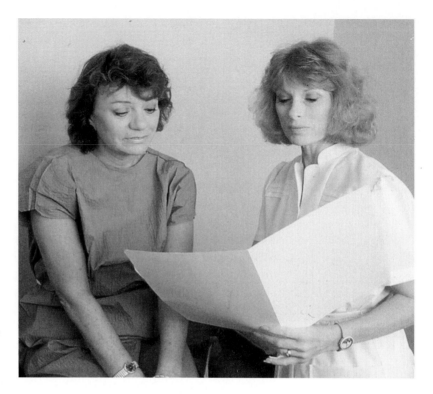

Frequently, the assistant may be authorized to obtain pertinent introductory information about the patient's problem.

The **history of present illness (HPI)** is an exact description of the following information pertaining to the illness:

- The symptoms that are troubling the patient.
- When the symptoms were first noted.
- The patient's opinion as to the cause of the illness.
- Possible influences by any external factors.
- Any remedies that the patient may have tried.
- Any medical treatment the patient may have been given.

The **past medical history (PMH)** includes any illnesses the patient has had in the past along with the treatments administered or operations performed. The past medical history also includes a description of any accidents, injuries, congenital problems, and allergies to medicines or other substances.

The **family history (FH)** consists of facts about the health of the patient's parents, siblings, and other blood relatives that might be significant to the patient's condition. This information is especially important in treating hereditary diseases.

The **social history (SH)** and marital history are included if they are pertinent to the patient's treatment. Information regarding the patient's eating, drinking, or smoking habits; the patient's occupation; and the patient's interests may be included.

In the **review of systems (ROS)**, the doctor reviews each body system with the patient (for example, the respiratory system and the genitourinary system) by asking specific questions about the functioning of each system and reviewing information on the patient's chart. Figure 8-3 shows an example of a clinical data sheet that includes a review of systems.

Name Laura Paulson   Telephone 555-7261

Date of Birth 3/1/--   Age 44

3/6/--   PROBLEM: Annual female exam for this 44-year-old
                    female.

          PMH: Tonsillectomy, age 3; wisdom teeth pulled,
                age 29.

          ALLERGIES: SULFA.

          CURRENT MEDICATIONS: None.

          FH: Dad died at age of 70 of multiple problems
                including carcinoma of larynx, stroke, and
                finally pneumonia. Mother is 66 and in
                good health. No siblings.

          SH: Completed 12th grade education. Homemaker.
                Does not smoke and never has. Denies alcohol.
                Has never taken birth control pills; has never
                received cortisone-type medications or blood
                transfusions.

          MARITAL HISTORY: Husband, 46 and in good health;
                            married 24 years. Three children
                            in good health.

          ROS: Skin, negative. Wears glasses; last eye exam
               this year. ENT, gets occasional sinusitis.
               Respiratory, negative. CV, no chest pain or
               palpitations. GI, negative. LMP, 2/6/--.
               Gravida III, Para III. Birth control method:
               used IUD for past 15 years. Musculoskeletal,
               occasional stiffness of elbows. Neuro,
               negative.

Figure 8-3   Clinical Data Sheet With Review of Systems (ROS)

Objective Information

The doctor's examination of the patient is sometimes recorded under the heading **"objective."** Results of the examination are dictated under the heading **"physical exam (PE),"** which often includes laboratory and X-ray results. A complete physical examination record is very detailed and follows a format in which findings for each of the major areas of the body are included under separate subheadings. Figure 8-4 shows an example of a clinical data sheet listing the results of a physical examination.

Name Laura Paulson   Telephone 555-7261

Date of Birth 3/1/--   Age 44

3/6/-- PROBLEM: Annual female exam for this 44-
                   year-old female.
PMH: Tonsillectomy, age 3; wisdom teeth
            pulled, age 29.
ALLERGIES: SULFA.
CURRENT MEDICATIONS: None.
FH: Dad died at age of 70 of multiple
            problems including carcinoma of larynx,
            stroke, and finally pneumonia. Mother is
            66 and in good health. No siblings.
SH: Completed 12th grade education.
            Homemaker. Does not smoke and never has.
            Denies alcohol. Has never taken birth
            control pills; has never received
            cortisone-type medications or blood
            transfusions.
MARITAL HISTORY: Husband, 46 and in good health;
                    married 24 years. Three
                    children in good health.
ROS: Skin, negative. Wears glasses; last eye
            exam this year. ENT, gets occasional
            sinusitis. Respiratory, negative. CV,
            no chest pain or palpitations. GI,
            negative. LMP, 2/6/--. Gravida III,
            Para III. Birth control method: used IUD
            for past 15 years. Musculoskeletal,
            occasional stiffness of elbows. Neuro,
            negative.
PHYSICAL EXAM:
GENERAL: Alert white female in no acute distress.
          BP, 118/82; P, 86; R, 24. Height, 65 in.
          Weight, 128 lb.
HEENT: Normocephalic. Ears, TMs are normal.
            Eyes, PERRLA; extraocular movements
            intact. Nose, patent. Throat, within
            normal limits.
NECK: Supple. Thyroid, not enlarged.
            Carotids,equal without bruits.
CHEST: Negative. Lungs, clear to A & P.
HEART: Regular sinus rhythm without murmurs.
ABDOMEN: Soft without masses, tenderness, or scars.
BACK: No CVA tenderness. Spine, straight.
EXTREMITIES: Within normal limits with fine
               varicosities bilaterally.
NEURO: Cranial nerves II-XII, grossly intact.
            Reflexes, equal bilaterally.
BREASTS: Fine lumps bilaterally; nothing
          suspicious.
PELVIC: Cervix, clean. IUD, present. Uterus
            anteverted and smooth; adnexa and vagina,
            within normal limits;
            rectovaginal,confirms.

Physical Exam

Figure 8-4   Clinical Data Sheet With Results of Examination (PE)

Figure 8-5   Clinical Data Sheet
With Assessment and Plan

The **assessment** is the doctor's interpretation of the subjective and objective findings, including any tests, X rays, or procedures that are performed. The term *assessment* is used interchangeably with the terms **diagnosis (Dx)** and **impression** and gives a name to the condition from which the patient is suffering. Sometimes the assessment is tentative, pending further developments. Occasionally, the doctor uses the phrase **rule out (R/O)** before a diagnosis, meaning that the diagnosis, while possible, is not likely and that further tests will be performed to be certain.

The **plan**, or treatment section, lists the following information regarding the doctor's treatment of the illness:

- Prescribed medications and their exact dosages.
- Instructions given to the patient.
- Recommendations for hospitalization or surgery.
- Any special tests that need to be performed.

Whenever an additional medication is prescribed or the treatment is changed in any way, a dated notation is entered in the patient's chart. See Figure 8-5 for an example of a clinical data sheet with the doctor's assessment and plan.

The patient's **prognosis**—the doctor's opinion of what the outcome of the illness will be; that is, the patient's chances of improvement or cure—is an important part of the record. This is often expressed simply as "good," "fair," "poor," or "guarded."

When transcribing, care must be taken with the use of abbreviations. Many doctors require the assistant to spell out the terms even though the dictator used abbreviations when dictating. If you are unsure about the abbreviation and you cannot find it in references, it may be acceptable to transcribe the abbreviation as dictated.

PROJECT 28   Keying a Physical Examination Report

Dr. Newman has handwritten the examination information for Thomas Baab on WP 52. He asks you to key this information onto Thomas's clinical data sheet. Then return the completed form to Mr. Baab's chart..

■ CHART FORMS

Many different types of printed forms are available from office supply companies for keeping patients' records. Specialists may have their own forms printed to fit their specialty. Most file folders are designed to accommodate 8 $^1/_2$- by 11-inch sheets, so this size is commonly used. Tape or staple smaller forms or reports to a standard-sized sheet before filing to avoid misplacing them.

Printed forms may have illustrations for the doctor to use in indicating the exact spot where a pathological condition was found. Small zeros may be used after some of the questions on a printed form to indicate "negative," meaning there is nothing to report. A reaction or a symptom that shows disease is present is called "positive" and is indicated on a printed form by a plus sign (+).

Shingled Forms

Some medical forms that are small or irregular in size have an adhesive strip across one edge so that they may be easily affixed to a standard 8 $^1/_2$- by 11-inch sheet. Such forms are called "shingled forms," and the procedure used to attach them to the patient's chart is called "shingling." When forms are shingled, the first report is attached at the bottom of the standard-sized sheet, and each succeeding report is then attached on top of the previous form in chronological order about an inch farther up the page in an overlapping pattern. Disadvantages of using the shingled format include the length of time needed to search for specific information, the difficulty in photocopying the information, and the difficulty in completing such forms using word processing software.

PROJECT 29 | Preparing a Medical Record for An Obstetrical Patient

Obstetrics (OB) is a medical specialty in which a specialized form is used to record data. WP 53 shows an obstetrical chart that has been started for Erin Mitchell. The OB form sent from Erin's former physician, Dr. Grace Tai, is on WP 54. Complete the patient's identification section on Dr. Newman's partially completed form. Then attach the two OB forms together, and place them in the patient's chart. Enter the following notation, dated October 14, on Erin's clinical data sheet: "Patient transferred from Dr. Tai. Please see OB record for H&P and pregnancy to date."

Progress Reports

Often the patient will be instructed to return for a recheck or a follow-up visit. The documentation for a follow-up visit is known as a **progress report**. The physician's objective findings concerning improvement or aggravation of the condition, any change in treatment or medication, and the patient's own report about the condition are recorded in the progress report.

■ **PROBLEM-ORIENTED MEDICAL RECORDS**

In a **problem-oriented medical record**, the doctor will often use a special form to list each problem (that is, each complaint or symptom). There are four essential components of data organization in the problem-oriented medical record.

Database

The database consists of the complete history of the patient, including the problem, history of present illness, past medical history, family history, social history, and review of systems, followed by information derived from a complete examination and routine diagnostic tests.

Problem List

The problem list is a running account of the patient's problems. It is referred to at each clinic visit. Using the list, the doctor can, at a glance, learn what problems the patient has had, how often they have appeared, and the treatment prescribed. This list saves time in that the doctor does not have to study the entire patient's chart before obtaining relevant information.

Initial Plan

Using the database and the problem list, the physician begins a treatment plan. That plan is detailed in the problem-oriented medical record.

Progress Notes

Subsequent visits are recorded by updating the problem list. This procedure helps assure that all problems are considered during a visit. Dates of examinations are listed on the master sheet. When a problem is resolved, the outcome is also stated on the master sheet. Progress notes are often recorded using the **SOAP** format:

S:	**S**ubjective findings
O:	**O**bjective findings
A:	**A**ssessment
P:	**P**lan

Figure 8-6 shows an example of a problem-oriented medical record in which the SOAP format is used.

```
Name  Eugene Pappas                                    Telephone 555-9256
Date of Birth 1/5/--                                   Age  29

3/7/--        PROBLEM 1:  Tonsillitis

              CHIEF COMPLAINT:  Sore throat x2 days.

              S: Sore Throat, fever, difficulty swallowing.
              O: Temperature, 101°.  Pharyngitis with
                 exudative tonsils.
              A: Tonsillitis
              P: 1. Throat culture.
                 2. 1.2 units CR Bicillin.
                 3. Recheck in 10 days.

                                        Mark Newman, M.D./tjo

3/17/-        PROBLEM 1

              S: Recheck.  Feels better.
              O: Temperature, normal.
              A: Problem 1 resolved.
              P: Saline gargles, if necessary.  Discharged.

                                        Mark Newman, M.D./tjo

7/6/-         PROBLEM 2:  Chip fracture lunate, left.

              S:  Pain in instep and tarsal bones.
              O:  Swelling and ecchymosis, left foot.
              A:  X ray shows ? undisplaced chip fracture of
                  lunate.
              P:  1.  Continue supportive shoe.
                  2.  Recheck PRN.

                                        Mark Newman, M.D./tjo

7/7/-         Telephone call from patient complaining of severe
              pain concerning Problem 2.  Advised to take Tylenol
              tab. 2 q4h PRN.
                                        tjo

7/13/-        PROBLEM 2

3/7/-
              S:  Recheck foot.  Pain minimal.
              O:  Swelling disappeared.
              P:  Discussed importance of foot care.

                                        Mark Newman, M.D./tjo
```

Figiure 8-6 Clinical Data Sheet
Showing SOAP Format

PROJECT 31 Transferring Information to a Clinical Data Sheet

Dr. Newman asks you to transfer the information from the house-call slip on Raymond Murray (WP 39) onto Raymond's clinical data sheet using the SOAP format.

■ MEDICAL REPORTS

All reports and correspondence pertaining to a patient are kept in the patient's folder.

One section of the patient's file might be designated for each of the various types of reports (for example, laboratory results or X-ray reports). The reports in each section are then filed chronologically with the most recent report in front. The kind and number of medical reports in the file depend on the patient's condition and the specialty of the attending physician.

Laboratory Findings

The results of laboratory tests may be written directly on the clinical data sheet, or a special report may be sent from the laboratory to be inserted into the patient's chart. Laboratory reports are always given to the doctor with the patient's chart. The doctor initials the report to indicate that it has been reviewed and may also add a notation regarding further instructions. The report is then filed in the patient's folder.

Entering Laboratory Reports

You have received the following telephone message regarding Gary Robertson and have given the message to Dr. Newman.

MESSAGE

TO Dr. Newman   **DATE** 10/16 **TIME** 4 p.m.

FROM Lab

PHONE

☐ PLEASE CALL   ☐ RETURNED YOUR CALL   ☐ WILL CALL AGAIN

REGARDING Gary Robertson

Urine culture from 10/14:

Enterobacter <100,000 colonies.

TAKEN BY lj

Dr. Newman asks you to transfer the information to a lab slip on WP 56 which you may initial for him and then file in Gary's chart. Dr. Newman's office procedure is to enter these lab results in the patients' charts on a plain sheet of paper labeled "LAB." Dr. Newman does not shingle reports. Arrange the reports from top to bottom, left to right.

You have also received and need to file the laboratory reports on WPs 55 and 56 for Thomas Baab, Monica Armstrong, David Kramer, and Gary Robertson.

X Rays

Patients' X-ray films are placed in special envelopes and filed in cabinets specially designed for storing them. If the patient is sent to a radiologist for X rays, the radiologist keeps the films and sends only a report of the findings to the referring doctor.

Biopsy Reports

A biopsy is made for diagnostic purposes. The specimen is examined by a pathologist in a laboratory. The results of the test are then sent to the referring doctor and are filed in the patient's chart.

Immunization Records

These records are permanent records noting the date of immunization for polio, diphtheria, pertussis, measles, and so forth. As subsequent boosters are administered, this information is recorded. This record is sometimes found stamped on the inside of the patient's file folder.

Medication Records

The medication record sheet lists names of, dosages of, and instructions for using prescribed medications. The nurse or doctor keeps this current by adding medications when they are prescribed and writing "discontinued" when medications are discontinued or dosages are changed.

Special Procedures

Since the results of many special procedures such as electrocardiograms are recorded on bulky tapes or forms, only the diagnostic portion of that information is entered in the patient's chart. A notation about the doctor's interpretation of the test results is also entered.

PROJECT 33 Entering a Procedure Note

Dr. Newman hands you the notes on WP 57 regarding the flexible sigmoidoscopy performed on Thomas Baab. Key this report onto Mr. Baab's clinical data sheet.

■ PRESERVING RECORDS

All medical records should be kept until the possibility of a malpractice suit has passed. This time period is determined by the state's statute of limitations.

Although most records are kept permanently, they are generally removed from the active file to inactive or closed storage. To save space, micrographics may be used for long-term storage. Medical information may be useful later if a son or daughter consults the physician for a problem similar to a parent's illness. Transfer, storage, retention, and disposal of records are discussed in Chapter 6.

■ OWNERSHIP

The ownership of medical records is addressed by the American Medical Association Judicial Council of Opinions and Reports. According to the council, medical notes made by a doctor are the doctor's property; however, with the patient's consent, the information may be transferred. The notes are for the doctor's use in the treatment of the patient. A fee may be charged for preparing complex medical reports, but information should not be withheld because of an unpaid fee. The physician is ethically obligated to furnish copies of office notes to any physician who is assuming responsibility for care of that patient.

■ QUALITY ASSURANCE

The medical record probably is the best measure of the quality of care given a patient. The medical assistant helps the physician maintain high standards of care by paying attention to the data that is entered in the medical record.

If the assistant is unsure about a word dictated (for example, it may be unclear whether it is *15* or *50* milligrams) or has a question regarding the correctness of what is heard when transcribing, the item should be flagged for the doctor's attention. The assistant should not interrupt the doctor if he or she is attending to other tasks at that time.

The assistant should make sure that each record contains the following:

- Dated notations describing the service received by the patient.
- Notations regarding every procedure performed.
- Accurate notations. An addendum by the physician should be made if a discrepancy occurs (for example, a previous notation about a condition may have stated "left side," while the latest notation states "right side").
- If necessary, a discharge summary regarding hospitalization before the patient arrives for a follow-up visit.

Credibility of the record is called into question when there is delayed filing of reports or the doctor's notes, incomplete files, illegible records, or alterations in the record.

A standard office procedure should be used to follow up on pending reports for X rays and other diagnostic procedures. A separate file marked "Pending Work" might be used, or a reminder might be placed in a tickler file.

Key Terms

The following terms appear in **boldface** type in this chapter. Do you recall what they mean? Refer to the chapter for definitions you need to review.

assessment
chief complaint (CC)
diagnosis (Dx)
family history (FH)
history of present
  illness (HPI)
impression
objective
past medical history
  (PMH)
physical exam (PE)

plan
problem-oriented
  medical record
prognosis (Px)
progress report
review of systems (ROS)
rule out (R/O)
SOAP
social history (SH)
subjective

Medical Vocabulary

The following medical terms were used in the projects and figures for this chapter. Review each term and its meaning.

adenopathy: disease or enlargement of a gland.
adnexa: surrounding structures.
angina: spasmodic pain due to lack of oxygen in the cardiac blood vessels.
bruit: an abnormal sound heard with a stethscope.
cervical: pertaining to the region of the neck.
COPD: chronic obstructive pulmonary disease.
costochondritis: inflammation of the cartilage around the ribs.
cyanosis: bluish discoloration of the skin.
cystitis: inflammation of the bladder.
Denver screen: profile for growth and development of a child.
disc margins: the area of the retina where the optic nerve and blood vessels enter.
dyspnea: difficulty in breathing.
dysuria: painful urination.
gallop: an abnormal heart sound.
gastroenteritis: inflammation of the stomach and the intestines.
hemoccult: blood in the stool.
hepatosplenomegaly: enlargement of the liver and the spleen.
lymphadenopathy: inflammation of the lymph glands or lymph nodes.
mammogram: a breast X ray.
obese: overweight.
otitis: inflammation of the ear.
pharynx: the throat.
supple: easily moveable.

tinea cruris: a fungal infection in the male perineal or groin area.
tonsillectomy: removal of the tonsils.

Topics for Discussion

1. You are keying the dictation of a medical report and the following situations occur:
   a. You are not able to hear clearly the dosage of medication, that is, whether it was 16 milligrams or 60 milligrams.
   b. The person dictating the report spells out a term, but you are quite certain the person has misspelled it.
   c. The chief complaint for the report is dictated as "numbness of fingers of the left hand"; however, positive findings for the "right hand" are dictated for the physical examination.
   d. The doctor states that the date is August 4. You believe the appointment was on August 2.
   e. You believe that you clearly hear the abbreviation *FFS*, but you don't know what the abbreviation means. Did you hear the abbreviation correctly?

2. Using a medical reference, define the following medical abbreviations:

A&P	HPI	RTC
BP	LMP	S1 and S2
CC	N&V	S/P
CPE	Pap	SH
Dx	PE	TMs
EKG	PERRLA	TPR, P, R
EOM	PE tubes	UA
FH	PMH	UC
F/U	PRN	URI
GI	RBC	VS
H&P	R/O	WBC
HEENT	ROS	

Role-Playing

1. You are taking information from a patient, and the patient refuses to tell you the problem. The patient says, "That's between the doctor and me." What do you do?
2. You have keyed several letters for the doctor. When placing them on the doctor's desk for signatures, you see that the desk is in disorder. What should you do?

Billing

OBJECTIVES

Upon completion of this chapter, you should be able to:

- Explain how fees are determined.

- Obtain necessary credit information about the patient.

- Compute charges and make the appropriate entries for services rendered, charges, and payments.

- Request payment for services rendered.

- Prepare effective collection letters.

One of the assistant's responsibilities is maintaining the doctor's financial records. This includes collecting fees for the services provided by the office to the patient. Therefore, it is necessary to know the amount of the charges, how to discuss fees with patients, how to handle payments, and how to record transactions.

Patients' accounts are handled differently from office to office in accordance with the needs of the practice and the available equipment. The doctor sets the fees for all procedures, medications, laboratory work, and X-ray services provided by the office. Changes in the fees are made only after consulting the physician. Only general rules for billing procedures are discussed in this chapter.

■ DETERMINING FEES

The physician tries to determine fees that are fair to the community and to the profession. *Current Procedural Terminology*, a publication of the American Medical Association, provides guidelines for the establishment of fees. According to this publication, fees should be based on the following factors:

- Amount of time required for the examination.
- Level of skill required in completing the examination.
- Knowledge needed to interpret and coordinate the examination and test results, as well as the risks involved.

Federal and state governments establish guidelines and monitor fees for specific patients, such as those on Medicare or those on public assistance.

Fee Schedules

The doctor has a **fee schedule** that lists procedures the doctor performs and the corresponding charges. Refer to this fee schedule to determine the total cost for each patient's visit (**services rendered**). This schedule should be posted where it is easily accessible to the assistant.

The assistant must know the policy of the office regarding financial arrangements: the charges when a reduction of the fee is possible, the acceptable minimal payment, and any other facts needed to deal efficiently with problems concerning patients' payments.

Discussion of the Fee

Patients who call to make a first appointment may inquire about the charges. Patients should be told that it is difficult to discuss exact charges prior to a visit because the charges will depend on the extent of the examination, the tests, and the type of treatment provided. Nonetheless, an estimate of the fee should be given.

Example

CALLER: I'm new in this area and don't have a doctor. What does Dr. Newman charge for an examination?

ASSISTANT: A routine office charge is approximately $40, but that amount depends on the treatments that are provided and the tests that are performed. It is the policy of this office that new patients establish credit by paying for the first visit at the time of the visit.

Ideally, the patient should be told the approximate cost of the procedures before treatment begins. Providing this information in advance will help avoid misunderstandings and will make collection of payments easier. It may be necessary for the assistant to explain the fee by calling attention to the time involved; the cost of medications or supplies; and the skill, knowledge, and experience of the physician. Either the doctor or the assistant can discuss the fee with patients. If the doctor discusses the fee with a patient, the assistant needs to know what has been discussed.

It is a fair assumption that a patient who inquires about charges before a visit is concerned about the price and should be shown every consideration. If a definite amount is quoted and this amount seems to worry the patient, the assistant can reassure the patient by saying that arrangements can be made to ease payment.

The fee for operations, maternity care, and other major procedures should be discussed in advance. The charge may be described as covering total care, which includes a specified number of visits or procedures. In discussing the fee with a patient, it is important to point out exactly what the fee covers, including office visits, X rays, special procedures, supplies, and follow-up care. In some cases, a letter composed by the assistant or the physician can be used to respond to inquiries about the physician's fee. An example of such a letter is shown in Figure 9-1.

PROJECT 34 Composing A Letter Quoting Fees

Erin Mitchell has asked Dr. Newman about his charges for obstetrical care. Dr. Newman asks you to write a letter to Erin explaining the usual charges, using the fee schedule on WP 58. (Note the different categories on the fee schedule. Keep the fee schedule in your Miscellaneous folder, and use it to determine and record charges for services rendered.)

Make the following changes concerning Erin's charges: The initial obstetrical physical examination was performed by Dr. Tai and will not be repeated. Because Erin's due date is approximately one month away, she will probably have four routine antepartum office visits, each with a hemoglobin and urinalysis, plus the delivery charge of $650. Any additional services would include additional charges. Use letterhead stationery, and date the letter October 17. File the completed letter in Erin's file.

MARK NEWMAN, M.D.

2235 South Ridgeway Avenue
Chicago, IL 60623-2240

Board Certified in Family Medicine

312-555-6022
FAX: 312-555-0025

September 15, 19--

Mr. and Mrs. Eli Burnett
7024 Yales Avenue South
Chicago, IL 60621-4207

Dear Mr. and Mrs. Burnett:

Recently you inquired about our OB charges. Dr. Newman's routine delivery fee is $650. A routine OB examination is $30, our Office Visit Focused charge. The postpartum examination is also the same charge.

The verification of pregnancy and the OB physical examination charges are not included in the $650 fee. Additional laboratory texts, X rays, injections, and so forth, will result in additional charges. These charges could include the following:

Urinalysis	$10.00
Hemoglobin	10.00
Newborn physical in hospital	35.00
Circumsion	75.00

Each charge will be entered onto your billing statement. Please verify your insurance coverage. Any amount not covered by your insurance will be your responsibility. We also ask that you pay the $650 delivery charge before delivery.

If you have further questions, please call me.

Sincerely,

Theresa J. Olssen

Theresa J. Olssen
Medical Assistant

Figure 9-1   Letter Explaining OB Charges

Whenever a patient consults the doctor, there is a charge but not necessarily a payment. Therefore, it is necessary to keep track of all **transactions**; that is, charges the patient incurs for office visits or for any other services—for example, X rays, laboratory tests, physical therapy treatments—and any payments the patient has made.

Charge Slips

A common method for recording the procedures is to use a **charge slip**, or charge ticket.

Charge slips may be reproduced in-house or purchased from a medical stationer. These slips save time since the doctor needs only to check each item performed. Most charge slips are tailored to the doctor's practice. Charge slips typically contain the following information:

- A checklist of procedures and their corresponding codes.
- A checklist of diagnoses and their corresponding codes.
- Space for additional information and instructions.
- A blank for the patient's previous balance.
- A blank for the total charges for the patient's visit.
- A blank for payment received.
- A blank for the patient's current balance.

The charge slip is initiated when the patient registers for the visit. The following procedures are then used to ensure that the proper billing information is recorded:

1. The charge slip is attached to the patient's chart.
2. As the doctor performs procedures, check marks are made in the appropriate boxes.
3. The doctor adds any pertinent instructions.
4. The diagnoses and corresponding codes are marked.
5. The charge slip is taken to the checkout area for the assistant to record the transaction in the appropriate manner.

Figure 9-2 on page 156 shows an example of a completed charge slip.

A charge slip is also commonly known as a **superbill**. Medical stationers supply superbills in triplicate—one copy for the doctor, one copy to be submitted to the patient's insurance carrier, and one copy for the patient. There is also a space for the patient's signature, which authorizes direct payment from the insurance company to the attending physician.

Patient's Ledger

The patient's **ledger** is a record that shows the professional services rendered to the patient, the charge for each service, payments made by the patient, and the balance owed by the patient. Transactions are recorded on the ledger card each time a service is performed to keep

| NO. | DATE | DESCRIPTION | CHARGE | CREDIT | | CURRENT BALANCE |
				PAYMENT	ADJ.	
	9/3	OVE/EKG	105 00	70 00		35.00

ITEM	FEE	ITEM	FEE	
New Patients:		**X rays:**		Wayne Elliot
99202 OV Focused (OVF)	___	71020 Chest	___	PATIENT
99203 OV Expanded (OVE)	___	73560 Knee Films	___	1257 W. School St.
Established Patients:		76091 Mammogram	___	PATIENT'S ADDRESS
99212 OV Focused (OVF)	___	72090 Scoliosis Film	___	Chicago, IL 60651-5571
99213 OV Expanded (OVE)	_40⁰⁰_	70210 Sinus	___	CITY STATE, ZIP
99214 OV Detailed (OVD)	___			self
99215 OV Comprehensive	___	**LABORATORY:**		RESPONSIBLE PERSON
House Call:		85022 CBC	___	
99352 HC	___	82465 Cholesterol	___	RELATIONSHIP
Hospital Visits:		85007 Differential	___	
99221 Initial HV	___	82270 Hemoccults x3	___	
99232 HV	___	85018 Hemoglobin (Hgb)	___	INSURANCE NAME CONTRACT NO.
Obstetrical/GU:		86308 Mono Test	___	401 Hypertension
54150 Circumcision	___	88156 Pap Smear	___	
59410 Delivery	___	89300 Semen Analysis	___	DIAGNOSIS
99433 Newborn Physical	___	80012 SMA-12	___	
59400 Total Delivery	___	86588 Strep Screen	___	NEXT APPOINTMENT
55250 Vasectomy	___	89060 Synovial Fluid	___	
Injections:		81000 Urinalysis (UA)	___	
J1030 DepoMedrol-40 mg	___	87086 Urine Culture (UC)	___	
J1040 DepoMedrol-80 mg	___	85048 WBC	___	
90701 DTP	___	85009 WBC with Diff	___	
90702 DT	___	87210 Wet Prep	___	
90724 Influenza	___	**Miscellaneous:**		
90707 MMR	___	93000 EKG	_65⁰⁰_	
90712 Oral Polio	___	45330 Flex Sig.	___	
90703 TT	___	A4550 Sterile Tray	___	

MARK NEWMAN, M.D.
2235 S. Ridgeway Avenue, Chicago, IL 60623-2240
312-555-6022   FAX 312-555-0025

Figure 9-2   Completed Charge Slip

the account current. The ledger may be typed, handwritten, or computerized. The billing account is arranged by family name, with all family members listed on the same account and all transactions recorded on one ledger file. Figure 9-3 shows an example of a ledger with the transactions for all the members of one family on a single form. Each family member is identified on the statement by a different number.

The copy of the ledger that is sent to the patient is called a **statement**, or bill. The statement may be either a photocopy of the ledger or a separate printout if a computerized ledger is used. Time is saved if the statements are mailed in window envelopes because the need to prepare envelopes is eliminated. Another means of saving time is the self-mailer. The bill is produced on a form that becomes the return envelope when folded properly. The patient can fold the bill according to the instructions, enclose the payment, and mail the resulting envelope.

Listing, or itemizing, the procedures on the ledger reminds patients when they visited the doctor and what services were performed. Some common procedures are listed using procedural codes to save space on the ledger form. Explanations of the codes are printed at the bottom of the form.

STATEMENT

MARK NEWMAN, M.D.
2235 South Ridgeway Avenue
Chicago, IL 60623-2240
312-555-6022   Fax 312-555-0025

Family
1. Wayne
2. Gwen
3. Emily
4. Rose
5.

Wayne Elliot
1257 West School Street
Chicago, IL 60651-5571

NO.	DATE	DESCRIPTION	CHARGE	CREDIT		CURRENT BALANCE
				PAYMENT	ADJ.	
1	9/3	OVE/EKG	105.00	70.00		35.00
2	9/15	Delivery	650.00			685.00
4	9/17	Newborn physical	35.00			720.00
3	9/17	OVF/Hgb	40.00	700.00		60.00

CBC—complete blood count
EKG—electrocardiogram
HC—house call
Hgb—hemoglobin
HV—hospital visit

INJ—injection
LAB—laboratory work
NP—new patient
OVD—office visit, detailed
OVE—office visit, expanded

OVF—office visit, focused
Pap—Pap smear
ROA—received on account
UA—urinalysis
UC—urine culture

Figure 9-3   Ledger Showing Family Transactions

The bill is generally sent to the patient who received treatment, although in some cases another person may be designated as the one responsible for receiving and paying the bill. In general, parents are responsible for the medical bills of minor children living in their home.

The **pegboard**, or write-it-once system of keeping patients' accounts, uses a pegboard to combine the daily summary record, a ledger card, and the charge slip (or superbill). The daily summary record is a journal in which all the transactions of the office are entered, including patients seen by the doctor, services rendered, charges, payments, and balances. After the daily summary, ledger, and charge slip have been properly aligned on the pegboard, an entry can be written once on the top of the form and it will appear in the correct position on the forms below.

Computerized Billing

Many computer software programs are available to handle patients' billing. Besides generating an itemized statement, a computerized billing system may include monthly reports summarizing the operation of the practice; amounts of money generated by various departments such as laboratory, X ray, and physical therapy; and amounts generated by individual physicians in the practice. Such programs are a

Prepare a ledger card for each patient who has an index card. Use the ledger forms on WPs 59 through 63. Note that some of the ledgers have been started for you. Photocopy the blank ledgers on WP 63 to use for the other patients. (You will need a total of 36 ledgers.) Key the information for each patient in the address section of the ledger. (Remember, the charges will be sent to the parent when the patient is a minor.) Use the fee schedule on WP 58 and the following information to update the ledgers.

Monica Armstrong	10/14:	OVF, CBC, SMA–12, UA, Hemoccults
	10/16:	Mammogram
Thomas Baab	10/15:	CPE (OV Comprehensive), UA, CBC, and SMA–12
	10/16:	Flex Sigmoidoscopy
Todd Grant	10/15:	OVE, EKG
David Kramer	10/14:	OVE (NP), UA, Hgb (Alan Mitchell's ledger)
Jeffrey Kramer	10/14:	OVF, Hgb, UA
Laura Lund	10/14:	OVD, Pap
Ardis Matthews	10/15:	OVE
Erin Mitchell	10/14:	OVE (NP), UA, Hgb
Raymond Murray	Previous balance, $75	
	10/12:	HC
Gary Robertson	10/14:	OVF, UA, UC

Post additional charges or payments daily to keep the accounts up to date. File the ledger cards alphabetically, clip them together, and keep them in your Miscellaneous folder.

valuable accounting tool for the physician, and the assistant should be familiar with their use.

Computer billing statements are printed in duplicate, with one copy for the patient's record and one copy to be forwarded to the insurance carrier. This statement contains all the necessary information for the insurance company and eliminates additional form processing for the assistant. A sample of a computer billing statement is shown in Figure 9-4.

■ ARRANGING FOR PAYMENT

The method of payment is arranged at the time of the patient's first visit. In most offices, a combination of methods is used and may include the following:

- Patients pay at the time of the visit by cash or check (some offices may accept credit cards).
- Bills are mailed to patients monthly or at the end of a procedure or hospital stay.
- Patients pay a fixed amount weekly or monthly until the bill is paid in full.

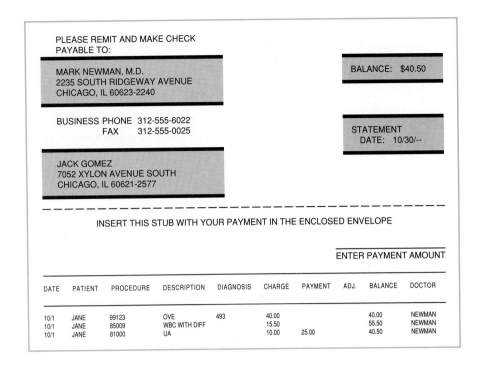

PLEASE REMIT AND MAKE CHECK
PAYABLE TO:

MARK NEWMAN, M.D.
2235 SOUTH RIDGEWAY AVENUE
CHICAGO, IL 60623-2240

BALANCE: $40.50

BUSINESS PHONE 312-555-6022
FAX 312-555-0025

STATEMENT
DATE: 10/30/--

JACK GOMEZ
7052 XYLON AVENUE SOUTH
CHICAGO, IL 60621-2577

- -

INSERT THIS STUB WITH YOUR PAYMENT IN THE ENCLOSED ENVELOPE

ENTER PAYMENT AMOUNT

DATE	PATIENT	PROCEDURE	DESCRIPTION	DIAGNOSIS	CHARGE	PAYMENT	ADJ.	BALANCE	DOCTOR
10/1	JANE	99123	OVE	493	40.00			40.00	NEWMAN
10/1	JANE	85009	WBC WITH DIFF		15.50			55.50	NEWMAN
10/1	JANE	81000	UA		10.00	25.00		40.50	NEWMAN

Figure 9-4 Computerized
Billing Statement

- Bills are sent to health insurance carriers.
- Some doctors work on a cash-only basis.
- A patient with a poor credit rating may be on a cash-only basis.

In many offices, the patient is given a charge slip to leave at the checkout desk. When the doctor is finished with the examination and treatment, the doctor should remind the patient to stop at the check-out desk on the way out of the office. The assistant should note the method of payment and make it clear to the patient that prompt payment is expected. Depending on the situation, one of the following statements might be used:

Example

Assistant: Our policy is payment at the time of the visit. Will you be paying by cash or check?

or

I note that your visit is covered by insurance. Please submit this claim as soon as possible.

or

Your insurance requires a copayment of $10 for today's visit. Will you be paying by cash or check?

On occasion, patients will respond with a reason why they are not able to pay at this time or why a previous balance has been left unpaid. The assistant should exercise good judgment about the person's ability and willingness to pay. Handling such situations is learned through practice and requires an understanding of human nature. Here are some examples of reasons patients may give for not paying a fee.

Example

> PATIENT: I'm sorry. I must have forgotten my checkbook.
> ASSISTANT: Our policy is payment at the time of your visit. Please send us your check as soon as you get home.

In full view of the patient, the assistant might put a stamp on a self-addressed envelope and give the envelope to the patient for mailing the check.

Example

> PATIENT: My insurance will cover this bill.
> ASSISTANT: Our policy is for the patient to pay the bill and then for the insurance company to reimburse the patient. We will fill out our portion of the insurance claim today, so the insurance company will be able to reimburse you promptly. The fee for today's visit is [amount].

In full view of the patient, the assistant could then turn the ledger card over to jot down brief notes regarding the account, including the date of the visit and when the patient intends to pay.

Cash Payments

The assistant must be careful to enter each cash payment in the patient's ledger and in the daily summary record. The patient's name, services rendered, charges, payment **received on account (ROA)**, and balances should be included.

Payments should be given to the assistant, not the doctor. A **receipt** must be given to the patient who pays cash. Copies of receipts are kept as permanent records. The patient should be advised to keep the receipt and a copy of the charge slip for income tax purposes in claiming medical deductions. If the patient pays by check, the canceled check is the receipt. An example of a receipt is shown in Figure 9-5.

Certain rules must be observed to safeguard money received. Cash, checks, and money orders should be kept in a secure location such as a locked drawer. Currency should be separated by denominations. Checks should be immediately stamped with a **restrictive endorsement**, which specifies "Pay to the order of..." or "For deposit only." To minimize the danger of theft, money should be deposited in the bank daily.

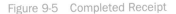

No. 566
To Wayne Elliot
Date 9/3/--
For Services
Amount $70⁰⁰

No. 566   September 3 19 --
Received from Wayne Elliot
Seventy and ⁰⁰/₁₀₀ ——————————— *Dollars*
FOR Services rendered
                    Theresa J. Olssen
$ $70 ⁰⁰/₁₀₀

Figure 9-5 Completed Receipt

Sending Statements

Although most bills are sent out once a month, a statement may be sent at the end of a procedure or upon discharge from the hospital. It is more efficient to send out statements monthly so that the doctor's bill can be paid along with the patient's other monthly bills. In large practices, however, **cycle billing** may be advantageous. Under this system, all accounts are divided alphabetically into groups, with each group billed on a different date. If cycle billing is used, the patient should be informed on the first visit approximately when the bill will be mailed. A definite pattern for sending bills should be established and maintained.

Example

ASSISTANT: I notice that you are in the billing cycle for the end of the month; those bills will be mailed in the next few days. The charges are payable within 30 days. We would appreciate prompt payment.

A patient may request not to have any correspondence sent to a particular address, for example, the home or business address. A notation to this effect should be made on the patient's ledger card and index card so this request will not be overlooked.

Payment Plans

For the patient who is unable to pay a medical bill in one lump sum, a schedule of payments, or contract, can be agreed upon by the patient and the assistant. The agreement should be in writing, and a copy of the plan should be given to the patient as a reminder of the commitment to pay the doctor. The amount to be paid weekly or monthly is stated in the agreement, and the agreement is used as a reference when corresponding with the patient about unpaid bills.

Example

ASSISTANT: We haven't received your payment for this past month. According to the agreement we made, your payment was due on the tenth of the month. Is there some reason we have not heard from you?

Health Insurance

Many patients carry health insurance that provides payment for a portion of their medical expenses. At the time of registration, ask new patients to show their health insurance cards. These cards usually state the type of insurance, the coverage provided, policy numbers, and the date of enforcement. Frequently, these cards are photocopied and the copies are entered into the patients' files for reference. The details of insurance and the assistant's responsibilities in this area are covered in Chapter 10 on health insurance.

Third-Party Liability

Sometimes a person other than the patient assumes liability, or responsibility, for the charges. The assistant must contact this third party for verification of financial obligation. Relatives, particularly children of aged parents, may say they will be responsible for payment of the bill, but this promise must be in writing. Oral promises are not legally binding. Once the patient is well, the relatives may forget the obligation to pay. A signed promise will greatly reduce the credit risk. A third party is not obligated by law unless he or she has signed an agreement to pay the charges.

Professional Courtesy

Medical etiquette prescribes that physicians treat colleagues and their immediate families free of charge or at a reduced cost. Most doctors carry health insurance that pays for a portion of their medical expenses; however, follow the policy of your employer regarding professional courtesy and billing. If the colleague being treated asks for a bill, it is proper to send one with a cover letter. Figure 9-6 shows an example of a letter explaining the office billing procedure to a colleague who has been extended professional courtesy.

Fee Adjustment

Should the need arise, the doctor can adjust the cost of any procedure; the doctor will then inform the assistant of the **fee adjustment**. Fees should not be reduced as a way to receive payment quickly and avoid collection procedures. In some cases, doctors' fees are adjusted to the financial situation of the patient. For example, a fee adjustment may be extended to a patient who cannot pay or who dies. The doctor must be careful in deciding to reduce or cancel a fee because such an action may be misinterpreted and even lead to a malpractice suit. If a

```
                    MARK NEWMAN, M.D.
                                        2235 South Ridgeway Avenue
                                            Chicago, IL 60623-2240
        Board Certified in Family Medicine        312-555-6022
                                              FAX: 312-555-0025


September 15, 19--



Evan Alexes, M.D.
46534 20th Avenue South
Chicago, IL 60621-8491

Dear Dr. Alexes:

We are pleased to provide professional services for you at no
charge.  If you have health insurance, we would appreciate
assignment of benefit for the covered services.  We will be glad
to process your insurance claim for you.

If laboratory and X-ray service are performed outside this
clinic, please check with the providers at the time of service
regarding their billing procedures.

Thank you for allowing us to participate in your care.

Sincerely,

Mark Newman

Mark Newman, M.D.

lj
```

Figure 9-6   Letter Explaining Professional Courtesy Billing Procedure

doctor chooses to reduce or cancel a fee, the decision must be in writing for the protection of the doctor.

In cases that involve a considerable sum, the patient may not be able to pay the fee and may have to seek financial assistance. The assistant should be acquainted with the local agencies to which a patient can be referred when financial assistance is needed.

CREDIT INFORMATION

Arranging a method of payment does not ensure the collection of the doctor's fees. Doctors sustain losses when they render services to patients who turn out to be bad credit risks. Precautions to ensure collections include obtaining as much information about a new patient as possible such as the following:

- The patient's occupation or the occupation of the person who is responsible for the bill.
- The patient's place of employment with the business address and telephone number.
- The name and telephone number of the person who referred the patient to the doctor.

Credit standing is also indicated by bank references and charge accounts. The patient's credit rating should be obtained if the doctor's fees are substantial and if the patient is not well known to the doctor.

Handling credit arrangements should be done tactfully and in a routine manner. If the credit arrangement is presented in the right spirit, no fair-minded patient will object. It is important, however, that the amount of the fee be agreed upon and that it be clearly understood what the fee will cover.

■ COLLECTION OF ACCOUNTS

As a general rule, at least one-third of the outstanding accounts should be collected each day. It is regrettable that patients are often slow and even delinquent in paying physicians. There are various reasons a patient might not pay a bill. For example, the patient may unintentionally or intentionally ignore the bill; the patient may not have the money to pay the bill; or the patient may be unwilling to pay the bill for a reason such as disagreeing with the amount of the bill. Other reasons for nonpayment of medical bills include a patient's excessive debt, unemployment, illness, disability, family problems, or marital problems.

The assistant must know how to handle patients' accounts properly to reduce the physician's losses from unpaid bills. The first step in the collection process is to collect payment at the time of the office visit, if possible. Then the assistant must keep accounts current and be aware of the status of each account.

Payments must be entered promptly so that at billing time there is no question about any balance due. Each month **delinquent accounts** (any unpaid accounts with a balance that is 30 days past due) should be "aged" to show their status in the collection process (that is, 30, 60, or 90 days past due). As in any business, interest may be charged on unpaid balances that are 30 days past due.

Office practices vary concerning how many reminders of past-due balances should be sent to a patient and how to send them out. A **dunning statement** is a written reminder about an overdue account. Some doctors attach a reminder to the bill stating that the account is overdue. The actual wording of this kind of reminder varies according to how long the account is overdue. Sample overdue messages are shown in Figure 9-7.

Other physicians may prefer a more personal approach. A brief, handwritten note on the monthly statement may prompt patients to settle past-due accounts faster. The following are examples of notations that may be written on overdue billing statements:

Example

Is everything okay? We missed your payment for last month. Please call us if we can help.

or

Just a reminder: According to my note concerning our telephone conversation of October 1, you promised to send us a

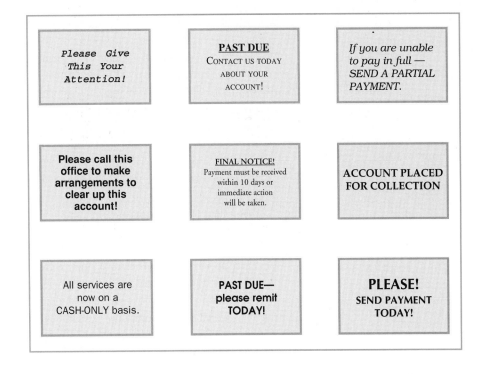

Figure 9-7 Overdue Reminder Stickers

payment by the 15th. If you need help regarding this bill, please contact us.

You might also want to give praise by adding a personal note on the statement following a payment.

Example

Thanks for your prompt payment.
—Linda

Guidelines for Payment

Management or the accounting department in every office must determine the **collection ratio** (total collections divided by net charges of the practice). The percentage will show the effectiveness of the collections (the higher the percentage, the more effective the collections). Management would then set the guidelines for payments—how much is to be collected daily, how much should be collected on each account, and so forth.

Course of Action

Every office needs to establish a course of action to be taken on overdue accounts. This might include having the assistant take the following steps with the person responsible for an overdue account:

1. Attach a reminder sticker to a statement for an account that is 30 days overdue.

2. Telephone the person responsible for payment of an account that is 45 days overdue.
3. Send a brief, signed, personal note written directly on a statement for an account that is 60 days overdue.
4. Again telephone the person responsible for payment of an account that is 75 days overdue.
5. Send a collection letter to the person responsible for payment of an account that is 90 days overdue along with the billing statement.
6. Send a more persuasive letter and/or telephone someone who has an account that is 90 days overdue and who has not responded to past contacts.

The doctor will need to establish the office policy regarding collection procedures, including when to send statements, reminders, and letters and when to take final action. Federal laws such as the Truth in Lending Act, Fair Credit Reporting Act, and Use of Telephone for Debt Collecting Act regulate credit and collections for businesses. Also, individual states may have laws that guide the collection process. The material in this chapter discusses only basic collection procedures.

Collection by Letter

The longer a bill remains unpaid, the less likelihood there is of collecting it. A bill should be followed up most vigorously after being overdue for three months.

Writing collection letters that bring results is a skill. Collection letters should be personal letters, not form letters. The letter should show that you are sincerely interested in the patient's problem and want to work out a solution. Collection letters should be brief, with short sentences. The letters should appeal to the patient's sense of pride and fair play, and to the desire for a good credit rating. The amount that is due should be stated clearly in each collection letter, and the patient should be asked to telephone the assistant to discuss the situation. Figure 9-8 shows two examples of effective collection letters.

Collection by Telephone

Another effective method of collection is to telephone the patient personally. A telephone call cannot be ignored as easily as a letter can. It also can be effective in reminding a person who has unintentionally forgotten to pay. Tact and experience are necessary in order to be effective in telephone collections.

Techniques of telephone collection include the following:

- Identify yourself.
- Be sure you are talking to the person who is responsible for payment of the account.
- Make the collection call in the evening, especially if the person who is responsible for payment of the accounts is out during the day.

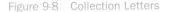

MARK NEWMAN, M.D.

2235 South Ridgeway Avenue
Chicago, IL 60623-2240
312-555-6022
FAX: 312-555-0025

Board Certified in Family Medicine

July 1, 19--

Mrs. Clair Munson
3492 Green Avenue South
Chicago, IL 60624-3422

Dear Mrs. Munson:

In reviewing our accounts, I find that you have an overdue
balance of $78.

As you are aware, all bills are due within 30 days of service.
Is there some reason we have not heard from you?

Please send us your check for $78 this week to clear your account
or contact our office immediately.

Sincerely,

Theresa J. Olssen

Theresa J. Olssen
Medical Assistant

MARK NEWMAN, M.D.

2235 South Ridgeway Avenue
Chicago, IL 60623-2240
312-555-6022
FAX: 312-555-0025

Board Certified in Family Medicine

August 1, 19--

Mrs. Clair Munson
3492 Green Avenue South
Chicago, IL 60624-3422

Dear Mrs. Munson:

It is Dr. Newman's policy to contact patients who have accounts
with balances that are 60 days overdue and who have not written
to or called our office to arrange a payment plan.

All we ask is that you cooperate in contacting us about your
overdue balance of $78 as soon as possible. We are certain that
we can work out a suitable payment plan.

Please send us your check for $78 this week to clear your account
or get in touch with us immediately to arrange a payment plan.

Sincerely,

Theresa J. Olssen

Theresa J. Olssen
Medical Assistant

Figure 9-8 Collection Letters

- Never call a patient at a place of employment to inquire about an unpaid bill.
- Always use a pleasant manner to reflect your confidence that the problem can be resolved.
- Ask to discuss the bill to determine whether the patient has any questions. This query should elicit some response, which is your cue to continue the rest of the conversation.
- Listen carefully.
- Do not show irritation in your voice or appear to be scolding the patient.
- Inform the person that you need to know why the bill has not been paid or why inquiries about the unpaid bill have not been answered.
- If the patient promises to pay, ask when you can expect a payment and for what amount. Then make a note about the conversation, saying, for example, "I am making a note in your account file that you promised to pay $100 on September 10. Is that correct?"

When collecting by telephone, always keep complete, accurate records of who said what, who promised to pay, how much was promised, and when the payment was promised. Note any unusual circumstances. Ask the person responsible for the bill to write down the arrangement.

If the person who promised over the telephone to pay the account does not follow through, telephone after 15 days to remind the person that the promise is overdue. At this point, another course of action may be to send a letter stating that the account will be terminated and sent to a collection agency if the person does not telephone or send payment within 10 days, or when the promise to pay is 30 days past due.

After updating the ledgers, you note that Suzanne Roberts has not made a payment for three months. There is a notation that a reminder note was sent on September 30 and a follow-up telephone call was made October 10. Write a letter in your name to Suzanne requesting payment. Use letterhead stationery, and date the letter October 20.

Terminated Accounts

A physician who finds it impossible to extract payment from a patient may decide to terminate the physician-patient relationship.

If a patient comes to the office requesting medical care after an account has been terminated, the doctor should be consulted and may decide to see the patient on a cash-only basis.

Collection by Agency

If the patient has not paid the bill after a reasonable time and routine collection procedures have failed, the doctor has two ways of attempting collection. The doctor can sue the patient and go to court, but this is a time-consuming and costly procedure. The other method is to turn the account over to a collection agency. Once an account has been turned over for collection, the office will have no further contact with the patient concerning billing. Approximately 40 to 50 percent of the amount due is lost when the account is turned over to an agency, and the longer the bill goes unpaid, the less money the doctor will receive when the account is finally settled.

There are various types of collection agencies, and a doctor will want to investigate an agency thoroughly to determine its reputation.

Collection From Estates

When a patient has died, a bill should be sent to the estate after a short interval. The probate department of the local government can provide the name and address of the person responsible for the deceased patient's debts.

Statute of Limitations

If the doctor fails to collect a fee within a certain period of time, the collection becomes illegal under the statute of limitations and no further claim on the debt is possible. Each state sets its own time limitation. The doctor should obtain legal counsel for advice concerning these statutes.

PERSONAL DEVELOPMENT PROJECTS

Key Terms

The following terms appear in **boldface** type in this chapter. Do you recall what they mean? Refer to the chapter for definitions you need to review.

charge slip
collection ratio
cycle billing
delinquent accounts
dunning statement
fee adjustment
fee schedule
ledger
pegboard

receipt
received on account
  (ROA)
restrictive endorsement
services rendered
statement
superbill
transactions

Topics for Discussion

1. Fracture care is sometimes charged as one lump fee to cover all visits, tests, and services connected with treating the fracture. Would this be considered a good policy from a billing standpoint? Alternatively, would it be preferable to itemize the visits, X rays, and other procedures separately?

2. Discuss how a collection telephone call should be handled when the patient expresses dissatisfaction with the care provided by the physician and states that a second opinion has been obtained and further care is being provided by another physician.

3. Explain the advantages and disadvantages of having patients pay a fixed amount every month.

Role-Playing

1. Wayne Elliot asks you why he was charged for two office visits when his daughters, Emily and Rose, were seen at the same time in the same room for the same problem—an earache.

2. Ellen Stevens, a newcomer to the community, telephones to ask what Dr. Newman charges for an office visit.

3. A new patient is checking out after seeing Dr. Newman. Ask for payment at the checkout desk.

SIMULATION 2

Today you will begin your second two–day simulation in Dr. Newman's office. The days are Tuesday, October 21; and Wednesday, October 22.

PROCEDURES

Review the "General Procedures" in Simulation 1. Follow the same instructions—under "Specific Procedures"—for Days 1 and 2 as you did in Simulation 1.

MATERIALS

The materials you will need are generally the same as those listed for Simulation 1. Pull the patients' charts and ledgers according to the appointment calendar, and put them in your To-Do folder.

Materials	Source

Appointment calendar

Card file

Supplies folder

To-Do folder

Day 1

Patients' charts and ledgers for October 21	
Telephone log	WP 64
Draft of a letter to Thomas Baab	WP 65
Letter from Dr. Tai	WP 66
X–ray and laboratory reports	WP 67
Charge slips	WP 69

Day 2

Patients' charts and ledgers for October 22	
X–ray and laboratory reports	WP 68
Charge slips	WP 70

Patients' folders

The following items have been added to the patients' folders (charts) since the last simulation:

Armstrong, Monica	Projects 30 and 32 Simulation 1: appointment card
Baab, Thomas	Projects 28, 32, and 33
Babcock, Sara	Project 30 Simulation 1: message
Grant, Todd	Project 30
Kramer, David	Projects 30 and 32
Kramer, Jeffrey	Simulation 1: registration form, release form, and index card Project 30 Simulation 1: message and appointment card
Lund, Laura	Project 30
Matthews, Ardis	Project 30
Mitchell, Erin	Projects 25 and 34 Simulation 1: registration form, release form, letter, index card, and appointment card
Murray, Raymond	Project 31
Roberts, Suzanne	Project 36
Robertson, Gary	Projects 30 and 32 Simulation 1: appointment card

Ledger cards for all current patients (Project 35)

Miscellaneous folder

Dr. Grace Tai	Simulation 1: index card

If you have not completed all the projects and do not have all these records set up in advance, talk with your instructor.

MEDICAL VOCABULARY

The following medical terms are used in Simulation 2. Review each term and its meaning.

anesthetized: having been subjected to anesthesia; having lost sensation or feeling.
atherosclerosis: hardening of the blood vessels caused by plaque deposits.
Betadine: brand name for a surgical antiseptic.
chronicity: a long duration of time.
condylar: pertaining to a rounded prominence on a bone.
diplopia: double vision.
disequilibrium: disturbance of balance.
ecchymosis: in a bruise, the seepage of blood into the tissues from broken vessels beneath the skin causing purple discoloration.
effusion: the release of fluid, which may collect in a cavity or joint.
exudate: fluid escaped from a blood vessel and deposited in body tissue.
gravida: a pregnant woman.
hematoma: a collection of clotted blood in body tissue.

hidradenitis: inflammation of a sweat gland.

hyperventilation: abnormal and excessive breathing.

inflammation: a local body response to tissue injury characterized by redness, heat, and swelling.

nausea: the feeling of having to vomit.

neuronitis: inflammation of a neuron.

nystagmus: a rapid, involuntary movement of the eyeball.

palpation: examination of a patient by touching.

pharyngitis: inflammation of the pharynx or throat.

phlegm: mucus secreted in the respiratory system.

proximal: nearest.

pustular: containing pus.

pyelonephritis: inflammation of the renal pelvis and kidney.

rhinorrhea: discharge of fluid form the nose; runny nose.

Romberg test: a test of equilibrium.

suppurative: producing pus.

tendinitis: inflammation of a tendon.

tinnitus: ringing in the ears.

tympanic membrane: eardrum.

valgus: a deformity in which a body part is away from the midline of the body.

varus: a deformity in which a body part is turned inward toward the midline of the body.

vestibular: pertaining to a space or a cavity.

Financial Responsibilities

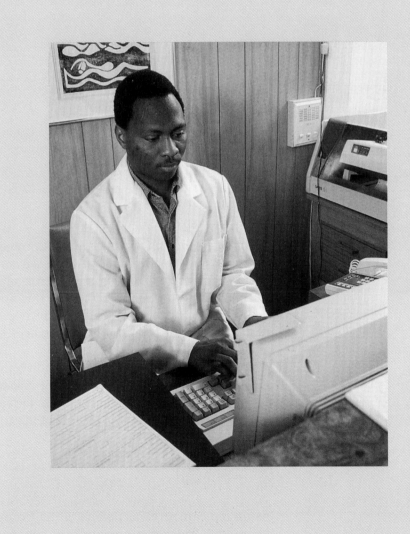

Health Insurance

Upon completion of this chapter, you should be able to:

- Discuss the assistant's role in processing insurance claims.

- Describe the various types of health insurance coverage.

- Define health insurance terms.

- Explain Medicare's Part A and Part B.

- Explain the purpose of the Medicaid program.

- Explain the purpose of workers' compensation insurance.

- Define *CHAMPUS* and *CHAMPVA*.

- Discuss the differences between HMOs, IPAs, and PPOs.

- Discuss the purpose of diagnostic and procedural coding.

- Process insurance claim forms in given situations.

- Explain the follow-up process for insurance claims.

Health insurance refers to insurance protection against medical care expenses. Because health insurance is a complex field, this chapter is meant only as an introduction to the role of the medical assistant. The assistant must be well informed on this subject, because duties will include many phases of health insurance. Patients ask many questions about health insurance and expect the assistant to know the answers.

Many patients do not pay doctors directly; instead, the doctors are paid by insurance companies. It is the assistant's responsibility to see that the doctor receives compensation for services. This responsibility is partly fulfilled by the processing of insurance claim forms.

■ TYPES OF INSURANCE COVERAGE

Insurance can be classified as either group insurance or individual insurance. Under group insurance, one master policy is issued to an organization or employer and covers the eligible members or employees and their dependents. Thus, all the members or employees have the same health care coverage. Group insurance provides better benefits with lower premiums than does individual insurance. Individual insurance applies only to the person taking out the policy and to that person's dependents. Because it is not obtained at a group rate, the cost is higher than for group insurance.

Following are descriptions of major types of health insurance coverage. A basic health insurance policy might include hospital, medical, and surgical insurance. A comprehensive insurance package would include several of the major types of insurance listed.

Hospital

Hospital insurance provides protection against the costs of hospital care. It generally provides a room allowance (a stated amount per day for a semiprivate room) with a maximum number of days per year. Special provisions are made for operating room charges, X rays, laboratory work, drugs, and other medically necessary items while the insured person is an inpatient. An *inpatient* is a person who is admitted to the hospital for a minimum of 24 hours.

Medical

Medical insurance covers benefits for outpatient medical care including physicians' fees for hospital visits and nonsurgical procedures. The term *medical* refers to the physician's costs. Special provisions are made for diagnostic services such as laboratory, X ray, and pathology costs. An *outpatient* is a person who receives medical care at a hospital or other medical facility but who is not admitted for more than 24 hours.

Surgical

Surgical insurance provides protection for the cost of a physician's fee for surgery, whether it is performed in a hospital, in a doctor's office, or elsewhere (such as a surgical center). Charges for anesthesia generally are covered by surgical insurance.

Outpatient

Outpatient insurance usually provides protection for emergency room visits and other outpatient divisions in a hospital or medical facility such as X ray, pathology, and psychological services.

Major Medical

Major medical insurance offers protection for large medical expenses, such as extensive injuries from a car accident, that go above and beyond the maximum established by a regular health insurance policy. There is usually an added cost for this type of insurance coverage.

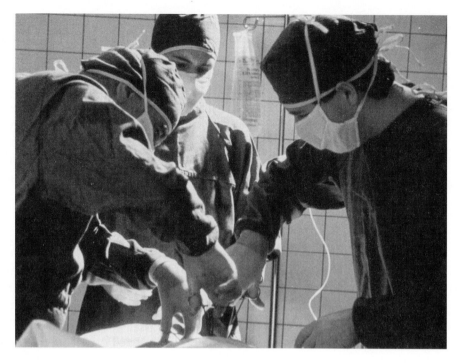

Surgical insurance typically covers charges for anesthesia as well as the cost of a physician's fee for surgery.

Dental Care

Insurance can be obtained to cover all or part of the costs of dental care.

Special Risk

A person can also obtain protection against a certain type of accident (for example, an airplane crash) or illness (for example, cancer) through **special risk insurance**.

■ INSURANCE TERMINOLOGY

The assistant must be familiar with basic insurance terminology in order to process insurance claims.

Carrier

An insurance **carrier** is the insurance company that provides the insurance benefits.

Provider

Whoever provides the health care for the patient is considered the **provider**. The provider may be a doctor, a clinic, or a hospital.

Coverage

Each health insurance policy must state the **coverage**—the extent of health benefits—for each type of insurance that is included in the policy.

Subscriber

A **subscriber**, the insured, or the policyholder is the person who takes out the insurance policy. The policy is in the subscriber's name and can cover the subscriber and the subscriber's dependents.

Contract

An insurance contract is a formal written agreement between the subscriber and the carrier stating details of the coverage. A **family contract** covers the subscriber, the subscriber's spouse, and the subscriber's unmarried dependents with some limitations, such as age of the dependents and/or student status. A **single contract** covers only the subscriber.

Premium

The rate charged for the insurance policy is known as the **premium**. Premiums are usually paid on a regular basis, for example, monthly or quarterly.

Deductible

Many types of insurance coverage have a **deductible** to help contain health care costs. The subscriber must incur a certain amount of medical expense before the insurance carrier will pay. For example, with a $300 deductible for outpatient insurance, the subscriber pays the first $300 of outpatient expenses in the current calendar year.

UCR Allowable Fees

An insurance carrier can state in an insurance contract that it will pay reasonable and customary fees, or usual, customary, and reasonable fees. These may be referred to as "R and C fees" or "UCR fees," respectively.

A **usual fee** is an individual provider's average charge for a certain procedure. For example, a general practitioner may consistently charge $30 for brief office visits. Such charges would be shown on the doctor's fee schedule and charge slip.

A **customary fee** is determined by what doctors with similar training and experience in a certain geographic location typically charge for a procedure. For example, the range for an appendectomy performed by surgeons in a certain metropolitan area might be from $875 to $1000. Therefore, a surgeon's charge of $900 would be considered a customary fee and would be covered by insurance. Another surgeon who charges $1200 for the same procedure would only receive $1000 in payment from the insurance carrier. The **reasonable fee** is the fee allowed or approved by the insurance carrier.

Coinsurance and Copayment

Coinsurance refers to an arrangement in which the subscriber and the insurance carrier share in covering a certain percentage of the medical care costs. Most major medical health plans have coinsurance plans. In an 80/20 coinsurance plan, the insurance carrier pays 80 percent of the medically necessary costs, while the subscriber is responsible for 20 percent.

Copayment refers to a contractual arrangement in which a person must pay a set fee for items such as $15 for every office visit or $8 for each prescription and so forth.

Assignment of Benefits

Physicians may choose to collect payment directly from the patient or to accept an **assignment of benefits**. When a physician accepts an assignment of benefits, the physician agrees to receive payment directly from the patient's insurance carrier. In this case, the patient signs an assignment of benefits statement on the insurance form (shown in Figure 10-1). This statement authorizes the insurance com-

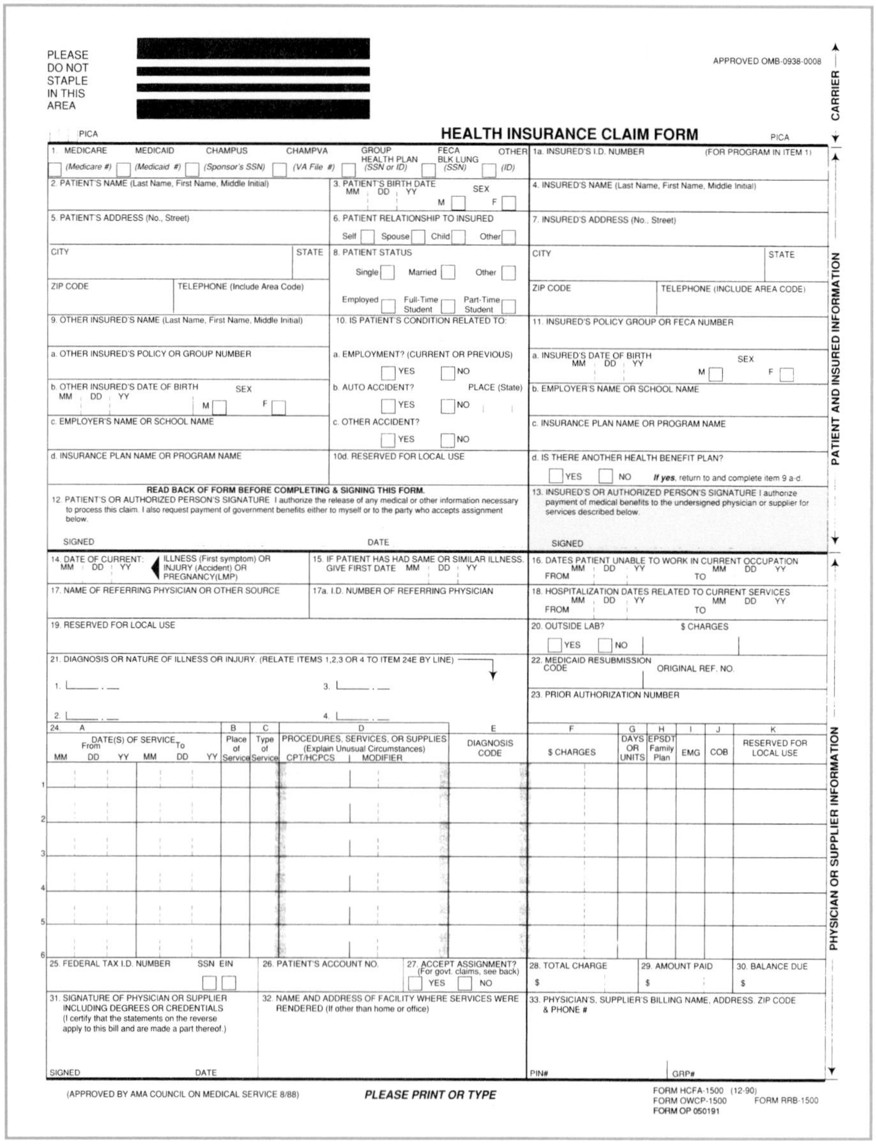
PLEASE DO NOT STAPLE IN THIS AREA

APPROVED OMB-0938-0008

CARRIER

PICA HEALTH INSURANCE CLAIM FORM PICA

1. MEDICARE (Medicare #) MEDICAID (Medicaid #) CHAMPUS (Sponsor's SSN) CHAMPVA (VA File #) GROUP HEALTH PLAN (SSN or ID) FECA BLK LUNG (SSN) OTHER (ID)

1a. INSURED'S I.D. NUMBER (FOR PROGRAM IN ITEM 1)

2. PATIENT'S NAME (Last Name, First Name, Middle Initial)

3. PATIENT'S BIRTH DATE MM DD YY SEX M F

4. INSURED'S NAME (Last Name, First Name, Middle Initial)

5. PATIENT'S ADDRESS (No., Street)

6. PATIENT RELATIONSHIP TO INSURED Self Spouse Child Other

7. INSURED'S ADDRESS (No., Street)

CITY STATE

8. PATIENT STATUS Single Married Other

CITY STATE

ZIP CODE TELEPHONE (Include Area Code)

Employed Full-Time Student Part-Time Student

ZIP CODE TELEPHONE (INCLUDE AREA CODE)

9. OTHER INSURED'S NAME (Last Name, First Name, Middle Initial)

10. IS PATIENT'S CONDITION RELATED TO:

11. INSURED'S POLICY GROUP OR FECA NUMBER

a. OTHER INSURED'S POLICY OR GROUP NUMBER

a. EMPLOYMENT? (CURRENT OR PREVIOUS) YES NO

a. INSURED'S DATE OF BIRTH MM DD YY SEX M F

b. OTHER INSURED'S DATE OF BIRTH MM DD YY SEX M F

b. AUTO ACCIDENT? PLACE (State) YES NO

b. EMPLOYER'S NAME OR SCHOOL NAME

c. EMPLOYER'S NAME OR SCHOOL NAME

c. OTHER ACCIDENT? YES NO

c. INSURANCE PLAN NAME OR PROGRAM NAME

d. INSURANCE PLAN NAME OR PROGRAM NAME

10d. RESERVED FOR LOCAL USE

d. IS THERE ANOTHER HEALTH BENEFIT PLAN? YES NO *If yes*, return to and complete item 9 a-d.

READ BACK OF FORM BEFORE COMPLETING & SIGNING THIS FORM.

12. PATIENT'S OR AUTHORIZED PERSON'S SIGNATURE I authorize the release of any medical or other information necessary to process this claim. I also request payment of government benefits either to myself or to the party who accepts assignment below.

SIGNED DATE

13. INSURED'S OR AUTHORIZED PERSON'S SIGNATURE I authorize payment of medical benefits to the undersigned physician or supplier for services described below.

SIGNED

PATIENT AND INSURED INFORMATION

14. DATE OF CURRENT: MM DD YY ILLNESS (First symptom) OR INJURY (Accident) OR PREGNANCY(LMP)

15. IF PATIENT HAS HAD SAME OR SIMILAR ILLNESS. GIVE FIRST DATE MM DD YY

16. DATES PATIENT UNABLE TO WORK IN CURRENT OCCUPATION MM DD YY FROM TO

17. NAME OF REFERRING PHYSICIAN OR OTHER SOURCE

17a. I.D. NUMBER OF REFERRING PHYSICIAN

18. HOSPITALIZATION DATES RELATED TO CURRENT SERVICES MM DD YY FROM TO

19. RESERVED FOR LOCAL USE

20. OUTSIDE LAB? YES NO $ CHARGES

21. DIAGNOSIS OR NATURE OF ILLNESS OR INJURY. (RELATE ITEMS 1,2,3 OR 4 TO ITEM 24E BY LINE)

1. 2. 3. 4.

22. MEDICAID RESUBMISSION CODE ORIGINAL REF. NO.

23. PRIOR AUTHORIZATION NUMBER

24. A DATE(S) OF SERVICE From MM DD YY To MM DD YY	B Place of Service	C Type of Service	D PROCEDURES, SERVICES, OR SUPPLIES (Explain Unusual Circumstances) CPT/HCPCS MODIFIER	E DIAGNOSIS CODE	F $ CHARGES	G DAYS OR UNITS	H EPSDT Family Plan	I EMG	J COB	K RESERVED FOR LOCAL USE
1										
2										
3										
4										
5										
6										

PHYSICIAN OR SUPPLIER INFORMATION

25. FEDERAL TAX I.D. NUMBER SSN EIN

26. PATIENT'S ACCOUNT NO.

27. ACCEPT ASSIGNMENT? (For govt. claims, see back) YES NO

28. TOTAL CHARGE $

29. AMOUNT PAID $

30. BALANCE DUE $

31. SIGNATURE OF PHYSICIAN OR SUPPLIER INCLUDING DEGREES OR CREDENTIALS (I certify that the statements on the reverse apply to this bill and are made a part thereof.)

SIGNED DATE

32. NAME AND ADDRESS OF FACILITY WHERE SERVICES WERE RENDERED (If other than home or office)

33. PHYSICIAN'S, SUPPLIER'S BILLING NAME, ADDRESS, ZIP CODE & PHONE #

PIN# GRP#

(APPROVED BY AMA COUNCIL ON MEDICAL SERVICE 8/88)

PLEASE PRINT OR TYPE

FORM HCFA-1500 (12-90) FORM OWCP-1500 FORM RRB-1500 FORM OP 050191

Figure 10-1 Insurance Form Authorization for Assignment of Benefits

pany to make direct payment to the doctor. If the doctor does not accept assignment, the assistant bills the patient, the patient collects from the insurance company, and then the patient pays the doctor.

Coordination of Benefits

A **coordination of benefits** (COB) clause in an insurance policy provides that a patient who has two insurance polices can have only a maximum benefit of 100 percent of the health costs. Thus, the patient does not benefit financially from being ill.

With coordination of benefits, one insurance carrier must be designated as the primary carrier. The most common method for determining the primary carrier in such a situation is the **Birthday Rule**. This rule states that if a dependent is covered by two policies, the policy of the subscriber with the earlier birthday in the calendar year is the primary policy. The secondary policy covers any remaining costs such as deductibles and coinsurance.

Release of Information

The patient must sign a **release of information** authorizing the release of medical information to an insurance company in order to process the claim. A sample release section from an insurance form is shown in Figure 10-2 on page 180.

PROJECT 37 Health Insurance Terms

On WP 71, match each health insurance term in Column 2 with the proper definition in Column 1. Be prepared to discuss your answers in class.

■ INSURANCE INFORMATION

The medical assistant must obtain complete and accurate information on a patient who comes into the doctor's office. Not only is this information helpful in facilitating the care of the patient, but also it is necessary for the processing of insurance claims. The information should be kept in the patient's chart and updated when necessary.

Identification Cards

If a patient has a health insurance plan, the assistant should ask to see the identification card (ID). This card states the name of the insurance policy, the subscriber's name, and the insurance policy number. This card should be photocopied and a current copy kept in the patient's file.

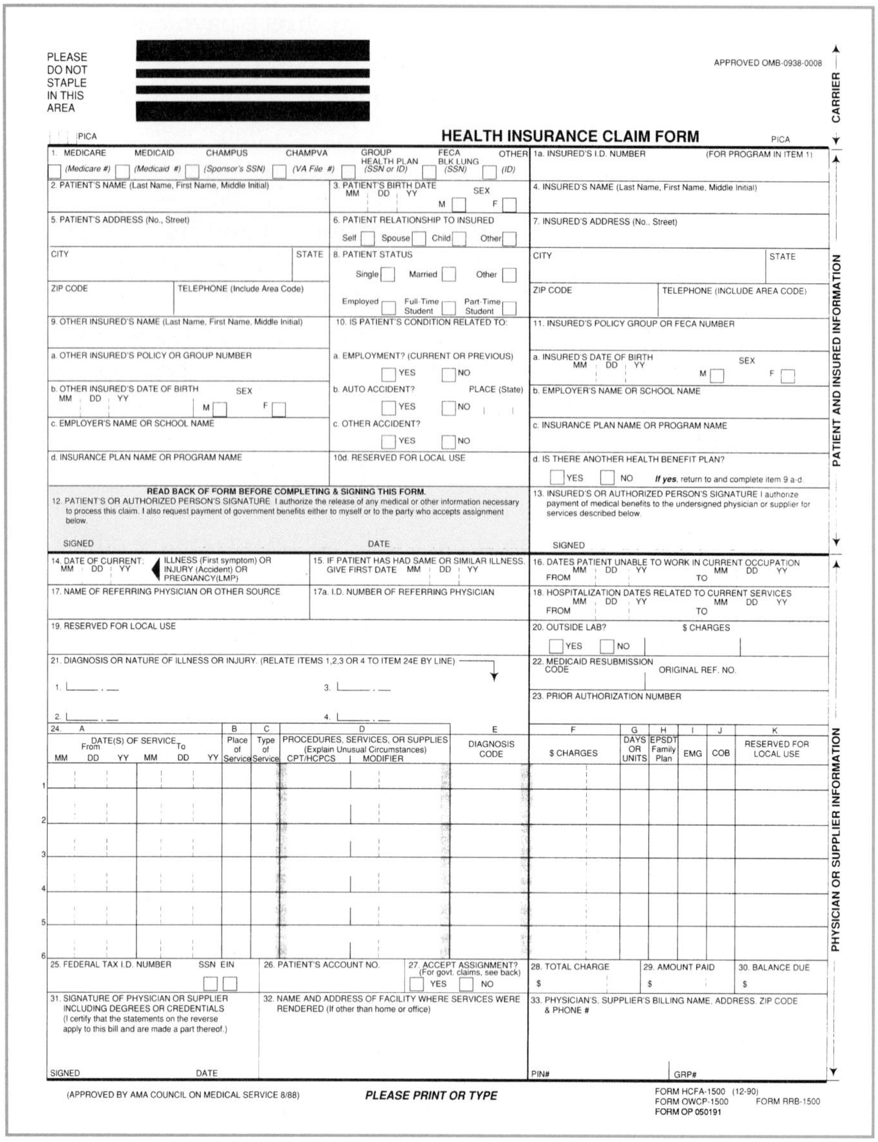

PLEASE DO NOT STAPLE IN THIS AREA

APPROVED OMB-0938-0008

CARRIER

PICA — HEALTH INSURANCE CLAIM FORM — PICA

1. MEDICARE (Medicare #) MEDICAID (Medicaid #) CHAMPUS (Sponsor's SSN) CHAMPVA (VA File #) GROUP HEALTH PLAN (SSN or ID) FECA BLK LUNG (SSN) OTHER (ID)

1a. INSURED'S I.D. NUMBER (FOR PROGRAM IN ITEM 1)

2. PATIENT'S NAME (Last Name, First Name, Middle Initial)

3. PATIENT'S BIRTH DATE MM DD YY SEX M F

4. INSURED'S NAME (Last Name, First Name, Middle Initial)

5. PATIENT'S ADDRESS (No., Street)

6. PATIENT RELATIONSHIP TO INSURED Self Spouse Child Other

7. INSURED'S ADDRESS (No., Street)

CITY STATE

8. PATIENT STATUS Single Married Other

CITY STATE

ZIP CODE TELEPHONE (Include Area Code)

Employed Full-Time Student Part-Time Student

ZIP CODE TELEPHONE (INCLUDE AREA CODE)

9. OTHER INSURED'S NAME (Last Name, First Name, Middle Initial)

10. IS PATIENT'S CONDITION RELATED TO:

11. INSURED'S POLICY GROUP OR FECA NUMBER

a. OTHER INSURED'S POLICY OR GROUP NUMBER

a. EMPLOYMENT? (CURRENT OR PREVIOUS) YES NO

a. INSURED'S DATE OF BIRTH MM DD YY SEX M F

b. OTHER INSURED'S DATE OF BIRTH MM DD YY SEX M F

b. AUTO ACCIDENT? YES NO PLACE (State)

b. EMPLOYER'S NAME OR SCHOOL NAME

c. EMPLOYER'S NAME OR SCHOOL NAME

c. OTHER ACCIDENT? YES NO

c. INSURANCE PLAN NAME OR PROGRAM NAME

d. INSURANCE PLAN NAME OR PROGRAM NAME

10d. RESERVED FOR LOCAL USE

d. IS THERE ANOTHER HEALTH BENEFIT PLAN? YES NO *If yes,* return to and complete item 9 a-d.

READ BACK OF FORM BEFORE COMPLETING & SIGNING THIS FORM.

12. PATIENT'S OR AUTHORIZED PERSON'S SIGNATURE I authorize the release of any medical or other information necessary to process this claim. I also request payment of government benefits either to myself or to the party who accepts assignment below.

SIGNED DATE

13. INSURED'S OR AUTHORIZED PERSON'S SIGNATURE I authorize payment of medical benefits to the undersigned physician or supplier for services described below.

SIGNED

PATIENT AND INSURED INFORMATION

14. DATE OF CURRENT: MM DD YY ILLNESS (First symptom) OR INJURY (Accident) OR PREGNANCY(LMP)

15. IF PATIENT HAS HAD SAME OR SIMILAR ILLNESS. GIVE FIRST DATE MM DD YY

16. DATES PATIENT UNABLE TO WORK IN CURRENT OCCUPATION FROM MM DD YY TO MM DD YY

17. NAME OF REFERRING PHYSICIAN OR OTHER SOURCE

17a. I.D. NUMBER OF REFERRING PHYSICIAN

18. HOSPITALIZATION DATES RELATED TO CURRENT SERVICES FROM MM DD YY TO MM DD YY

19. RESERVED FOR LOCAL USE

20. OUTSIDE LAB? YES NO $ CHARGES

21. DIAGNOSIS OR NATURE OF ILLNESS OR INJURY. (RELATE ITEMS 1,2,3 OR 4 TO ITEM 24E BY LINE)

1. ___ . __ 3. ___ . __

2. ___ . __ 4. ___ . __

22. MEDICAID RESUBMISSION CODE ORIGINAL REF. NO.

23. PRIOR AUTHORIZATION NUMBER

24. A DATE(S) OF SERVICE From MM DD YY To MM DD YY	B Place of Service	C Type of Service	D PROCEDURES, SERVICES, OR SUPPLIES (Explain Unusual Circumstances) CPT/HCPCS | MODIFIER	E DIAGNOSIS CODE	F $ CHARGES	G DAYS OR UNITS	H EPSDT Family Plan	I EMG	J COB	K RESERVED FOR LOCAL USE
1										
2										
3										
4										
5										
6										

25. FEDERAL TAX I.D. NUMBER SSN EIN

26. PATIENT'S ACCOUNT NO.

27. ACCEPT ASSIGNMENT? (For govt. claims, see back) YES NO

28. TOTAL CHARGE $

29. AMOUNT PAID $

30. BALANCE DUE $

31. SIGNATURE OF PHYSICIAN OR SUPPLIER INCLUDING DEGREES OR CREDENTIALS (I certify that the statements on the reverse apply to this bill and are made a part thereof.)

SIGNED DATE

32. NAME AND ADDRESS OF FACILITY WHERE SERVICES WERE RENDERED (If other than home or office)

33. PHYSICIAN'S, SUPPLIER'S BILLING NAME, ADDRESS, ZIP CODE & PHONE #

PIN# GRP#

PHYSICIAN OR SUPPLIER INFORMATION

(APPROVED BY AMA COUNCIL ON MEDICAL SERVICE 8/88)

PLEASE PRINT OR TYPE

FORM HCFA-1500 (12-90) FORM OWCP-1500 FORM RRB-1500 FORM OP 050191

Figure 10-2 Insurance Form Authorization for Release of Information

Essentials for Completing Claim Forms

It is of the utmost importance to complete claim forms accurately. Forms that are incomplete will be returned for correction. The basic information that is required on most claim forms includes the following items:

- Contract numbers—that is, the group number and the subscriber number from the current ID card.
- The patient's complete name, date of birth, sex, and relationship to subscriber.
- The subscriber's complete name, address, date of birth, and employer.
- Information on a secondary carrier—subscriber's name, date of birth, and employer.
- Information about whether the condition is job-related or accident-related and whether it is an illness or injury.

- The patient's account number (if your facility assigns numbers to patients).
- Complete ICD-9-CM diagnostic codes for the submitted claim.
- Information about the provider—name, address, identifying codes, and signatures.
- A statement of services rendered, which should include dates, procedural codes, charges, and total charges.

The assistant must use procedural and diagnostic codes to submit the claim.

Current Procedural Terminology, Fourth Edition (**CPT-4**), published by the American Medical Association, lists standard five-digit codes for procedures.

The *CPT-4* is divided into six sections: Evaluation and Management (EM) codes that denote the different categories of visits (office, hospital inpatient, consultation, etc.) for new and established patients; Anesthesiology; Surgery; Radiology; Pathology and Laboratory; and Medicine. Each section starts with *"Guidelines,"* which list any necessary modifiers, that is, further explanations, to obtain more accurate code numbers. Also, an alphabetic index is provided in the back of the book.

The CPT codes are used by insurance companies to identify services rendered. The procedure codes are then compared with the stated diagnoses to determine whether the procedures were medically necessary.

There are currently three levels of procedural codes:

- Level I includes all CPT codes except for anesthesiology.
- Level II includes the codes assigned by the **HCFA** (Health Care Financing Administration) for services not in the CPT system. This alphanumeric coding system is called the **HCPCS** (HCFA Common Procedures Coding System). HCPCS provides codes for services such as specific injections, drugs, and solutions; chiropractic services; dental procedures; ambulance services; durable medical equipment and supplies.
- Level III is used if there is no uniform national code for a procedure. In this instance, an alphanumeric code beginning with *W, X, Y,* or *Z* may be assigned by the local office handling Medicare claims.

Diagnostic codes are obtained from the *International Classification of Diseases*, Ninth Edition, Clinical Modification (**ICD-9-CM**).

Universal HCFA-1500 Claim Form

Although each insurance company may have its own insurance form, the American Medical Association has devised a form to standardize insurance claims and eliminate the great difference in claim forms and procedures. Known as **"HCFA-1500 Form,"** this standardized form, which is shown in Figure 10-3, on page 182, can be used for both group and individual claims and by many government-sponsored plans.

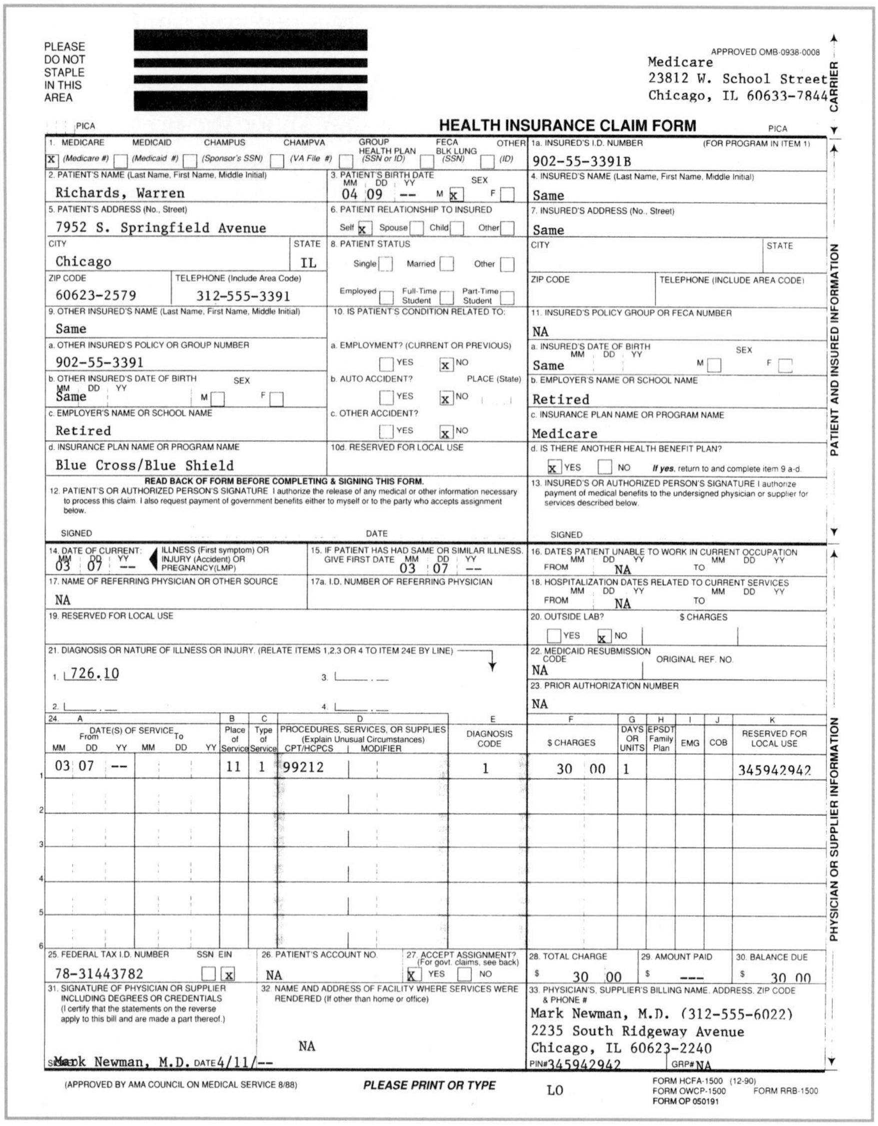

PLEASE DO NOT STAPLE IN THIS AREA

APPROVED OMB-0938-0008

Medicare
23812 W. School Street
Chicago, IL 60633-7844

CARRIER

PICA — HEALTH INSURANCE CLAIM FORM — PICA

1. MEDICARE [x] (Medicare #) MEDICAID [ ] (Medicaid #) CHAMPUS [ ] (Sponsor's SSN) CHAMPVA [ ] (VA File #) GROUP HEALTH PLAN [ ] (SSN or ID) FECA BLK LUNG [ ] (SSN) OTHER [ ] (ID)
1a. INSURED'S I.D. NUMBER (FOR PROGRAM IN ITEM 1): 902-55-3391B

2. PATIENT'S NAME (Last Name, First Name, Middle Initial): Richards, Warren
3. PATIENT'S BIRTH DATE MM DD YY: 04 09 -- SEX M [x] F [ ]
4. INSURED'S NAME (Last Name, First Name, Middle Initial): Same

5. PATIENT'S ADDRESS (No., Street): 7952 S. Springfield Avenue
6. PATIENT RELATIONSHIP TO INSURED: Self [x] Spouse [ ] Child [ ] Other [ ]
7. INSURED'S ADDRESS (No., Street): Same

CITY: Chicago STATE: IL
8. PATIENT STATUS: Single [ ] Married [ ] Other [ ]; Employed [ ] Full-Time Student [ ] Part-Time Student [ ]
CITY STATE

ZIP CODE: 60623-2579 TELEPHONE (Include Area Code): 312-555-3391
ZIP CODE TELEPHONE (INCLUDE AREA CODE)

9. OTHER INSURED'S NAME (Last Name, First Name, Middle Initial): Same
10. IS PATIENT'S CONDITION RELATED TO:
11. INSURED'S POLICY GROUP OR FECA NUMBER: NA

a. OTHER INSURED'S POLICY OR GROUP NUMBER: 902-55-3391
a. EMPLOYMENT? (CURRENT OR PREVIOUS) [ ] YES [x] NO
a. INSURED'S DATE OF BIRTH MM DD YY: Same SEX M [ ] F [ ]

b. OTHER INSURED'S DATE OF BIRTH MM DD YY: Same SEX M [ ] F [ ]
b. AUTO ACCIDENT? PLACE (State) [ ] YES [x] NO
b. EMPLOYER'S NAME OR SCHOOL NAME: Retired

c. EMPLOYER'S NAME OR SCHOOL NAME: Retired
c. OTHER ACCIDENT? [ ] YES [x] NO
c. INSURANCE PLAN NAME OR PROGRAM NAME: Medicare

d. INSURANCE PLAN NAME OR PROGRAM NAME: Blue Cross/Blue Shield
10d. RESERVED FOR LOCAL USE
d. IS THERE ANOTHER HEALTH BENEFIT PLAN? [x] YES [ ] NO *If yes,* return to and complete item 9 a-d.

READ BACK OF FORM BEFORE COMPLETING & SIGNING THIS FORM.
12. PATIENT'S OR AUTHORIZED PERSON'S SIGNATURE I authorize the release of any medical or other information necessary to process this claim. I also request payment of government benefits either to myself or to the party who accepts assignment below.
SIGNED DATE
13. INSURED'S OR AUTHORIZED PERSON'S SIGNATURE I authorize payment of medical benefits to the undersigned physician or supplier for services described below.
SIGNED

PATIENT AND INSURED INFORMATION

14. DATE OF CURRENT: ILLNESS (First symptom) OR INJURY (Accident) OR PREGNANCY(LMP) MM DD YY: 03 07 --
15. IF PATIENT HAS HAD SAME OR SIMILAR ILLNESS. GIVE FIRST DATE MM DD YY: 03 07 --
16. DATES PATIENT UNABLE TO WORK IN CURRENT OCCUPATION FROM NA TO

17. NAME OF REFERRING PHYSICIAN OR OTHER SOURCE: NA
17a. I.D. NUMBER OF REFERRING PHYSICIAN
18. HOSPITALIZATION DATES RELATED TO CURRENT SERVICES FROM NA TO

19. RESERVED FOR LOCAL USE
20. OUTSIDE LAB? [ ] YES [x] NO $ CHARGES

21. DIAGNOSIS OR NATURE OF ILLNESS OR INJURY. (RELATE ITEMS 1,2,3 OR 4 TO ITEM 24E BY LINE)
1. 726.10 2. 3. 4.
22. MEDICAID RESUBMISSION CODE: NA ORIGINAL REF. NO.
23. PRIOR AUTHORIZATION NUMBER: NA

24. A DATE(S) OF SERVICE From MM DD YY	To MM DD YY	B Place of Service	C Type of Service	D PROCEDURES, SERVICES, OR SUPPLIES (Explain Unusual Circumstances) CPT/HCPCS MODIFIER	E DIAGNOSIS CODE	F $ CHARGES	G DAYS OR UNITS	H EPSDT Family Plan	I EMG	J COB	K RESERVED FOR LOCAL USE
03 07 --		11	1	99212	1	30 00	1				345942942

25. FEDERAL TAX I.D. NUMBER: 78-31443782 SSN [ ] EIN [x]
26. PATIENT'S ACCOUNT NO.: NA
27. ACCEPT ASSIGNMENT? (For govt. claims, see back) [x] YES [ ] NO
28. TOTAL CHARGE $ 30 00
29. AMOUNT PAID $ ---
30. BALANCE DUE $ 30 00

31. SIGNATURE OF PHYSICIAN OR SUPPLIER INCLUDING DEGREES OR CREDENTIALS (I certify that the statements on the reverse apply to this bill and are made a part thereof.)
SIGNED Mark Newman, M.D. DATE 4/11/--
32. NAME AND ADDRESS OF FACILITY WHERE SERVICES WERE RENDERED (If other than home or office): NA
33. PHYSICIAN'S, SUPPLIER'S BILLING NAME, ADDRESS, ZIP CODE & PHONE #
Mark Newman, M.D. (312-555-6022)
2235 South Ridgeway Avenue
Chicago, IL 60623-2240
PIN# 345942942 GRP# NA

PHYSICIAN OR SUPPLIER INFORMATION

(APPROVED BY AMA COUNCIL ON MEDICAL SERVICE 8/88) PLEASE PRINT OR TYPE LO FORM HCFA-1500 (12-90) FORM OWCP-1500 FORM RRB-1500 FORM OP 050191

Figure 10-3 Completed HCFA-1500 Form

Note that HCFA-1500 form is divided into two parts: (1) patient and insured (subscriber) information (Items 1–13) and (2) physician or supplier information (Items 14–33). The basic information required to complete the form and the sources of that information are shown in Figure 10-4.

Remember to complete all necessary blanks when filling out an insurance claim form to show that the item was not overlooked; use a dash or the letters *NA* ("Not Applicable") for items that do not require any information. All claim forms should be keyed or generated using computer software designed for completing forms. Keep a photocopy or printout of the claim for the patient's chart and for insurance follow-up.

After a claim has been completed and sent to the insurance company, write the date and "Submitted to insurance" after the last entry on the patient's ledger. A copy of the ledger is also sent to the patient for billing. The patient or other designated person is still responsible for the complete charge, even if insurance is involved.

HCFA-1500 FORM GUIDELINES

ITEM NO.	DESCRIPTION	RESOURCE
1,1a	Type of insurance and insured's ID number	ID card
2, 3, 5, 6	Patient's name, DOB, address, telephone number, and relationship to insured	Chart, patient's registration form
4, 7	Insured's name and address (Same)	Chart
8	Patient's status	Chart
9, 9a–d	Other insured's name and information—policies that supplement the primary carrier	Chart
10a–c	Patient's condition related to	Chart
11, 11a–d	Primary carrier information	Chart
12	Release of information may have signature on *Authorization for Release of Medical Information Statement*—"patient's signature on file"	Patient's and/or insured's signature
13	Authorization of payment of benefits to provider ("patient's signature on file" if have previously signed authorization on file)	Patient's and/or insured's signature
14	Date of current illness (first-symptom date), injury (accident date), or pregnancy (LMP)	Chart
15	First date of same or similar illness	Chart
16	Dates patient unable to work	Chart
17, 17a	Referring physician and ID number (PIN—provider individual number)	Chart, insurance manual
18	Hospitalization dates	Chart
19	Reserved for local carriers' specified information	Insurance manual
20	Usage of outside lab	Ledger/chart
21	ICD-9-CM diagnostic codes	Chart and code books
22	Only used on Medicaid claims	Medicaid procedures
23	Prior authorization number	Contact carrier
24A–G	Services rendered—one procedure per line, maximum of six lines on one claim	Chart, charge slip, ledger, coding books
24A	Dates of procedures	
24B	Place of service codes: 11 Office 12 Patient's home 21 Inpatient hospital 22 Outpatient hospital 23 Hospital emergency room 24 Ambulatory surgical center 25 Birthing center 26 Military treatment center 31 Skilled nursing facility 32 Nursing facility 33 Custodial care facility 34 Hospice 41 Land ambulance 42 Air or water ambulance 51 Inpatient psychiatric facility 52 Federally qualified health center 53 Community mental-health center 54 Intermediate care facility/mentally retarded 55 Residential substance abuse treatment 56 Psychiatric residential treatment center 61 Comprehensive inpatient rehabilitation 62 Comprehensive outpatient rehabilitation 65 End-stage renal disease treatment	

Figure 10–4 HCFA-1500 Guideline Chart

24C	Type of service codes:	
	1 Medical care A Used DME 2 Surgery F Ambulatory surgical center 3 Consultation H Hospice 4 Diagnostic X ray L Renal supplies/home 5 Diagnostic laboratory M Alternate payment for maintenance 6 Radiation therapy N Kidney donor 7 Anesthesia V Pneumococcal vaccine 8 Surgical assistance Y Second opinion on elective surgery 9 Other medical services Z Third opinion on elective surgey 0 Blood or packed RBC	
24D	CPT and/or HCPCS codes	
24E	Diagnosis code—relate the procedure codes to the appropriate diagnosis (i.e., 1, 2, 3)	
24F	Charges for each service	
24G	Number of times the procedure was given	
24H	Leave balnk	
24I	Check if hospital medical emergency existed	
24J	Leave blank	
24K	Physician's PIN number	Doctor's information
25	Employer's federal tax ID number (EIN)	Doctor's information
26	Patient's account number—if patient known as a number	Chart/ledger
27	Accept assignment	Doctor's information
28, 29, 30	Total, amount paid, balance due	Ledger
31	Signature of physician and date	
32	Name and address of outside facility used other than home or office	Chart/ledger
33	Provider's billing name, complete address, and telephone number—include PIN and GRP numbers (group number assigned by carrier)	

Figure 10-4 *(cont'd.)*

Also after the claim has been completed, it should be noted on the insurance claim register as shown in Figure 10-5.

Keep a generous supply of insurance forms in the office, and be aware of the various time limits for submitting claims.

Computerized Claims

There are many software programs available that provide automatic transfer of the necessary data onto the insurance claim form. The last portion of this text uses Medisoft, a software program that transfers the patient's and the subscriber's information, charges, procedural and diagnostic codes, and so forth onto an insurance claim form.

E-claims (electronic claims) provide transfer of the insurance data via a modem or computer disk. Most of the major insurance carriers and programs such as Medicare have an E-claim option. E-claim pro-

Name of Patient	Insurance Carrier	Contact Person	Claim Date	Amounts		Follow-Up Data (Date)	Differences Between Received and Payment
				Sent	Payment		
Richards, Warren	Medicare	Jeff Parson 555-9920	04/11/--	30.00	22.40	--	7.60--adjusted

STATEMENT

MARK NEWMAN, M.D.
2235 South Ridgeway Avenue
Chicago, IL 60623-2240
312-555-6022   Fax 312-555-0025

Family
1. Warren
2.
3.
4.
5.

Warren Richards
7952 S. Springfiled Ave.
Chicago, IL 60623-2579

NO.	DATE	DESCRIPTION	CHARGE	CREDIT		CURRENT BALANCE
				PAYMENT	ADJ.	
1	3/7/--	OVF	30.00			30.00
—	4/11/--	Submitted to Medicare	——			30.00
—	5/1/--	ROA Medicare	——	22.40	7.60	— 0 —

Figure 10-5   Insurance Claim Register and Ledger

grams have the capability to indicate incomplete or inaccurate data immediately, thus giving the user the opportunity to correct the data.

The use of computerized claims speeds up payments and ensures a greater degree of accuracy.

Follow-Up for Claims

The assistant must conduct a follow–up on all submitted claims, using the insurance claims register. The time line to do the follow-up varies according to the insurance carrier and insurance program and may vary from one or more months from date of submission. Experience with insurance will enable the assistant to know when follow-up on a claim is necessary.

The **EOB** (Explanation of Benefits) is a report from the carrier that explains the reimbursement of a claim. The EOB states uncovered benefits, deductibles, copayment responsibilities, and other reasons for any noncoverage in the claim.

There are many reasons for rejection of an insurance claim. For example, there might be a missing diagnosis, an item incorrectly coded, procedures not matching the diagnosis, or missing information about the patient or provider. The assistant must take care to process and complete insurance claims accurately to ensure prompt and precise compensation for the doctor.

■ INSURANCE PLANS

To provide protection for hospitalization and medical expenses, various prepaid medical care plans have been established. Some are private, such as Blue Cross and Blue Shield, and some are government-sponsored, such as Medicare, Medicaid, CHAMPUS, and CHAMPVA.

Blue Cross and Blue Shield

Blue Cross and Blue Shield plans or combinations of both are non-profit, prepaid, medical care plans that provide insurance benefits. The National Association of Blue Shield Plans provides guidance and membership standards for the plans. Both plans provide health care to their subscribers through participating providers who agree to accept the plans' payments for services. The Blue Cross plan typically covers hospitalization expenses, the Blue Shield plan primarily covers medical services.

The coverage of these plans varies from state to state, so the assistant should contact the local representatives to obtain information about types of contracts and how to process claims. Check with a local directory to obtain the necessary information.

Medicare

In 1965 Congress passed the Medicare health insurance bill to provide medical care for persons aged 65 and over. **Medicare** is divided into two parts—Part A, hospitalization insurance; and Part B, medical insurance.

Hospitalization Insurance. *Part A*, Medicare's hospitalization insurance, provides coverage of medically necessary services for an inpatient in a hospital or an extended-care facility such as a nursing home. Medically necessary services for a Medicare inpatient include such items as a semiprivate room, an operating room, drugs, and laboratory and X-ray tests. The Medicare patient is responsible for a deductible for each benefit period (a spell of illness that ends when a patient has been out of the hospital or other facility for 60 consecutive days). The 1995 deductible was $716 per benefit period.

Hospitalization insurance also provides coverage in a skilled nursing facility following a hospital stay for a limited time with a coinsurance status. Also, home health care benefits and hospice care are covered under the hospitalization insurance.

Register the doctor's office on the Medicare newsletter mailing list to keep abreast of the frequent changes in Medicare regulations, and check with your state's Medicare agent (the insurance company designated to handle Medicare) to obtain current information on claims processing.

Medical Insurance. *Part B*, Medicare's medical insurance, helps the patient pay for items such as doctor's services, outpatient services, medical services and supplies, and home health care benefits.

Each year the patient must meet a deductible, which in 1995 was the first $100 for covered services. After the deductible, Medicare covers 80 percent of the Medicare allowable charge for medically necessary services. The patient is responsible for the remaining 20 percent.

A doctor who accepts assignment on Medicare cases agrees to receive direct payments from Medicare for only the amounts allowed by Medicare for medical services. The difference between what Medicare allows and what is charged is written off (that is, not collected) by the office. The amount written off is considered an adjustment to the patient's bill. This adjustment is marked on the ledger as a reduction from the total bill.

The following example shows how a payment for a typical case would be handled by a patient with Medicare coverage, assuming 1995 figures.

Example

Charles Parish, who sprained an ankle, went to visit the doctor for medically necessary services. This was the patient's first visit of the year.

The following charges resulted from the sprained ankle: February 2, total $225; February 9, total $72; and February 23, total $85.

Medicare allowed the entire charge, and Mr. Parish paid the deductible and coinsurance on February 23.

Total bill	$382.00
Less: Patient's deductible	−100.00
	$282.00
Less: Patient's 20% coinsurance	− 56.40 (20% of $282)
Medicare's share—80% after deductible	$225.60

Mr. Parish thus had to pay a total of $156.40 ($100 deductible + $56.40 coinsurance).

In order to establish an annual Medicare fee schedule, Congress commissioned a Harvard research project to establish the Medicare Resource-Based Relative Value Scale (RBRVS) reimbursement system. The RBRVS considers the physician's expenses, professional liability expenses, and overhead (practice) expenses in a complicated formula with a national conversion factor.

Dr. Newman uses the HCFA-1500 Form for all claims except workers' compensation. Prepare a Medicare claim form for Florence Sherman's October 21 and 22 services using her index card and chart.

The following numbers are used in Dr. Newman's processing of insurance claims. (Mark them on the fee schedule for future use.)

PIN (Provider Identification Number)   345942942
EIN (Employer's Tax ID number)   78-31443782

In processing insurance claims, you will need to obtain procedure codes from *CPT-4* and HCPCS and diagnostic codes from *ICD–9-CM*. If these references are not available, consult your instructor.

Use WP 72, date the claim October 24, and mark on Florence's ledger that the claim was submitted. File the completed form in your Miscellaneous folder.

Medicaid

A separate section of the Medicare law provides assistance for health care free of charge or at a low rate for the indigent (people who already receive some type of government aid). Each state formulates its own **Medicaid** program following some federal guidelines. The program is financially sponsored by both state and federal governments. Because programs vary in coverage and benefits from state to state, the assistant must contact the Medicaid state office through the state department of health or welfare to obtain current information.

The patient cannot be billed for differences between the doctor's usual charges and the allowed Medicaid charge; therefore, a separate Medicaid fee schedule should be maintained. However, services that are not covered can be billed to the Medicaid patient.

■ CHAMPUS AND CHAMPVA

The armed forces has a comprehensive insurance program to provide for the health care of service families in the following eligible categories: active duty, retired, or survivors. **CHAMPUS** (Civilian Health and Medical Program of the Uniformed Services) provides medical care and hospitalization in civilian hospitals and from civilian physicians for mainly those on active duty, retired, or survivors when there are no available government medical facilities. Participation by providers is voluntary. The provider must submit the claim and accept the CHAMPUS reimbursement amount as payment in full.

Like most other insurance plans, CHAMPUS is a cost-sharing program that has deductible payments and coinsurance payments. The assistant should check with the state CHAMPUS office to obtain current coverage rates and procedures.

CHAMPVA (Civilian Health and Medical Program of the Veterans Administration) is similar to CHAMPUS; it covers spouses and dependent children or survivors of service-related disabled veterans. Check the patient's CHAMPUS identification card for the responsible person's proper status and identification numbers.

■ WORKERS' COMPENSATION INSURANCE

Each state has its own **workers' compensation** laws to guarantee that an employee who is injured or who becomes ill in the course of employment will have adequate medical care and an adequate means of support while unable to work. The employer must obtain insurance against workers' compensation liability and is liable whether or not the employee is at fault for an accident or injury. The operation of workers' compensation insurance is under the jurisdiction of the state department of labor or under that of a special industrial commission.

The assistant must verify with the employer that a patient who claims workers' compensation was indeed injured or became ill in the course of employment. The doctor must submit a report, usually within 48 hours, to the workers' compensation insurance carrier, which notifies the Workers' Compensation Board. The report must include the patient's case history, symptoms, complete medical findings, tentative diagnosis, prescribed treatment, and length and extent of disability or injury. There are different categories of disabilities, such as permanent, temporary, or partial. These categories are defined by the state and administered by its department of labor. A sample workers' compensation initial report is shown in Figure 10-6 on page 190.

Progress reports on the case must be filed regularly until the patient is released from care by the doctor. The final report must be designated as such, indicating that the patient has recovered fully from the work-related disability.

Clinical notes of work–related illness or injury should be separate from other medical services or labeled *"workers' compensation."* Copies of workers' compensation reports are kept in the patient's chart for future reference. Copies may be necessary to document the treatment provided by the doctor if the dispute comes before an arbitration board or court.

PROJECT 39 Processing a Workers' Compensation Report

Cheng Sun, a cabinetmaker, was injured on the job at Billings, Inc., on October 21. Billings, Inc., is located at 7645 W. Monroe Street, Chicago, IL 60644-5519, and the company's telephone number is 555-8149. Billings has its workers' compensation insurance through Northstar Insurance, 9080 N. Central Avenue, Chicago, IL 60635-4428, and their telephone number is 555-9980.

The state office that regulates workers' compensation is Workers' Compensation, 2804 South Ridgeway Avenue, Chicago, IL 60623-7781, and their telephone number is 555-9962.

Submit an initial workers' compensation form using WP 73 for the services rendered. Date the form October 24. File the completed form in your Miscellaneous folder. Note the Workers' Compensation address for future use.

WORKER'S COMPENSATION BOARD

PLEASE PRINT OR TYPE — INCLUDE ZIP CODE IN ALL ADDRESSES — CLAIMANT'S SS # MUST BE ENTERED BELOW

ATTENDING PHYSICIAN'S 48-HOUR REPORT

WCB CASE NO. (If known)	CARRIER CASE NO. (If Known)	DATE OF INJURY AND TIME	ADDRESS WHERE INJURY OCCURRED (City, Town or Village)	SOCIAL SECURITY NUMBER
		10/7/-- 10:30 a.m.	1442 N. Pulaski Road Chicago, IL 60651-1489	336-72-5225

INJURED PERSON	NAME Jason Stephens	AGE 51		ADDRESS 712 N. Ridgeway Ave. Chicago, IL 60624-7125	APT. NO.
EMPLOYER	Abbott Memorial Library			1442 N. Pulaski Rd., Chicago, IL 60651-1440	
INSURANCE CARRIER	Nelson Casualty, Limited			878 N. Sawyer Ave., Chicago, IL 60624-8766	

HISTORY

1. State how injury occurred and give source of this information. (If claim is for *occupational disease*, include occupational history and date of onset or related symptoms).

Patient states that he fell off a ladder while taking down a

high bookshelf. Has pain in right upper arm.

2. Is there a history of unconsciousness? [ ] YES [X] NO — If "Yes," for how long? — Were X-Rays taken? [X] YES [ ] NO

3. Was patient hospitalized? [ ] YES [X] NO — If "Yes," state name and address of hospital:

4. Was patient previously under the care of another physician for this injury? [ ] YES [X] NO — If "Yes," enter his name and address, and reason for transfer under "Remarks" (Item 10).

DIAGNOSIS

5. Describe nature and extent of injury or disease and specify *all* parts of body involved:
Subjective: Pain in upper arm. Objective: Bruises on torso, hip, and thigh.

Upper arm swollen. Assessment: X rays revealed fractured right humerus,

midshaft, nondisplaced.

TREATMENT

6. Nature of treatment:
Arm sugar-tong splinted and strapped to the body. Avoid use of arm.

Date of your first treatment:
10/7/-- — If treatment is continuing, estimate its duration. Six weeks

If treatment is not continuing, is this your final report? [ ] YES [ ] NO — If "Yes," state date of last treatment:

DISABILITY

7. May the injury result in permanent restriction, total or partial loss of function of a part or member, or permanent facial, head or neck disfigurement? [ ] YES [X] NO

8. Is patient working? [ ] YES [X] NO — Is patient disabled? [ ] YES [X] NO — If "Yes," estimate duration of disability: Six weeks

CAUSAL RELATION

9. In your opinion, was the occurrence described above the competent producing cause of the injury and disability (if any) sustained? [X] YES [ ] NO

REMARKS

10. Enter here additional information of value, requests for authorization, etc.:

11. Medical testimony is occasionally required. If your testimony should be necessary in this case, please indicate the days of the week (and hours) most convenient to you for this purpose: _____

Dated: 10/8/--	Typed or printed name of Attending Physician: Mark Newman, M.D.		Address 2235 S. Ridgeway Ave. Chicago, IL 60623-2240
WCB Rating Code SJ	WCB Authorization No. 381075	Telephone No. 555-6022	Written Signature of Attending Physician *Mark Newman, M.D.*

C-48   ANSWER ALL QUESTIONS. AVOID USE OF INDEFINITE TERMS

Figure 10-6 Worker's Compensation Initial Report

■ ALTERNATIVE HEALTH CARE PLANS

In recent years, several different types of alternative health care plans have emerged, giving patients a broader choice in the type of insurance coverage they can carry.

Health Maintenance Organizations

A popular alternative to traditional insurance programs is the **HMO** (health maintenance organization), which is a medical center or a designated group of physicians that provides medical services to subscribers for a monthly or an annual fee. The subscriber to an HMO plan is able to obtain health care on a regular basis with unlimited medical attention and minimal coinsurance payments. Thus, HMOs encourage subscribers to take advantage of preventive health care services in an attempt to make health care coverage more cost-efficient.

Preferred Provider Organizations

The **PPO** (Preferred Provider Organization) contracts to perform services for PPO members at specified rates. These rates, or fees, are generally lower than the fees charged to regular patients. The PPO gives subscribers a list of PPO member-providers from which subscribers can receive health care at PPO rates. If a patient chooses to receive treatment from a provider who is not in the PPO network, the patient has to pay any difference between the PPO's rate and the outside provider's rate.

Each physician in a practice may be a member of more than one PPO, and all the doctors in the practice may not necessarily belong to the same PPOs.

Individual Practice Associations

An Individual Practice Association (**IPA**) represents providers who have formed an organization to provide prepaid health care to individuals and/or groups who purchase the coverage. Subscribers must exclusively use the affiliated members of the IPAs, such as designated doctors, pharmacies, and hospitals.

Key Terms

The following terms appear in **boldface** type in this chapter. Do you recall what they mean? Refer to the chapter for definitions you need to review.

assignment of benefits	hospital insurance
Birthday Rule	*ICD–9–CM*
carrier	IPA
CHAMPUS	major medical
CHAMPVA	insurance
coinsurance	Medicaid
coordination of benefits	medical insurance
(COB)	Medicare
copayment	outpatient insurance
coverage	PPO
CPT–4	premium
customary fee	provider
deductible	reasonable fee
E-claim	release of information
EOB	single contract
family contract	special risk insurance
HCFA	subscriber
HCFA–1500 form	surgical insurance
HCPCS	usual fee
HMO	workers' compensation

Topics for Discussion

1. Contact your state's department of health or department of welfare to obtain current information on the Medicaid program for your state. Discuss the benefits available to Medicaid recipients in your state.
2. Invite a representative of the local Blue Cross and/or Blue Shield organization to speak on processing claims.

Role-Playing

1. Ellen Schwanberg does not understand her hospital bill. She is a Medicare patient and is unsure why she must pay a $100 deductible and a $30 co-payment. She asks you to look at the bill and explain it to her.
2. Joseph Provost has not paid his bill and asks whether you have received payment from his insurance company. (The form was mailed; payment is to be made to the patient.)

Financial Records

OBJECTIVES

Upon completion of this chapter, you should be able to:

- List the essential records in a doctor's office.
- Prepare a daily journal.
- Maintain a monthly summary record.
- Explain the different check endorsements.
- Write checks using appropriate techniques.
- Prepare a deposit slip.
- Reconcile a bank statement.
- Prepare a petty cash voucher.
- Prepare payroll records.

The doctor's time and medical expertise are perhaps the most valuable assets to a medical practice. Therefore, it is important for the medical assistant to relieve the physician of many of the financial responsibilities in a practice so that the doctor can make the best use of the available time. The assistant must maintain accurate financial records in order for the doctor to have a record of all transactions, to be able to prepare tax records, and to be able to determine whether the practice is operating at a profit or a loss.

Financial data must be accumulated, analyzed, and summarized to determine the financial standing of the business. The accounting for a doctor's practice can be done on a cash basis or an accrual basis. If the practice operates on a cash basis, charges for services are not recorded as income until payment is received and expenses are not recorded until paid. Under the accrual method, income is recorded when earned, whether or not payment is received, and expenses are recorded when they are incurred.

Records must be available to the Internal Revenue Service (IRS) at all times, and all source documents must be kept for tax purposes. The assistant must, therefore, have a working knowledge of tax regulations and of the accounting process in order to be responsible for the recording aspects of accounting.

A variety of accounting software packages can be used to perform any office accounting system on the computer. Such accounting software can be used to prepare all of the financial records, including the charge slips, ledgers, daily journals, monthly summaries, and annual summaries. Most packages also provide the user with monthly, quarterly, and yearly financial comparisons so that decisions can be made concerning collections and disbursements. The assistant is responsible for inserting accurate information to update these records continually.

Daily Journal

The **daily journal** is used to record daily fees charged and payments received. It is referred to as a "day sheet" or a "daily earnings record." It is the journal for accounts receivable and cash receipts. Fees charged and payments received must be recorded promptly on the daily journal, whether done manually or on a computerized system. A typical daily journal is shown in Figure 11-1.

It is necessary to have an accurate balance of accounts, and this is obtained through completion of the section labeled "Accounts Receivable Control," which is shown at the bottom of the daily journal. **Accounts receivable** refers to the balance due from patients on current accounts. The charges are added and the payments are subtracted from the balance of the previous day to get the current accounts receivable balance. Balancing the journal should be done at the end of the day or as early as possible the next day.

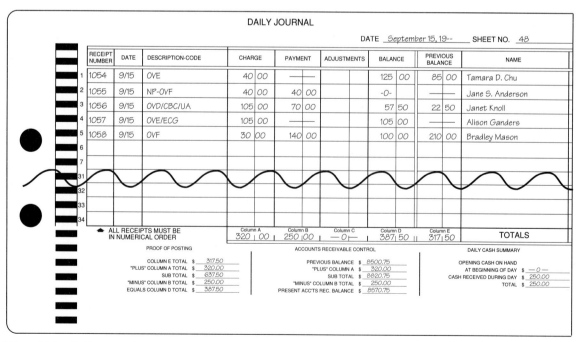

Figure 11-1   Daily Journal

There is also a section labeled "Proof of Posting," which is typically in the lower left corner of the daily journal. Completing this section does not prove that the correct amounts were necessarily charged; it only proves that the columns balance.

The Section labeled "Daily Cash Summary" in the lower right corner is used to account for the daily cash flow.

Pegboard Accounting

A system that can be used in a small office is the **pegboard accounting** system, or "write-it-once" system. Forms for the pegboard are made with holes on the left side to fit over pegs. Three forms are essential to the operation of the pegboard system: numbered charge/receipt slips, patients' ledgers, and the daily journal, which is the record of accounts receivable and cash receipts.

The charge/receipt slips are shingled over the daily journal. The patient's ledger is aligned between the daily journal and the charge/receipt slip. The information (patient's name, services rendered, charge, payment, and balance) is written on the top form (the charge/receipt slip) and appears at the same time on the patient's ledger card and the daily journal.

Because of the way the system operates, postings can be made to the ledger cards in the patient's presence, the patient can receive the bill immediately, and the ledger card is always up to date—ready for use as a monthly billing statement. In addition, every charge slip is accounted for because the slips are entered in the daily journal in numerical sequence.

The pegboard or "write-it-once" system can be used with encounter forms, or superbills, that include insurance codes for medical procedures.

The daily journal for October 22 has been started for you on WP 74. Complete journals for October 22 and October 27, using WPs 74 and 75. Follow these instructions in preparing daily journals.

1. Enter the patients' names on the daily journal as they are listed in the appointment book.
2. Using the ledgers, enter the previous balance for each patient.
3. Post the transactions (charges and payments) to the ledgers and to the daily journal.
4. Compute the current balance from the day's charges and payments for each patient.
5. Total Columns A, B, C, D, and E.
6. Complete the Proof of Posting section.
7. Compute the current accounts receivable balance (by completing the Accounts Receivable Control section), and post it onto the next daily journal.
8. Complete the Daily Cash Summary section.

Note that no deposits were made on the days during which this project took place. Charges and payments (by check) for October 27 are as follows:

Doris Casagranda, OVF; paid entire bill
Jeffrey Kramer, no show (not entered)
Marc Phan, OVE; paid $25
Sarah Morton, OVE, scoliosis X ray; paid $80
Randy Burton, OVE, DTP, oral polio; paid $65
Cheng Sun, chest X ray, UA, SMA–12, CBC, hemoccults; paid $50

File all financial items in your Miscellaneous folder.

Computer Summaries

Each practice may have software designed to generate an analysis of items that are of importance to that practice, such as separating office charges from lab and X ray charges or listing an individual doctor's transactions. Some samples of different summary options available in a medical accounting software program are shown in Figure 11-2. Sample *(a)* shows a patient day sheet. Sample *(b)* shows a daily summary by procedure codes. Sample *(c)* shows a summary of payments used to make a deposit. Sample *(d)* displays a practice analysis showing how many procedures were performed.

Spreadsheet capabilities in a software program allow the office to customize a format for inserting data and calculations. The designer decides how many columns and rows are needed for the necessary data and inserts formulas for the calculations. Spreadsheets simplify such tasks as creating expense reports, producing profit and loss statements, budgeting, and so forth.

```
                    Mark Newman, M.D.                    101495
                    PATIENT DAY SHEET                     Page 1
                        10-14-95

Entry   Date   Document Location-Diagnosis      Prov Code          Amount


(ARMSTMO0)      Armstrong, Monica
1      10-14-95 951014   3-                       1  99212           30.00
2      10-14-95 951014   3-                       1  85022           20.00
3      10-14-95 951014   3-                       1  80012           30.00
4      10-14-95 951014   3-                       1  81000           10.00
5      10-14-95 951014   3-                       1  82270           15.00
6      10-14-95 951014   3-                       1  76091           80.00
        Previous Balance      Today's Charges   Today's Receipts   Total Balance
             $0.00                 $185.00            $0.00           $185.00

(KRAMEAN1)      Kramer, Jeffrey
7      10-14-95 951014   3-                       1  99212           30.00
        Previous Balance      Today's Charges   Today's Receipts   Total Balance
             $0.00                  $30.00            $0.00            $30.00
         -
```

Figure 11-2 Examples of Computer Summaries

(a)

```
                        Mark Newman, M.D.                    101495
                        PROCEDURE DAY SHEET                   Page 2
                           10-14-95

    Entry  Date   Pat #   Document Location-Diagnosis    Debits  Credits

                Total of 82465            Qty:    1      $10.00

    (85018    )   HEMOGLOBIN (Hgb)

    12   10-14-95 MITCHAL1 951014    3-                   10.00
    15   10-14-95 MITCHAL2 951014    3-                   10.00
    28   09-24-95 DAYTOTH0 950924    3-                   10.00
    35   09-24-95 MENDEAN0 950924    3-                   10.00
    78   10-21-95 MITCHAL1 951021    3-                   10.00
                Total of 85018            Qty:    5      $50.00

    (85022    )   CBC

    2    10-14-95 ARMSTM00 951014    3-                   20.00
    21   10-15-95 BAABTH00 951015    3-                   20.00
    27   09-24-95 DAYTOTH0 950924    3-                   20.00
    33   09-24-95 MENDEAN0 950924    3-                   20.00
    47   07-18-95 MATTHEA1 950718    3-                   20.00
                Total of 85022            Qty:    5      $100.00
                _____
```

(b)

```
                        Mark Newman, M.D.                    101495
                        PAYMENT DAY SHEET                     Page 1
                           10-14-95

    Entry  Date   Pat #   Document Location-Diagnosis    Receipt Amount

    (1        )

    29   09-24-95 DAYTOTH0 950924    3-                          50.00
    41   04-22-95 MATTHEA1 950422    3-                          75.00
                Total  of 1               Qty:    2            $125.00

    (INS      )

    68   10-08-95 SHERMFL0 951008    3-                         200.00
                Total  of INS             Qty:    1            $200.00

    TOTAL OF RECEIPTS FOR DEPOSIT                               $325.00
```

(c)

```
                        Mark Newman, M.D.                    101495
                        PRACTICE ANALYSIS                     Page 1
                           10-14-95

    Code      Procedure          Amount   Qty  Average   Cost    Net

    76091     MAMMOGRAM
              Account:           80.00    1    80.00     0.00   80.00

    80012     SMA-12
              Account:           30.00    1    30.00     0.00   30.00

    81000     URINALYSIS (UA)
              Account:           40.00    4    10.00     0.00   40.00

    82270     HEMOCCULTS x3
              Account:           15.00    1    15.00     0.00   15.00

    85018     HEMOGLOBIN (Hgb)
              Account:           20.00    2    10.00     0.00   20.00

    85022     CBC
              Account:           20.00    1    20.00     0.00   20.00

    87086     URINE CULTURE (UC)
              Account:           10.00    1    10.00     0.00   10.00

    88156     PAP SMEAR
              Account:           35.00    1    35.00     0.00   35.00

    99202     OV FOCUSED (OVF)
              Account:           80.00    2    40.00     0.00   80.00

    99212     OV FOCUSED (OVF)
              Account:           90.00    3    30.00     0.00   90.00

    99213     OV EXPANDED (OVE)
              Account:           40.00    1    40.00     0.00   40.00


    Total Charges               $460.00  18
    Total Standard Receipts       $0.00   0
    Total Insurance Receipts      $0.00   0
    Total Standard Debit Adj      $0.00   0
    Total Standard Credit Adj     $0.00   0
    Total Insurance Debit Adj     $0.00   0
    Total Insurance Credit Adj    $0.00   0
    Total of Entries            $460.00  18

    Total Receivable          $2,785.00
```

(d)

■ ACCOUNTS PAYABLE

Office expenses, including payments for supplies, equipment, services, and salaries, are referred to as **accounts payable**. These payments should be made by check. This ensures that there are complete, accurate records of all money that is received and disbursed.

Checks must be very carefully written in order to prevent error or fraud. It is easy to forget to fill in the stub or check register or to enter the wrong amount. For this reason, the check stub or register should be completed before writing the check itself.

The date and *payee* (the name of the person to whom the check is made out) are entered on the stub, or register. Then the purpose of payment is recorded. The previous balance and any deposits made since the last check was written are added together, and the total is entered on the proper line. The amount of the check being issued is subtracted from this total, and the new balance is recorded. An example of a completed check with stub is shown in Figure 11-3.

Note the following special points about writing checks:

1. Write the name of the payee in full, starting at the extreme left of the line.
2. Draw a line from the end of the name to the dollar sign ($).
3. Write the amount in figures directly after the dollar sign.
4. Write the amount in words starting at the extreme left end of the designated line. After the dollar amount, write the word *and*, followed by the cents amount. The cents amount should be written as a fraction.
5. Draw a line from the fraction to the word *Dollars*.

Never sign the doctor's name yourself; the check can only be signed by the authorized person (known as the "drawer"), even in an emergency situation. In order to save time, you may fill out the stub and the check, but have the drawer sign the check.

PROJECT 41   **Preparing Checks**

Checks and check stubs have been completed for October 1 on WP 76. Remove WP 76 and the blank checks on WPs 77 and 78. Staple them together along the left edge to form a checkbook. Note that the checks are numbered consecutively and the last completed check stub shows the current bank balance.

Prepare checks for the October 3, 6, 7, and 8 disbursements, which are listed below. Enter the following deposits into the checkbook on the appropriate stubs: October 3, $370; October 6, $300; and October 8, $350.

October 3, National Medical Supplies: tweezers—$18.50.

October 3, Graphic Designs: two reams of paper—$24.00.

October 6, Plainview Lab: specimen tubes—$32.99.

October 7, Chicago Telephone Co.—$163.21.

October 8, Dr. Newman dinner with Dr. Arnold: entertainment—$75.00.

Place the completed checks in your Miscellaneous folder.

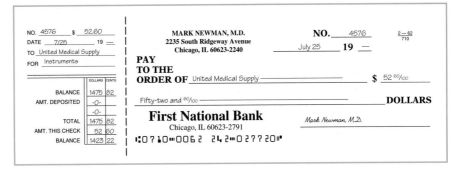

```
NO. 4576    $ 52.60          MARK NEWMAN, M.D.              NO.  4576        2—62
DATE  7/25      19 —      2235 South Ridgeway Avenue                         710
TO United Medical Supply      Chicago, IL 60623-2240       July 25    19 —
FOR  Instruments          PAY
                          TO THE
                          ORDER OF  United Medical Supply ———————  $ 52 60/100
              DOLLARS CENTS
BALANCE         1475  82  Fifty-two and 60/100 ————————————————— DOLLARS
AMT. DEPOSITED  -0-
                -0-       First National Bank        Mark Newman, M.D.
TOTAL           1475  82  Chicago, IL 60623-2791
AMT. THIS CHECK   52  60
BALANCE         1423  22  ⑈0710⑈0062 242⑈027720⑈
```

Figure 11-3   Check With Check Stub

■ MONTHLY SUMMARY

A **monthly summary** consists of records such as those shown in Figure 11-4. Figure 11-4*(a)* shows the daily charges and payments for the entire month, enabling the doctor to have monthly and yearly totals to date. Figure 11-4*(b)* shows the distribution of disbursements in various common categories. By using forms such as these, the doctor can determine monthly and yearly expenditures and net earnings.

SUMMARY FOR MONTH August   **YEAR** 19—

DAY OF MONTH	CHARGES (COLUMN "A")		PAYMENTS (COLUMN "B")		MISCELLANEOUS SUMMARIES					
1										
2										
3										
4	85	75	24	50						
5	370	20	178	50						
6	110	00	25	75						
7	560	75	370	80						
8	-0-		295	75						
9										
10										
11	150	80	210	00						
12	435	75	250	75						
13	342	50	183	55						
14	521	75	331	85						
15										
16										
17										
18	92	50	115	75						
19	522	80	321	55						
20	140	00	150	75						
21	475	20	352	80						
22										
23										
24										
25	87	50	70	15						
26	425	75	315	15						
27	115	85	82	50						
28	560	75	410	75						
29										
30										
31										
TOTAL FOR MONTH	4,997	85	3,690	85						
BROUGHT FORWARD	37,530	15	35,120	75						
GRAND TOTAL	42,528	00	38,811	60						

SUMMARY OF EXPENSE (From Reverse Side)

	AMOUNT	
DRUGS AND PROFESSIONAL SUPPLIES	193	37
LAB EXPENSE	275	00
SALARIES	480	00
OFFICE RENT AND MAINTENANCE	500	00
LAUNDRY SERVICE	43	07
ELECTRICITY, GAS, WATER	85	50
TELEPHONE	75	80
DUES AND MEETINGS	150	00
OFFICE EXPENSES (SUPPLIES, ETC.)	69	12
PROFESSIONAL INSURANCE		
BUSINESS TAXES		
INTEREST PAID		
ENTERTAINMENT	70	00
Other	55	30
TOTAL FOR PRESENT MONTH	1,997	16
FORWARDED FROM PREVIOUS MONTH	11,792	74
GRAND TOTAL	13,789	90

MONTHLY BALANCES

For the Present Month

TOTAL RECEIPTS (COL. B)	3,690	85
TOTAL EXPENSE	1,997	16
NET EARNINGS	1,693	69

For the Year To Date

GRAND TOTAL RECEIPTS	38,811	60
GRAND TOTAL EXPENSE	13,789	90
NET EARNINGS	25,021	70
ACCOUNTS RECEIVABLE (FROM LAST DAY SHEET OF THE MONTH)		

$ 3,116.45   CHECKED BY MB

Year 19—   Month August   PART A   MONTHLY SUMMARY SHEET

Figure 11-4 *(a)* Monthly Summary Showing the Daily Charges and Payments

EXPENDITURES FOR THE MONTH

DRUGS AND PROFESSIONAL SUPPLIES			SALARIES			DUES AND MEETINGS			ENTERTAINMENT			OTHER		
DAY	ITEM	AMOUNT	DAY	ITEM	AMOUNT	DAY	ITEM	AMOUNT	DAY	ITEM	AMOUNT	DAY	ITEM	AMOUNT
8/12	Surgical supplies	75 15	8/8	Molly Benson	240 00	8/15	AMA	150 00	8/15	Dr. Newman	35 00	8/13	Wilson Repair	55 30
	(disposable						(yearly dues)						(typewriter)	
	needles)		8/22	Molly Benson	240 00				8/22	Dr. Newman	35 00			
8/28	Surgical supplies	35 80												
	(sponges, etc.)													
8/29	Eastern Pharmacy	82 42												
	(drugs)													
							TOTAL	150 00		TOTAL	70 00		TOTAL	55 30
						OFFICE EXPENSES (SUPPLIES, ETC.)								
						8/5	Holbert's	24 12						
							(envelopes)							
						8/15	Post Office	45 00						
							(stamps)							
				TOTAL	480 00									
			OFFICE RENT AND UPKEEP											
			8/1	Falcon Realty	500 00					TOTAL			TOTAL	
									NONPROFESSIONAL EXPENSES					
	TOTAL	193 37							DAY	SOURCE	AMOUNT			
LAB EXPENSE				TOTAL	500 00									
8/15	KJ Lab Supply	275 00	**LAUNDRY SERVICE**											
	(disposable		8/15	Jason's Linen	15 75									
	items)		8/29	Jason's Linen	27 32		TOTAL	69 12						
						PROFESSIONAL INSURANCE								
				TOTAL	43 07		TOTAL			TOTAL				
ELECTRICITY, GAS, WATER						**BUSINESS TAXES**			**NONPROFESSIONAL RECEIPTS**					
8/28	Consolidated Elec	85 50							DAY	SOURCE	AMOUNT			
	TOTAL	85 50					TOTAL							
TELEPHONE						**INTEREST PAID**								
8/5	Chicago Teleph.	75 80												
	TOTAL	275 00		TOTAL	75 80		TOTAL						TOTAL	

ALL TOTALS TO BE TRANSFERRED TO PART A

(Right margin: Year 19___ Month August PART B MONTHLY SUMMARY SHEET)

Figure 11-4 (b) Monthly Summary Showing the Distribution of Disbursements

PROJECT 42   Preparing a Monthly Summary

Insert the total charges and payments from the daily journals you completed for October 22 and 27 onto the partially completed Part A of the Monthly Summary Sheet on WP 79.

Using the information from Project 41, transfer the check amounts to Part B of the Monthly Summary Sheet in the appropriate categories.

Place the Monthly Summary Sheet in your Miscellaneous folder.

■ BANKING

All money, whether cash or checks, that is received in the office should be deposited in the bank promptly. The assistant is responsible for various banking duties, including preparing deposits and reconciling bank statements.

Endorsements

All checks received should be endorsed immediately so there is no possibility of their being lost, stolen, or forgotten. There are three types of endorsements that can be used.

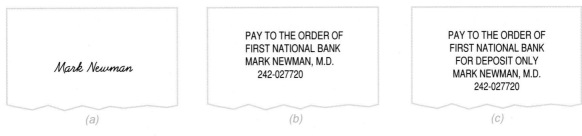

(a)   (b)   (c)

Figure 11-5   Samples of (a) a Blank Endorsement, (b) a Full
Endorsement, and (c) a Restrictive Endorsement

A **blank endorsement** has only the signature of the person to whom the check is payable. Once a check is endorsed in this way, it can be cashed by anyone. Therefore, blank endorsements are not used in business.

A **full endorsement** indicates the person, company, account number, or bank to whom the check is being transferred, followed by the payee's name.

A **restrictive endorsement** is the safest and most commonly used endorsement in business. It limits the use of the check by specifying to whom the money should be paid and the money's purpose, such as "For deposit only." The restrictive endorsement is convenient for business use, since the assistant can rubber-stamp the check and deposit it without obtaining the doctor's signature. Figure 11-5 shows examples of the three types of endorsements.

PROJECT 43   Preparing Receipts and Updating Financial Records

Today is October 28. Monica Armstrong has a CPE (OV Comprehensive), a Pap smear, and a flexible sigmoidoscopy; she pays $150 in cash for these services. Complete a receipt for her using one of the receipts on WP 80. All appropriate information should be included on the blanks provided on the receipt form. (Remember to number the next available receipt.) Remove all the remaining receipts, staple them together, and place them in your Supplies folder.

Other transactions today include the following:

Erin Mitchell—OVF, Hgb, and UA.

Gary Robertson, discharged from hospital—six HVs from October 22 to October 28.

Complete the daily journal for October 28 using WP 81, update the ledger cards for each of the patients in this project, and enter appropriate amounts into the monthly summary.

Place daily journal, Monthly Summary Sheet, and receipt in your Miscellaneous folder.

Deposits

Before the cash and checks received during the day can be deposited in the bank, a deposit slip such as the one shown in Figure 11-6 on page 202 must be prepared. Deposit tickets furnished by the bank are printed with the depositor's name and account number. The total amount of currency—bills and coins—is entered on the first line. Each check is listed separately. Some banks prefer to have each check identified by a number or bank name.

Figure 11-6 Deposit Slip

The total amount of cash and checks being deposited is entered on the appropriate line. The amount of the deposit is then entered on the first unused checkbook stub, or check register.

PROJECT 44 Preparing a Deposit Slip

Before Dr. Newman leaves the office on October 28, he asks you to deposit the money received on October 27 and October 28.

Prepare a deposit slip for these receipts using one of the blank deposit slips on WP 82.

Remove the remaining deposit slips, clip them together, and place them in your Supplies folder.

Enter the amount of the deposit in the checkbook.

Place the completed deposit slip in your Miscellaneous folder.

Bank Reconciliation

Each month the bank submits a statement of the checking account such as the one shown in Figure 11-7. This statement shows the beginning balance, total credits (deposits added to the account during the month), total debits (checks paid out of the account during the month), any service charges that were issued, and the resulting new balance.

The statement balance must be compared with the checkbook balance to determine whether there is a difference between the balances. This is known as reconciling the bank statement, or **bank reconciliation**. Many banks print a reconciliation form such as the one shown in Figure 11-8 on page 204 on the back of the monthly account statement showing the necessary steps in the reconciliation.

The first step in the reconciliation process is to compare the canceled checks returned by the bank with the items listed on the bank statement. Some banks do not return canceled checks with the bank statement, and the listing of checks on the statement must be used for reference.

Next, compare the checks listed on the bank statement with the checkbook stubs to verify that check numbers and amounts agree. Deductions such as service charges are explained on the bank statement and must now be recorded in the checkbook.

First National Bank
Chicago, IL 60623-2791

STATEMENT OF
ACCOUNT NUMBER
242 027720
CLOSING DATE ITEMS
JUNE 25   12

MARK NEWMAN, M.D.
2235 SOUTH RIDGEWAY AVENUE
CHICAGO, IL 60623-2240

PERSONAL CHECKING ACCOUNT STATEMENT

BEGINNING BALANCE	(+) TOTAL CREDITS	(-) TOTAL DEBITS	(-) SERVICE CHARGE	(=) NEW BALANCE
2,592.74	1,030.00	919.06		2,703.68

CHECKS & OTHER DEBITS		DEPOSITS & OTHER CREDITS	DATE	BALANCE
	2.54	165.00	6/2	2,755.20
		100.00	6/4	2,855.20
	97.00		6/5	2,758.20
	450.00		6/6	2,308.20
		120.00	6/9	2,428.20
	29.37		6/11	
	13.00			2,385.83
		85.00	6/12	2,470.83
	7.00	210.00	6/16	2,673.83
	15.62		6/17	2,658.21
		90.00	6/18	2,748.21
	37.98	185.00	6/23	
	65.12			2,830.11
	145.00		6/24	
	15.00			2,670.11
	41.43	75.00	6/25	2,703.68

SYMBOLS

C = CORRECTION	DM = DEBIT MEMO	RI = RETURN ITEM	ST = SAVINGS TRANSFER
CM = CREDIT MEMO	OD = OVERDRAFT	SC = SERVICE CHARGE	

Figure 11-7   Bank Statement

Any checks that were written but not yet paid by the bank (and therefore are not included with the statement) are called "outstanding checks." List the outstanding checks on the reconciliation form as shown in Figure 11-8 on page 204.

Next, deposits recorded in the checkbook must be compared with credit notations on the bank statement. A deposit entered in the checkbook but not recorded by the bank at the time the statement was made is known as a "deposit in transit."

If the checking account earns interest, then the interest must be recorded as a credit (similar to a deposit) in the checkbook.

Complete the reconciliation form following the given directions. If the final amount on the reconciliation statement does not agree with that in the checkbook, compare the monthly statement with the checkbook again in the following ways:

- Recheck the deposits entered on the bank statement with the ones entered in the checkbook.
- Confirm that all service charges shown on the statement are entered in the checkbook and properly deducted.
- Make sure no check has been drawn that has not been recorded in the checkbook.

CHANGE OF ADDRESS ORDER
TO CHANGE YOUR ADDRESS, PLEASE COMPLETE THIS FORM;
THEN CUT ALONG DOTTED LINE, AND MAIL OR BRING TO THE BANK.

NEW ADDRESS:

NUMBER
AND STREET _____

CITY _____ STATE AND ZIP CODE _____ NEW PHONE NUMBER _____

DATE _____ CUSTOMER'S SIGNATURE _____

OUTSTANDING CHECKS	
NUMBER	AMOUNT
	125 00
	18 65
	22 19
	48 90
TOTAL	214 74

TO RECONCILE YOUR STATEMENT AND CHECKBOOK

1. DEDUCT FROM YOUR CHECKBOOK BALANCE ANY SERVICE OR OTHER CHARGE ORIGINATED BY THE BANK. THESE CHARGES WILL BE IDENTIFIED BY SYMBOLS AS SHOWN ON FRONT.

2. ARRANGE ENDORSED CHECKS BY DATE OR NUMBER AND CHECK THEM OFF AGAINST THE STUBS IN YOUR CHECKBOOK.

3. LIST IN THE OUTSTANDING CHECKS SECTION AT THE LEFT ANY CHECKS ISSUED BY YOU AND NOT YET PAID BY US.

TO RECONCILE YOUR STATEMENT AND CHECKBOOK		
LAST BALANCE SHOWN ON STATEMENT	2,703	68
PLUS: DEPOSITS AND CREDITS MADE AFTER DATE OF LAST ENTRY ON STATEMENT	130	00
SUBTOTAL	2,833	68
MINUS: OUTSTANDING CHECKS	214	74
BALANCE: WHICH SHOULD AGREE WITH YOUR CHECKBOOK	2,618	94

Figure 11-8 Reconciliation Section of the Bank Statement

- Compare all checks with the stubs to make sure the amounts agree.
- Review the list of outstanding checks to see whether an old check is still outstanding.
- Recheck all addition and subtraction.

When the checkbook is reconciled, make a notation to that effect in the checkbook on the last-used stub or register line.

PROJECT 45 **Reconciling a Bank Statement**

Reconcile the bank statement that appears on WP 83 using your checkbook stubs for October. The reconciliation form is on the back of the statement.

Place completed form in your Miscellaneous folder.

■ PETTY CASH

A **petty cash** fund is established to pay small expenses that cannot readily be paid by check, such as cab fare, stamps, payments to messengers, and delivery charges. Each time a payment is made from the petty cash fund, an entry needs to be made in the petty cash register or a voucher needs to be completed if the office uses the voucher system. This provides a record of expenses and ensures that only authorized payments are made from the fund. A sample petty cash register is shown in Figure 11-9*(a)* ,and a petty cash voucher is shown in Figure 11-9*(b)*.

The amount of petty cash required for the office over a short period of time, such as a month, is estimated. A check for the estimated amount is then drawn, payable to the person responsible for the petty cash fund. The check is cashed, and an assortment of small bills and coins is obtained. The money is kept in a secure place, such as a locked metal cash box in a drawer.

At the end of the month or when the amount of cash is low, the fund is replenished. The total disbursements are determined from the petty cash register. The remaining cash in the fund is counted. The two amounts should add up to the original amount of the fund; this procedure is called "proving the petty cash fund." A check is then drawn to bring the petty cash fund back to its original amount.

Example

The original amount of the petty cash fund was $100. According to the petty cash register, expenses were $89.75. Thus, there should still be $10.25 in cash. The assistant counts the cash as verification and then draws a check for $89.75. The amount of the petty cash on hand is brought back up to $100 after the check is cashed.

The expenses should then be recorded in the appropriate columns on the monthly summary sheet. They may be entered as petty cash.

PETTY CASH REGISTER FOR MONTH OF July 19— Page 8

DATE	DESCRIPTION	VOU. NO.	TOTAL AMOUNT	DISTRIBUTION OF CHARGES: Postage Exp.	Donation Exp.	Travel Exp.	Office Sup. Exp.	Misc. Exp.	ACCOUNT	AMOUNT
	AMOUNTS FORWARDED									
1	Total in fund $100									
1	Office supplies	26	18 00				18 00			
7	Postage due	27	3 50	3 50						
8	Daily newspaper	28	2 50					2 50		
11	Postage stamps	29	13 00	13 00						
17	UNICEF	30	10 00		10 00					
21	Office supplies	31	7 50				7 50			
21	Daily newspaper	32	2 50					2 50		
24	Cab fare	33	13 00			13 00				
			70 00	16 50	10 00	13 00	25 50	5 00		
	Balance $ 30									
	Replenish fund $ 70									
	Balance $100									

(a)

No. _______ Amount _______________

PETTY CASH VOUCHER

_____________ 19 _______

For _______________________________

Charge to ___________________________

Approved by _______________ Received by _______________

(b)

Figure 11-9 Petty Cash *(a)* Register and *(b)* Voucher

■ PAYROLL

Federal regulations require that an employer withhold taxes from an employee's gross earnings and that the employer also pay certain payroll taxes. Employers must withhold amounts for federal and state income taxes and social security (Federal Insurance Contributions Act, or **FICA**).

Income Tax Withholding

Each employee must complete an Employee's Withholding Allowance Certification (Form W-4), which states the number of claimed exemptions. Actual amounts to be withheld for federal and state income taxes are determined from wage-bracket tables supplied by the IRS; the amount withheld depends on the amount earned, the number of claimed exemptions, and the current tax rate. The IRS can provide the wage-bracket tables for various payroll cycles, such as daily, weekly, biweekly, semimonthly, or monthly.

FICA Tax

In addition to income tax, the federal government requires that employers deduct a certain amount for social security, which is divided into two separate payroll taxes—one helps finance Medicare and the other pays for social security benefits. These amounts are a percentage of the employee's gross pay, regardless of the number of claimed exemptions. For example, the law could set this amount at 6.2 percent of the first $60,600 earned by an employee during the year for social security and 1.45 percent for Medicare with no earning limit. (The IRS—by phone or through one of its publications—or the doctor's accountant can advise you of the current rate.) Congress can change this amount, so you must obtain information on a yearly basis.

Payroll Records

The government requires that each employer keep records of the amount paid to each employee and the amounts withheld for tax purposes. A typical format for these records is shown in Figure 11-10.

An employee's individual earnings record must contain that employee's social security number, address, number of claimed exemptions, gross salary earned, net salary paid, income taxes withheld, FICA taxes, and state and local income taxes deducted, if applicable. The column labeled "Other" is used to indicate certain deductions that are required by law or that might be made under an agreement with the employer. For example, many employers will deduct, with the employee's permission, amounts for savings bonds, insurance, union dues, or other purposes. All amounts deducted are held in trust by the employer and must be remitted to the proper authority. When the payroll check is written, the gross wage amount is entered in the proper column of the monthly summary sheet.

INDIVIDUAL EMPLOYEE'S EARNINGS RECORD

Name Molly Benson

Address 5985 West Park Ave.

City Chicago, IL 60650

Telephone 555-4251

Social Security No. 301-48-7122

Marital Status Single

No. of Allowances 1

Birthdate 5/29/52

Position M.A. (part-time)

Monthly Rate

Weekly Rate $120

Overtime Rate $10/hour

Period Ending	Hours Worked	Gross Earnings			Deductions							Net Pay		Accumulated Earnings (Gross)	
		Regular	Overtime	Total	FICA	Federal Withholding	State Withholding	City Withholding	Insurance	Other	Total				
June 13	24	240 00		240 00	14 71	25 20	5 04				44 95	195 05	2,400 00
June 27	24	240 00		240 00	14 71	25 20	5 04				44 95	195 05	2,640 00
July 11	24	240 00		240 00	14 71	25 20	5 04				44 95	195 05	2,880 00
July 25	24	240 00		240 00	14 71	25 20	5 04				44 95	195 05	3,120 00
Aug. 8	24	240 00		240 00	14 71	25 20	5 04				44 95	195 05	3,360 00
Aug. 22	24	240 00		240 00	14 71	25 20	5 04				44 95	195 05	3,600 00
Sept. 5	24	240 00		240 00	14 71	25 20	5 04				44 95	195 05	3,840 00
Sept. 19	24	240 00		240 00	14 71	25 20	5 04				44 95	195 05	4,080 00
Oct. 3	24	240 00		240 00	14 71	25 20	5 04				44 95	195 05	4,320 00

Figure 11-10 Individual Employee's Earnings Record

Depending on the amount involved, the employer must remit amounts deducted from employees' retained earnings to the government each month, or at least each quarter (every three months). In addition to the amount for FICA taxes kept from employees' pay, the employer is obligated to contribute a matching FICA contribution for each employee.

When an employer remits money to the government for these holdings, a report is completed. Instructions for filling out such reports should be obtained from the IRS, because the details change from year to year.

PROJECT 46   Preparing Salary Check and Record

Prepare Linda Jenson's salary check for the two weeks ending October 24. She is paid biweekly (every two weeks) at a salary of $450 weekly. Her withholdings for the two–week period are as follows: federal income tax withholding is $117, state income tax withholding is $15.20, FICA is 7.65 percent of her salary, and insurance coverage is $42. Today's date is October 28.

Complete Linda's individual earnings record on WP 84. Enter the gross amount of her biweekly salary on the monthly summary sheet.

Place the individual earnings record and the Monthly Summary Sheet in your Miscellaneous folder.

Key Terms

The following terms appear in **boldface** type in this chapter. Do you recall what they mean? Refer to the chapter for definitions you need to review.

accounts payable

accounts receivable

bank reconciliation

blank endorsement

daily journal

FICA

full endorsement

monthly summary

payee

pegboard accounting

petty cash

restrictive endorsement

spreadsheet

Topics for Discussion

1. You have tried several times to reconcile the bank statement for the office checking account, and the checkbook will not balance with the bank statement. Describe what action you should take.

2. The office where you work does not keep petty cash vouchers. The cash box is conveniently located in a desk drawer in the reception area, and you notice that several employees take change from the cash box. Discuss why there needs to be a better control of the petty cash.

3. You learn that there is a position similar to yours available in the neighboring office. That office pays employees according to their production in addition to a base salary. Discuss whether you should consider changing jobs.

Role-Playing

1. From a conversation during a break, you learn that a new employee is making the same salary as you are. You have been employed in this same office for two years. The new employee asks about your salary. How should you respond?

2. Mr. Bennet asks whether Dr. Newman gives a discount when fees are paid at the time of service. How would you answer his question?

SIMULATION 3

Today you will begin your third simulation in Dr. Newman's office. The days are Wednesday, October 29; Thursday, October 30; and Friday, October 31.

PROCEDURES

Review the "General Procedures" in Simulation 1 for handling simulations. Follow the same instructions given in Simulation 1 under "Specific Procedures"—for Days 1 through 3.

MATERIALS

The materials you will need are generally the same as those listed for Simulation 1. Each day, pull the patients' charts and ledgers according to the appointment calendar, and put them in your To-Do folder.

Materials	Source
Appointment calendar	
Card file	
Supplies folder	
All the usual supplies are in the folder plus the following:	
Fee Schedule	Project 34
Blank receipts	Project 43
Deposit slips	Project 44
Miscellaneous folder	
Daily journal for October 22	Project 40
Daily journal for October 27	Project 40
Checkbook	Project 41
Checks 4700 through 4708 (completed)	Project 41
Monthly summary sheet for October	Projects 42, 43, 46
Receipt for Monica Armstrong	Project 43
Daily journal for October 28	Project 43
Deposit slips	Project 44
Bank Statement	Project 45
Employee earnings record	Project 46
Check 4709 (completed)	Project 46

To-Do folder

Day 1

Patients' charts and ledgers for October 27–29	
Daily journal for October 29	WP 85
To–Do list	WP 86
Telephone log	WP 87
Charge slips for October 29	WP 88
Insurance form	WP 89

Day 2

Patients' charts and ledgers for October 30	
Daily journal for October 30	WP 90
X–ray and laboratory reports	WPs 91 and 92
Incoming checks (8)	WPs 93 and 94

Day 3

Daily journal for October 31	WP 95
Draft of a letter to Dr. Miller-Young	WP 96
Charge slips	WP 97

Patients' folders

The following items have been added to the patients' folders (charts) since the last simulation:

Sherman, Florence	Project 38
Sun, Cheng	Project 39
Ledger cards for all current patients.	

If you have not completed all the projects and do not have all these records set up in advance, talk with your instructor.

MEDICAL VOCABULARY

The following medical terms are used in Simulation 3. Review each term and its meaning.

ASHD (arteriosclerotic heart disease): hardening of the arteries.

candida: a type of fungal infection.

cerumen: earwax.

CHF (congestive heart failure): inability of the heart to pump blood adequately.

CVA (costovertebral angle): the region where the ribs meet the vertebrae; also, the region of the kidney.

discrepancy: the quality or state of being at variance.

DPT: diphtheria, pertussis, and tetanus (whooping cough).

dyspepsia: indigestion.

endocervical: situated within the cervix.

erosion: a reddened area produced by tissue deterioration.

erythematous: characterized by increased redness.

etiology: the cause of a disorder.

fetor: a strong, offensive odor.

gastritis: inflammation of the mucous lining of the stomach.

iliac crest: a prominence of the hip bone.

jaundice: yellowish skin color.

labile: unstable.

lateral malleolus: the protruding, rounded bone on the outer aspect of the ankle.

malar: pertaining to the cheekbone.

menometrorrhagia: vaginal bleeding during menstruation or between the menstrual periods.

MI (myocardial infarction): heart attack.

para: a woman who has given birth (used in combination); for example, a *tripara* is a woman who has given birth to three children.

pectoralis major muscle: a large muscle in the anterior region of the chest.

pruritic: pertaining to or marked by itching.

scoliosis: curvature of the spine.

serous otitis media: a collection of fluid in the middle ear.

thyromegaly: an enlargement of the thyroid gland.

triceps: a muscle in the posterior region of the upper arm.

varicella: chicken pox

Professional Activities

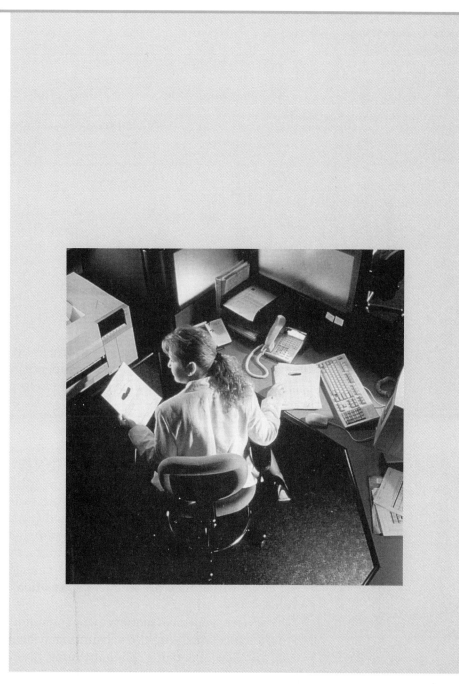

Office Management

Upon completion of this chapter, you should be able to:

- List four activities performed by a medical management consultant.

- Describe six items of information found in a patient information brochure.

- State the information typically found in a personnel manual, or an employee handbook.

- Begin the development of an office procedures manual.

- Explain the use of an outside service file.

- Discuss organization of the medical assistant's work area.

- Discuss safety in the office regarding floors, electric cords, fire hazards, and furniture.

- Discuss the assistant's responsibility toward housekeeping duties, laundry, maintenance, supplies, and the patients' waiting room.

Among the varied duties to be performed by the medical assistant is managing the office, including the supervision of office maintenance. Professional assistance is available to help plan the management of the office and its staff.

■ MEDICAL MANAGEMENT CONSULTANTS

Doctors do not have the time to devote to managing an office; they delegate that responsibility to the medical assistant. To manage an office efficiently, the assistant may require help from an accountant, a lawyer, an insurance representative, and a time-management expert. Organizations that specialize in office management are run by experts such as these; they are known as **"medical management consultants."**

For a fee, a medical management consultant will spend several days in the office analyzing the accounting system, appointment scheduling and flow of patients, filing methods, and work habits of the entire staff, including the doctors. After every detail of the operation has been studied, the consultant will make recommendations for changes. Recommendations may include changing the appointment system to accommodate patients and/or doctors better, or devising alternate methods for collection of payments, suggesting ways to reduce office expenses, and implementing comprehensive training for office personnel.

Business advice specifically offered to the doctors may include counseling about:

- Investment.
- Advantages and disadvantages of buying, renting, or leasing office space and equipment.
- Taxes.
- Incorporating the business.
- Estate planning.

The consultant is almost certain to suggest the use of a patient information brochure, a personnel manual, an employee handbook, or an office procedures manual.

■ MONTHLY PLANNING

A monthly planning calendar can be purchased from stationers (this can be an erasable board or a tear–off sheet) or created on a computer software program. It can be utilized for recording office-related information and activities such as staff members on duty, vacations, and upcoming meetings or events. The calendar should be placed in an area accessible to all office employees. An example is shown in Figure 12-1.

MONTHLY PLAN-IT BOARD

MONTH November   YEAR 19--

SUNDAY	MONDAY	TUESDAY	WEDNESDAY	THURSDAY	FRIDAY	SATURDAY
		1	2	3 Greg (lab) gone from 2-4	4	5
6	7	8	9	10 staff meeting 11-12 with lunch	11	12
13	14	15	16 Dr. Newman at National Convention	17	18	19
20	21	22	23	24	25	26
27	28	29	30			

Figure 12-1   Monthly Plan-It Board

Also, many computer software packages provide an electronic calendar. Electronic calendars can be daily, weekly, or monthly and can be used for tracking the schedule of each physician or that of everyone who works in the office.

■ PATIENT INFORMATION BROCHURE

A **patient information brochure** provides the patient with vital information about the practice. It should not take the place of a personal orientation for new patients conducted by the medical assistant, but it does provide the patient with a valuable written reference. Before you obtain professional assistance in designing the brochure, assemble the information you want to include. Follow these general rules:

1. Make the brochure visually appealing. An attractive layout and an open design with plenty of white (blank) space are critical. For example, avoid crowded columns of words; they give the page a gray look.
2. Make the brochure easy to read. Whenever possible, use words people know rather than technical terms.
3. Thank the patient for taking a moment to read about the office staff and the health care services provided.
4. Provide basic information about the doctors and the staff. For example, "Dr. Steiner is our pediatrician; Dr. Nguyen specializes in illnesses affecting the lungs."
5. Provide information about emergency care. For example, tell patients to use the 911 telephone number in life-threatening medical situations. Inform patients that the office has a 24-hour telephone service that provides instructions in emergency situations.
6. State routine office hours.
7. List special services provided by the clinic, such as special classes or medical testing programs.
8. Provide brief instructions about medication refills and insurance forms. Explain the office's remittance policy and provide some basic information about professional fees.
9. Include a statement such as the following at the end of the brochure: "If you have any questions about our clinic, please telephone us at xxx– xxxx."

■ PERSONNEL MANUAL

The **personnel manual**, or **employee handbook**, provides employees with information about the work environment at the medical facility. This includes office policies regarding punctuality, proper attire, smoking, and safety. The manual should also contain information about working hours, overtime procedures, holidays, sick time, vacation time, salaries, procedures for filing a complaint or grievance, and termination. Having a personnel manual enables the employee to refer to specific guidelines about employment practices at the office.

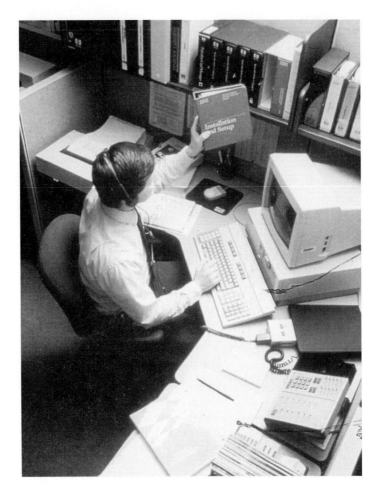

Reviewing the office procedures manual helps the office to operate smoothly.

OFFICE PROCEDURES MANUAL

An aid to efficient office routine is an **office procedures manual**, which can be made by the medical assistant. This manual serves as a reminder of the various tasks that have to be done and how to do them. It helps to keep the office running smoothly during an assistant's temporary absence due to illness or vacation, and it aids in training a substitute or successor.

The best place to keep the manual is in a loose-leaf binder with tab divisions. You can then write the different sections as each job is defined and easily make revisions by substituting new pages.

First, write an outline to determine the subjects to be included in the manual. Subheadings may be cross-referenced.

Common office tasks should be listed and described in various sections of the procedures manual. The section on patients' care will probably constitute a major portion of it. Other major sections of the manual may describe the daily routine and specific procedures. Sections may be added at a later time.

Sample forms should be included whenever they are referred to; the source for replenishing the supply of such forms should also be given. Also, much useful information can be organized as charts and

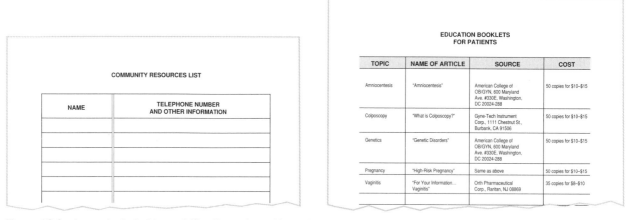

Section 4: HANDLING RECORDS

PATIENTS WHO HAVE MOVED

Procedure:

DECEASED PATIENTS

Procedure:

TRANSFER OF RECORDS

Procedure:

SUPERVISION OF FILING SYSTEM

Procedure:

COMMONLY PERFORMED PROCEDURES

NAME OF PROCEDURE _____

USUAL TIME REQUIREMENT _____

SUPPLIES AND INSTRUMENTS:

PATIENT PREPARATION:

SPECIAL INSTRUCTIONS:

COMMUNITY RESOURCES LIST

NAME	TELEPHONE NUMBER AND OTHER INFORMATION

EDUCATION BOOKLETS FOR PATIENTS

TOPIC	NAME OF ARTICLE	SOURCE	COST
Amniocentesis	"Amniocentesis"	American College of OB/GYN, 600 Maryland Ave. #330E, Washington, DC 20024-288	50 copies for $10–$15
Colposcopy	"What is Colposcopy?"	Gyne-Tech Instrument Corp., 1111 Chestnut St., Burbank, CA 91506	50 copies for $10–$15
Genetics	"Genetic Disorders"	American College of OB/GYN, 600 Maryland Ave. #330E, Washington, DC 20024-288	50 copies for $10–$15
Pregnancy	"High-Risk Pregnancy"	Same as above	50 copies for $10–$15
Vaginitis	"For Your Information... Vaginitis"	Orth Pharmaceutical Corp., Raritan, NJ 08869	35 copies for $8–$10

Figure 12-2   Items Included in an Office Procedures Manual

tables. Figure 12-2 shows examples of items that might be included in an office procedures manual to help the staff conduct office business more efficiently.

Following are suggestions for a manual as it might be set up for an office shared by several doctors with a number of employees. Many of these procedures could be separated into smaller tasks that might require a separate page.

Personnel

List the duties and responsibilities of each position in the office, stating especially whether some of the duties overlap or whether employees substitute for one another during absences.

Daily Routine

One section should describe the medical assistant's routine in detail.

- List the duties to be performed to prepare the office each morning before patients arrive. These include: checking the neatness of the office, calling the answering service or checking the answering machine for messages, processing incoming and outgoing mail, pulling charts for the day's appointments, preparing the day's appointment schedule, and checking to see that the examination rooms are ready to be used.
- List assignments of work stations for the assistants if such assignments are rotated.
- List other routine tasks the assistant is responsible for during the day. These include: preparing correspondence and patients' records, filing patients' records, maintaining financial records, and completing insurance forms.
- List routine duties the assistant performs at the close of each day such as locking desks and files, covering equipment, and preparing the telephone answering machine if one is used.

Transferring Patients' Records

In a separate section, explain the procedures for transferring patients' records.

- State which staff member is responsible for handling the transfer.
- List what can and cannot be transferred.
- Describe procedures for photocopying records to be transferred.
- Describe procedures for faxing records to be transferred.
- Describe procedures for recording when and what information was transferred.
- Describe the procedure for filing the release of information form.

Using the Telephone

Telephone procedures can be covered in another section.

- Designate the preferred greeting for answering the telephone.
- Explain the triage procedure.
- List the procedure for obtaining information about patients over the telephone.
- Provide suggestions for referring a patient to a physician on call, the hospital emergency room, another facility, and sources of financial assistance.

Scheduling Appointments

The procedures for scheduling appointments may comprise another section.

- List each doctor's time commitments, including office hours, hospital hours, teaching schedule, and time spent on research.
- Note which doctors have special scheduling requests, such as no more than two physicals in the morning or no complete physicals for Monday mornings or Friday afternoons.
- List the procedure for canceling and rescheduling appointments.
- List what information about patients is required for scheduling an appointment.
- List the standard length of time required for various procedures such as 1 hour for complete physicals, $1/2$ hour for school physicals, and so forth.

Providing Information for New Patients

Describe the information to be provided to patients who are new to the practice. Include the following:

- Office hours.
- Emergency care procedures.

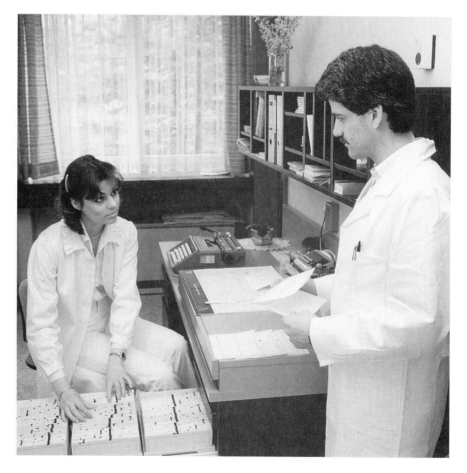

The assistant's work area needs to be organized for easy access to business and personnel records.

- Hospitals affiliated with the office and their addresses, telephone numbers, and visiting hours.
- The standard procedure for obtaining medication refills.

Filing

In a section on filing, give detailed information about the office practices.

- Describe the method of filing used, different filing sections (active, inactive, closed, transient), and where each section is located.
- Indicate the length of time records are to be kept in active files.
- If color is used as a filing aid, indicate what each color designates.
- Describe the preferred arrangement of documents in the patients' chart, including medication sheets, doctors' progress notes, laboratory reports, X-ray reports, special procedures notes, correspondence, and hospitalization summaries.
- List the types of medical reports that must be attached to a patient's chart before a physician reviews the chart.
- Describe follow-up procedures for test results and the transfer of patients' records.

Billing

In a section on billing, provide a sample ledger and explain the method of billing. The name, address, and telephone number of any accounting service used should be noted.

Collections

The steps established by the office in the standard collection process can be explained here. It is also useful to show sample collection letters and to provide a sample of the form used to track the collection process for a patient.

Processing Insurance Forms

Treatment of insurance forms may require a separate section.

- Include detailed instructions for handling each insurance account, for completing each type of form, and for billing patients who have insurance.
- Provide general information about each insurance carrier, including the address, the contact person, and the telephone number.
- List the approximate turnaround time for processing claims for each insurance carrier.

Forms and Supplies

A separate section on forms and supplies may be needed.

- Include an example of each form and item of stationery used in the office, listing the names, addresses, and telephone numbers of suppliers for ordering purposes. Also note how long it takes for stationery and supply orders to be filled.
- List the same information for supplies the doctor uses and any brand names preferred, the quantity usually ordered, and the last price paid. Note how long it takes for orders to be filled.
- Include an **inventory** chart—a list of office forms and supplies that can be used to keep track of quantities on hand.

Equipment

In a separate section, include an inventory of all office equipment. List the names, addresses, and telephone numbers of equipment manufacturers, dealers, and local repair services.

The assistant must check service contracts for equipment used in the practice to ensure that everything is in good working order.

PROJECT 47 Starting a Procedures Manual

Prepare several pages for your office procedures manual. Some of the information you need can be obtained from previous chapters. Several suggestions for topics are given below. You may add any other pages you choose at any time.

1. Inventory the chart forms used by Dr. Newman. Staple a sample of each form onto a separate page of the procedures manual. Locate each form (or one similar to it) in a stationery supply catalog. List the supplier information, quantity ordered, and current price. If a form is produced in-house, estimate the cost of producing the form. (Obtain stationery supply catalogs from your instructor.)

2. Describe the collection procedure, including the initial billing process, follow-up process, and

steps used for collection of accounts that are 60, 90, and 120 days overdue.

3. Design a form for taking inventory of office periodicals. (List any magazines that might be used in a waiting room.)

4. Design a form that patients can use to suggest topics for a patient information brochure. (Obtain sample brochures from your instructor or from local health agencies.)

5. Design a form for tracking the collection process, and explain how it is to be used.

File these items in your Miscellaneous folder.

◼ OUTSIDE SERVICES

In addition to referring patients to other physicians, every doctor has occasion to refer patients to outside agencies for care or for renting or purchasing medical supplies. Patients often ask where they may obtain specific health services. Names, addresses, and telephone numbers of those to whom the doctor might refer patients need to be easily accessible in an **outside service file**.

A card file using tabs as subject guides may be practical for storing information about such organizations. Another efficient approach is to store this information by subject in a computer database. The services listed might include the following:

- Convalescent homes and nursing homes.
- Dentists and dental specialists.
- Health insurance organizations.
- Home health care agencies.
- Laboratories.
- Medical employment pool for temporary staffing of medical personnel.
- Medical specialists for referrals.
- Medical supply companies.
- Pharmacies.
- Social service agencies.
- Welfare agencies.

ORGANIZATION

The medical assistant's desk, work area, and filing cabinets should be organized in such a way that they suit the needs of the practice and facilitate the work of the assistant.

The Assistant's Desk

One drawer may be set aside for personal items such as purse or wallet and tissues. An adequate supply of all stationery items should be stored in the desk. Pencils, erasers, paper clips, appointment cards, and other items that are used every day should be placed neatly and methodically in the drawers and kept in the same place at all times. Letterhead stationery, blank stationery, envelopes, patients' chart forms, and any other frequently used forms should be kept in a desk organizer near the keyboarding area. Copy paper and copying supplies should be easily accessible near the copying machine. The top of the desk should remain neat and clear of all unnecessary items.

An efficient way for the assistant to organize work is by using colored folders. For example, a blue folder might contain letters that have been finished and are ready for the doctor's signature, a yellow folder might contain records or documents to be filed in patients' charts, a red folder might contain work that needs follow-up, and a green folder might contain messages.

Business Records

In addition to patients' medical records, the assistant must store documents and papers pertinent to the running of the office, such as leases, insurance policies, tax reports, bank statements, and bills. These documents are referred to as business records. An office safe is advisable for some of the more important business documents such as office leases and insurance policies. Others will need to be systematically filed. Bills should be placed in a folder marked "Unpaid Bills" as soon as they are received.

When merchandise is delivered, an invoice usually accompanies it. A monthly statement is sent for regular deliveries. Both should be checked carefully—the invoice with the merchandise received and the bill with the invoice. If supplies are returned, a credit memorandum should be requested. This credit also must appear on the monthly statement. Paid bills should be filed appropriately, since they may have to be produced at an income tax audit.

Personnel Records

Each employee will have a separate personnel file containing information such as the application form and letter, résumé, employment agreement, performance evaluations, and attendance record. These are confidential records and should be stored in a locked drawer.

Each doctor will have a personal file that should contain additional information regarding, for example, licenses (state, narcotic, or workers' compensation registration), social security information, and identification numbers. There should be a list of the doctor's affiliations with organizations, medical societies, and hospitals along with a list of the doctor's continuing educational requirements. Notations should be made about license and membership renewal fees, including the due dates and any identifying numbers.

■ MAINTENANCE

It may be the medical assistant's responsibility to attend to the details involved in keeping the space used by the practice tidy and clean. For cleaning and janitorial services, the office may contract with a private company or maintain its own staff. Even if an outside contractor is employed, specific duties may be assigned to the regular office staff.

Waiting Room

The patients' waiting room should be checked by the assistant first thing in the morning. The patient's first impression of the office is very important, and the waiting room is the first place a patient enters. Patients associate a well-kept, cheerful room with a practice that is managed efficiently. Plants help to create a pleasant atmosphere, but they must be properly tended. Reading material should be up to date and in good condition. If children are among the doctor's patients, a few toys and games will help keep them occupied. Be sure that any toys available for children's use are safe and can be used without supervision. Sometimes there is a children's area set off from the rest of the waiting room. Keep all sharp instruments and all medicines out of children's reach.

Burned-out light bulbs, torn curtains, finger marks on window panes, pictures hanging askew, dead plants, stained tables, and the like give the patient a bad impression of the office, even if the waiting room is otherwise clean.

When the last patient leaves for the day, office personnel must check to see that electric equipment and lights are turned off and that the outside door is locked.

Cleaning Contractors

Generally, a cleaning contractor or department is responsible for daily cleaning and special weekly, monthly, or annual jobs. The medical assistant may monitor the cleaning personnel to ensure that the work is performed properly. Figure 12-3 shows some suggested daily, weekly, and periodic tasks.

Other jobs that must be attended to regularly include:

- Discarding old and torn magazines.
- Replacing light bulbs.
- Checking inventory of paper supplies, paper cups, bathroom tissue, and soap.

Laundry

Linen may consist of doctors' white coats, laboratory coats for nursing personnel, examination gowns, sheets, pillowcases, towels, and drapes. These items may be the property of the practice and thus sent out to be laundered, or they may be rented from a linen-supply company. Disposable items are frequently purchased in place of washable linens. The assistant may want to compare the expense of purchasing disposable linens versus the purchase and upkeep of conventional linens. Environmental issues should be considered when comparing costs.

Safety

The practice will carry personal liability insurance to cover any personal injuries that occur in the office as a result of an accident, such as that caused by slipping or falling. Malpractice insurance does not cover accidents or other injuries not connected with medical treatment. The assistant must make sure that safety guidelines are followed in the office.

DAILY	WEEKLY	PERIODICALLY
Clean floors.	Polish or vacuum furniture.	Clean draperies and blinds.
Vacuum carpets.	Clean mirrors and pictures.	Clean upholstery.
Clean drinking fountains.	Brush lamp shades.	Clean windows.
Straighten magazine rack.	Scrub and wax floors.	Clean fixtures.
Clear sidewalks, if needed.		
Empty wastebaskets.		
Wash all sinks and basins.		
Dust.		
Clean lavatories.		

Figure 12-3   Suggested Office Maintenance Tasks

Floors. Floors should never be so highly polished that they are slippery. Small rugs should be anchored by rubber pads, large rugs or carpets must be securely fastened to the floor, and any tear must be mended. Anything that is spilled must be mopped up quickly. Signs that caution people about wet floors should be used to prevent slipping.

Electric Cords. Cords must not be strung across an aisle; neither must they block the way between desks or tables. Special plastic coverings are available for use when a cord must run along the floor. For the protection of children, outlets should be covered.

Fire Hazards. Fire alarm systems should be checked regularly. Fire extinguishers should be strategically located and checked at regular intervals. Wall sockets must not be overloaded.

Furniture. Lack of space may cause people to bump into corners of tables and desks. Open drawers invite mishaps. Pulling out file drawers too far can result in the cabinet's tipping over if it is not bolted to the floor.

■ SUPPLIES

In every office, there are many different kinds of supplies, so inventories are essential. Items that are frequently taken for personal use, such as pens, pencils, soap, thermometers, rubber gloves, cellophane tape, self-adhesive notes, and printer ribbons, may disappear faster than their normal office use would indicate. Personal use of such items

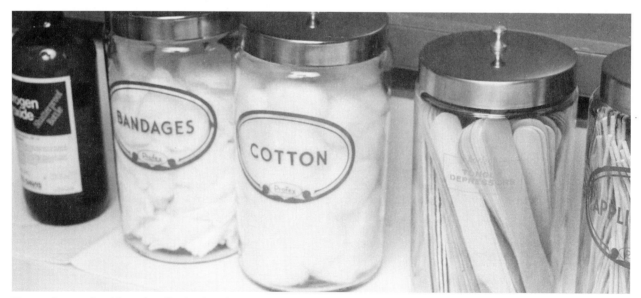

The assistant should continually check to be sure that necessary supplies are available.

will be discouraged if employees know the items are accounted for in inventory control.

The medical assistant may be responsible for ordering supplies; storing supplies; and monitoring their use, cost, and quality. A standard ordering procedure should be instituted to avoid running out of supplies. Supplies should be ordered when the stock runs low, not when the supply runs out.

The supply inventory should be checked weekly. An efficient method of inventory control is to use a form that indicates the quantity in stock for each item. A notation is made on the form each time an item is taken from the stock. Another method of inventory control is to note when the next-to-the-last item is taken from the supply or when the last box of a certain supply is opened and to place a new order then.

The main categories of medical office supplies include desk supplies, stationery supplies, maintenance supplies, and medical supplies. Nursing personnel are often responsible for maintaining medical supplies such as medications, dressings, gloves, and examination supplies. In some offices, however, the assistant may be responsible for ordering these, in addition to other supplies used in the office.

Key Terms

The following terms appear in **boldface** type in this chapter. Do you recall what they mean? Refer to the chapter for definitions you need to review.

employee handbook
inventory
medical management
  consultants
office procedures
  manual

outside services file
patient information
  brochure
personnel manual

Topics for Discussion

1. Discuss the advantages of having a task list when giving an orientation to a new employee.
2. Give suggestions for ways to lower office expenses.
3. Discuss the effects on job performance and office morale when employees participate in determining work assignments.

4. Office work is generally considered to be relatively free of accidents. Describe the kinds of accidents that may occur in a medical office.

Role-Playing

1. Your office employs a person for general office maintenance. Use the suggested work schedule in this chapter as a guideline for discussing this job with the maintenance person.
2. You have been asked to write an office procedures manual in the office where you work. Obtain a job description from each employee in the clinic to include in the procedures manual.
3. As a medical assistant, you have been asked to manage the office. Explain to the doctor or supervisor that you need the assistance of a medical management consultant.

Professional Reports

Upon completion of this chapter, you should be able to:

- Locate materials in a library using the card catalog, microfiche, or online computerized database.

- Proofread a document.

- Key a manuscript to be submitted for publication.

- Prepare a bibliography.

- Assist in maintaining a professional reference library in the doctor's private office.

- Discuss an inventory system for reprint materials.

Many physicians are involved in writing articles, books, and speeches. From time-to-time, the doctor may have to prepare a medical case history of particular interest or reports of a special investigation for presentation to colleagues. A doctor engaged in research work may do extensive writing in order to communicate findings to the scientific community. Whether it is for a lecture, an article, or a book, you may be required to assist in assembling information, preparing the manuscript, and, in the case of publication, performing editorial duties.

ASSEMBLING INFORMATION

The doctor may be involved with research in a wide variety of areas, including investigating clinical procedures, instruments, or drugs; conducting experiments; and studying pathological conditions. Such research may occur well before the publication of any findings. The assistant may become involved in the initial stages of research through obtaining material for the doctor's reports at a library.

Using the Library

Medical assistants and other health care professionals have access to medical libraries located in hospitals and universities. The librarian will be able to provide information about use of the library and about the types of materials available.

Libraries are organized to make information easily obtainable. The **card catalog** is an index of books available in the library and can help the researcher locate materials quickly. Every book in the library is cataloged by subject, author, and title. In many large libraries, the catalog is available on computer, which makes locating books even more efficient. Figure 13-1 shows how the same book may be cataloged in four ways, with four different cards.

Many libraries provide access to all of the materials in the local library system (which may include college libraries, city libraries, and

```
          LIBRARY OF CONGRESS CATALOGING-IN-PUBLICATION DATA

① Shtasel, Philip.  1925-
          Medical tests and diagnostic procedures; a
② patient's guide to just what the doctor ordered/Philip
  Shtasel—1st ed.
③         316 p.; 25 cm.

④         ISBN 0-06-016245-7

          1. Function tests (medicine)—popular works.  2.
⑤ Diagnosis—popular works.  3. Patient education.  I.
  Title.

⑥ RC82.S554 1990        ⑦ 616.075 dc20        ⑧ 89-45716
```

① Author's name
② Title, authors, publication information
③ Text pages and book size
√ International Standard Book Number (ISBN)
⑤ Subject entry
≈ Library of Congress classification number
Δ Dewey decimal number
⑧ Card serial number

```
                              TITLE

① MEDICAL TESTS AND DIAGNOSTIC PROCEDURES: a patient's
  guide to just what the doctor ordered.
② Philip Shtasel.  1925-

          Medical tests and diagnostic procedures:  a
  patient's guide to just what the doctor ordered./Philip
  Shtasel.

③ 1st ed. New York:  Harper & Row, c 1990.

④ xix,  316 p.; 25 cm.

⑤ 616.075 SHT
```

① Title
② Author's name
③ Publication information
√ Text pages and book size
⑤ Dewey decimal number

```
                           SUBJECT
① MEDICAL TESTS
②         Medical tests and diagnostic procedures:  a
  patient's guide to just what the doctor ordered.

③ Philip Shtasel.  1925-

          Medical tests and diagnostic procedures:  a
  patient's guide to just what the doctor ordered./Philiip
  Shtasel.

④ 1st ed. New York:  Harper & Row, c 1990.

⑤ xix,  316 p.; 25 cm.

⑥ 616.075 SHT
```

① Subject
② Title
③ Author's name
√ Publication information
⑤ Text pages and book size
≈ Dewey decimal number

```
                           AUTHOR
① Philip Shtasel.  1925-
②         Medical tests and diagnostic procedures:  a
              patient's guide to just what the doctor
              ordered.

          1st ed. New York:  Harper & Row, c 1990.
③             xix,316 p.; 25 cm.

          Includes index.
          1. Function tests (medicine).  2. Diagnosis.  3.
④ Patient Education.  4. Physical examinations.
          I. Title:  Medical tests and diagnostic procedures:
          a patient's guide to just what the doctor ordered.
          [Medical tests and diagnostic procedures].

⑤ 616.075 SHT
```

① Author
② Title
③ Publication information, text pages and book size
√ Subject and title cross-references
⑤ Dewey decimal number

Figure 13-1   One Book Indexed on Four Card Catalogs

so forth) through the use of a microfiche reader, a card catalog, or an online computer database. The librarian can also provide information regarding the use of each resource including various indexes, larger computer-based retrieval systems, and reference sources of recently published medical books.

Medical journals and periodicals contain most of the current medical literature. The assistant should use the indexes available in a medical library to obtain information from these sources. The *Index Medicus*, published by the National Library of Medicine, contains a monthly bibliography of medical reviews. *MEDLARS (Medical Literature Analysis and Retrieval Systems)* is one collection of medical and health science information available in a computerized database.

Books in Print is another valuable reference source for the researcher. It is a listing of all books currently in publication.

Abstracts

A doctor who is writing an article on a certain topic will first make a survey of work already published on that same subject. The assistant can help in this research by locating the literature and by providing **abstracts** (summaries) of pertinent information.

An abstract is a brief summary of an article, book, or case history. The *Journal of the American Medical Association (JAMA)* and most of the other medical and scientific journals contain abstracts of articles. An abstract gives the purpose of the article and summarizes the main ideas and conclusions. After reading an abstract, the doctor can decide whether the article needs to be studied more thoroughly.

■ PREPARING A MANUSCRIPT

Before written material is sent to a publisher, it goes through several steps, beginning with a **rough draft** and proceeding to the final, keyed **manuscript**. Steps in this process vary according to each doctor's preference. One writer may start by making an outline, jotting down main headings and subheadings. The rough draft may then be a filled-in, keyed outline. Another doctor may make voluminous notes and hand them to the assistant to be keyed. In any case, the rough draft is always the first complete and consecutive keying of the document.

Drafts

The draft should be double-spaced or triple-spaced, with generous margins on both sides. This spacing leaves ample room for additions and corrections. The most common proofreaders' marks for making changes to keyed drafts are shown in Figure 13-2 on page 230. A very practical system for keeping various drafts separated is to use different-colored paper for each draft.

Figure 13-2 Proofreader's Marks

Mark	Meaning	Example		Mark	Meaning	Example
∧	Insert word	add it		#	Insert a space	add so it
—	Omit word	and so it			Insert a space	and so it
....	No, don't omit	and so it		⌒	Omit the space	10 a.m.
\	Omit stroke	and so it		—	Underscore this	It may be
/	Make letter small	And so it			Move as shown	it is not
≡	Make a capital	if he is		∪	Join to word	the port
≣	Make all capitals	I hope so		word	Change word	and if he
	Move as indicated	and so		○	Make into period	to him.
=	Line up, even up	TO: John		⬭	Don't abbreviate	Dr. Judd
‖	Line up, even up	‖ If he is		○	Spell it out	① or ② if
ss [	Use single spacing	and so it		¶	New paragraph	If he is
∪	Turn around	had it so		∨	Raise above line	Hale says
ds [	Use double spacing	and so it		+#↑	More space here	It may be
=	Insert a hyphen	white-hot		−#↑	Less space here	If she is
	Indent — spaces	If he is		2#	2 line spaces here	It may be
∼	Bold	He is not		—	Italicize	It may be

Final Drafts

Authors frequently send copies of a manuscript to colleagues for suggestions or advice before submitting the **final draft** (manuscript) for publication. After the writer reviews the suggested changes and edits the rough draft, the manuscript is prepared.

Most publishers prefer to edit manuscripts and produce books using computers, so a copy of the manuscript on disk is usually required. At least one photocopy of the manuscript must be kept by the author.

Professional journals usually state guidelines for submitting materials for publication in the periodical. These specifications may state that the text should be double-spaced and should have margins of at least 1 inch on all sides. All pages should contain the same number of lines. Word processing software enables the user to establish formats that provide a document with uniform margins and page length. This uniformity also helps the writer and the editor estimate the number of words in the manuscript.

The title is centered in all-capital letters 2 inches from the top edge of the first manuscript page, followed by the author's name, degree, official title, and the institution where the author is employed. The body of the article should begin three lines below the author's name and title.

No page number is placed on the first page; subsequent pages are consistently numbered either at the top center, at the top right-hand corner, or at the bottom in the center. Manuscript pages are numbered consecutively, not by chapters.

Headings and Special Treatment of Words

Headings are used throughout the text to alert and guide the reader to new subjects. Main headings should be flush with the margin so that they will not be overlooked. Subheadings may begin with the paragraph indention and may be underscored. Words that are to be emphasized should appear in italics or underscored. Foreign words should appear in italics or underscored, but not medical terms in common use.

Quotations

When published material is quoted in an article or a book, either enclose the material in quotation marks or indent it from both margins to set it off from the text. If the quotation is brief, quotation marks are acceptable.

Footnotes and Endnotes

Footnotes and endnotes may be used to refer to sources of information the author wishes to cite in researching the work or to give the sources of quotations. With word processing software, **footnotes** can be printed at the bottom of the manuscript page on which the reference is made. **Endnotes** can be printed on a separate page at the end of the article. Use *The Gregg Reference Manual* to find examples of footnote and endnote formats; also be sure to follow any special style preferences of your employer in formatting footnotes and endnotes. Figure 13-3 shows examples of footnotes and endnotes.

PROJECT 48 Keying From a Rough Draft

A rough draft of the beginning of a manuscript appears on WPs 98 through 101. Rekey this draft in final form. In addition to the corrections shown, there are a number of errors in spelling and punctuation that must be corrected.

Store the finished copy in your Miscellaneous folder.

New employees may be hired on a probationary basis for a three-month period during which the employee or the employer may terminate the employment at any time. At the end of this probationary period, there is a **performance evaluation.**[1]

[1]. Karonne J. Becklin and Edith M. Sunnarborg, *Medical Office Procedures*, 3rd ed., Glencoe/McGraw-Hill, Westerville, Ohio, 1992, p. 241.

(a)

ENDNOTES

[1]. Karonne J. Becklin and Edith M. Sunnarborg, *Medical Office Procedures*, 3rd ed., Glencoe/McGraw-Hill, Westerville, Ohio, 1992, p. 241.

(b)

Figure 13-3   Examples of *(a)* Footnotes and *(b)* Endnotes

Illustrations

If photographs, tables, or graphs accompany the article, they should be handled carefully. Do not paste or mount any illustrative matter in the manuscript. Keep the illustrations separate, with a reference to the appropriate page of the manuscript. Photographs must be glossy prints, and captions should be on a separate piece of paper, not on the prints.

Bibliographies

All references used by the writer, including those cited in footnotes and endnotes, are compiled at the end of a chapter or at the end of the book under the heading "References" as a **bibliography**.

A complete reference contains all the information needed for the reader to find the book or article quickly. Bibliographic entries are listed alphabetically by author. If there is no author, alphabetize the references by title. The words *The* and *A* are disregarded in determining alphabetic sequence. If there is more than one author for the same reference, only the first author's name is inverted (last name first). If there is more than one entry by the same author, the author's name is replaced by a long dash (six hyphens) in all the entries for that author. The entries for this author are then alphabetized by title.

A periodical reference requires the name of the author, title of the article in quotation marks, name of the journal (underscored or in italics) in which the article appears, volume number and date of the issue, and page numbers on which the article begins and ends. See Figure 13-4 for a sample bibliography. The sequence of information varies somewhat with different publishers. Consult the publisher for the desired style.

Editing and Proofreading

When a manuscript has been accepted for publication, the author is notified and new tasks begin. The manuscript usually will be edited by the publisher, and the author will approve the edited manuscript, making any necessary final revisions.

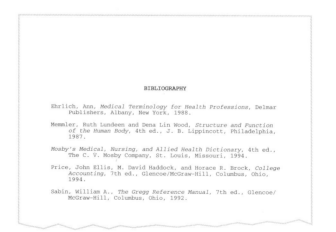

BIBLIOGRAPHY

Ehrlich, Ann, *Medical Terminology for Health Professions*, Delmar Publishers, Albany, New York, 1988.

Memmler, Ruth Lundeen and Dena Lin Wood, *Structure and Function of the Human Body*, 4th ed., J. B. Lippincott, Philadelphia, 1987.

Mosby's Medical, Nursing, and Allied Health Dictionary, 4th ed., The C. V. Mosby Company, St. Louis, Missouri, 1994.

Price, John Ellis, M. David Haddock, and Horace R. Brock, *College Accounting*, 7th ed., Glencoe/McGraw-Hill, Columbus, Ohio, 1994.

Sabin, William A., *The Gregg Reference Manual*, 7th ed., Glencoe/McGraw-Hill, Columbus, Ohio, 1992.

Figure 13-4   Bibliography Style

After a manuscript has been prepared, the proof (sometimes called the "galley proof") is sent to the author to be proofread for corrections. The proof needs to be carefully read for typographical errors and checked against the original manuscript to ensure that all material is in its proper place.

If the author or assistant is responsible for checking page proofs, they must be checked for proper pagination, insertion of footnotes and references, page makeup, and so forth. Publishers typically provide authors with guidelines for making changes on proofs.

■ MEDICAL JOURNALS

Most medical societies publish their own journals. For example, the American Medical Association publishes about a dozen periodicals on special subjects in addition to the official organ of the society, the *JAMA*, which includes articles relating to all aspects of the field of medicine. Other medical journals are published by hospitals, by universities, or independently. Most specialties have journals with articles concerned only with that particular specialty.

Journals can be bound for permanent reference, since they contain much valuable information. Most journals publish an index for the entire volume in the last number of each volume, although volumes may not correspond to the calendar year and may vary in the length of time covered. This index should be bound together with the journals in the appropriate volume.

A record should be kept of all journal subscriptions in the office. This record could be kept in the procedures manual, with a notation indicating the frequency of publication and the subscription price. The renewal information might also be kept in a tickler file.

Reprints

Doctors can inform colleagues about their work by lecturing and/or writing about it. If the doctor presents a paper at a medical meeting, it is usually published in the official publication of the society or in another medical journal. However, the article may be submitted to a journal without having first been presented at a meeting.

Doctors may receive a limited number of **reprints** of the article free from the publisher; additional copies are available at cost. These reprints are sent by the doctor to other professionals interested in the same or allied fields. A record should be kept of reprints sent and acknowledged by colleagues.

Sometimes a doctor may want a reprint of a designated article. Then a letter must be written requesting a reprint from the author or the publisher. A second note, acknowledging receipt of the reprint, should be sent after the reprint has been received. Incoming reprints should be date stamped and promptly acknowledged either on a printed form made for this purpose or by letter.

A designated area should be set aside for the storage of reprints, such as a certain shelf in a storage area. To allow for easy retrieval, a record should be maintained of all reprints stored in the office. One method of indexing reprints in storage is to include a form in the procedures manual on which the author, title, and source of the reprint can be noted.

■ REFERENCES AND RESOURCES

The assistant should be familiar with a variety of reference books and must know where to find various types of information. Following is a list of commonly used reference sources. Keep in mind that these references must be revised periodically so that the information they contain is up to date; the most recent edition should always be consulted.

- Dictionaries, general and medical: Provide spelling, pronunciation, definitions, syllabication, capitalization, hyphenation, and plural forms.
- Synonym and antonym references (thesauruses): Give the most appropriate word for a certain idea. (Many words have approximately the same meaning, but a certain shade of difference may exist between them.)
- Secretarial reference books: Provide information on grammar, punctuation, writing style, document formatting, and other subjects.
- Drug references: Give up-to-date information on medications, their brand and generic names, their manufacturers, and other information such as recommended dosages.
- State and local medical directories: Provide credential information about medical colleagues and contain information such as the correct spelling of names, the office addresses, and the telephone numbers of physicians. Such directories may be used to compile a list of consulting physicians.

PERSONAL DEVELOPMENT PROJECTS

Key Terms

The following terms appear in **boldface** type in this chapter. Do you recall what they mean? Refer to the chapter for definitions you need to review.

abstracts	footnotes
bibliography	manuscript
card catalog	reprints
endnotes	rough draft
final draft	

Topics for Discussion

1. Compile for Dr. Newman a list of JAMA articles on the use of treatments employing laser technology. He suggests that you begin your research at the hospital's library.
2. Key a bibliography from handwritten notes. Some of the information is incomplete because it is missing the year of publication and author. How will you find the correct information to complete this task?

Role-Playing

1. You notice that a large stack of journals and reprints has accumulated on Dr. Newman's desk so that little room is left for the doctor to work. Dr. Newman has indicated that he is looking through this material for research information. Propose a method of organizing this material for Dr. Newman.
2. Two hours remain until the office closes for the day, and you have at least two hours of transcription to complete for patients seen today. Dr. Newman is actively involved with health care issues in government, and he often asks you to help prepare reports and correspondence to legislators on these issues. Today, he stops at your desk and asks you to key a six-page handwritten report before you leave this afternoon. How would you handle this situation?

Medical Meetings and Travel Arrangements

Most physicians hold memberships in several professional societies. This provides them with an opportunity to meet with colleagues, further their education, and keep informed of new developments in the medical, political, and manufacturing fields.

■ MEDICAL SOCIETIES

There are national, state, and local medical societies, and most doctors are members at all three levels.

The national medical association is the American Medical Association (AMA). It is an organization that promotes the advancement of medicine and health care, sponsors medical research, recommends health care activities, and promotes medical education. The AMA publishes one of the most widely distributed journals in the world, the weekly *Journal of the American Medical Association (JAMA)*.

The AMA holds an annual general convention. The program consists of business meetings at which members discuss and vote on matters of policy and scientific sessions devoted to the presentation of medical reports. Commercial exhibitors—manufacturers of drugs, instruments, nutritional products, medical books, office technology, and related items—also display their merchandise. The medical assistant who has the opportunity is urged to visit such a commercial exhibit. It will prove fascinating and informative.

In addition to the AMA, there are a number of national societies such as the American College of Surgeons and the American Psychiatric Association that represent other medical specialties and health care fields.

The societies publish their membership lists annually. The current membership list is a useful reference, especially if the doctor is an active participant in committee work within an organization.

A great deal of work is involved if the physician is an officer of a society or a member of a special committee. The secretary of a society, for example, prepares the **agenda** (the order of business for a meeting), compiles the membership list, attends to publicity, and records the minutes of the meetings. The treasurer of a society is responsible for collecting membership fees and handling all disbursements. The program committee plans and prepares the programs for all society meetings, usually a year in advance. The publication committee arranges for the publication of manuscripts read at the society meetings.

Participation by the physician in a society involves much interaction with other members, governmental agencies, and institutions, including a variety of correspondence. The assistant will be asked to complete many detailed assignments for the physician, including sending out notices of meetings, preparing agendas for meetings, and making travel arrangements.

■ MEDICAL SOCIETY MEETINGS

National and state societies hold meetings once or twice a year, but local societies usually hold monthly meetings.

The date and place of the next meeting of a national or state society is decided a year in advance of the meeting. This information is published in the national or state journal, and notices of the meeting are sent to organization members well in advance of the date set. The meeting information should be entered on the appointment calendar when the notice of the meeting arrives.

Local medical society meetings are generally held in the same location on certain days of the month. Meeting dates and programs are published in the local medical journal or newsletter. The dates should be marked on the appointment calendar, and a memorandum should be prepared and given to the doctor a few days in advance of the meeting.

If a special meeting is called to discuss an important business matter or a new development, an announcement of the meeting is sent to each member. A sample of a meeting announcement is shown in Figure 14-1 on page 238.

THE CHICAGO MEDICAL SOCIETY

PROGRAM COMMITTEE MEETING

Tuesday, December 2, 19—
7:30 p.m.

UNIVERSITY HOSPITAL
5500 North Ridgeway Avenue
ROOM 254C

Figure 14-1 Meeting
Announcement

PROJECT 49 Preparing An Announcement

Dr. Newman has decided to hold a staff meeting with all employees. He asks you to prepare an announcement on November 3 and post it in various locations throughout the office. The meeting will be held on November 10 from 11 a.m. to noon in the conference room. Lunch will be provided.

Make a notation on the file copy that the announcement was posted in the laboratory, in the X–ray department, in the nurses' station, and at the front desk.

File the announcement in your Miscellaneous folder.

Preparing for Meetings

Either the secretary of the organization or the committee chairperson is responsible for making the following arrangements for a meeting:

- Selecting and reserving the room (which involves speaking with managers of several possible sites and then confirming the reservation). The manager must be told the number of people attending the meeting and its scheduled length.
- Obtaining a speaker, inviting the speaker to the meeting, and confirming the speaker's acceptance of the invitation. The speaker's credentials should be obtained for the introduction.
- Arranging for the luncheon, the dinner, or other refreshments. This may include obtaining sample menus, making appropriate selections, and confirming the number of reservations.
- Noting the date and time of the meeting on the appointment calendar.
- Preparing and mailing the meeting agenda or notice of the meeting, and keeping a copy with a notation of the mailing date. Notices of the meeting should be mailed at least one week but

not more than two weeks prior to the meeting date. Agendas are generally mailed in advance to allow members time to prepare for the business of the meeting.

■ Keeping a record of all society members who are contacted regarding the meeting, noting names, telephone numbers, dates, and any special reasons for contacting them.

A sample agenda is shown in Figure 14-2. Note the large amount of white space, which enables members to make notes on the agenda regarding the meeting.

The assistant may be asked to perform last-minute duties for a meeting, including checking the room for the following:

■ Appropriate temperature.

■ An adequate number of chairs.

■ A writing board with marking pens or a chalk board with chalk and an eraser.

■ A podium and microphone.

■ Audiovisual equipment.

■ Fresh water.

■ An electronic or computer writing pad and appropriate pointer.

Agendas and other handouts should be ready for distribution before the meeting. The assistant may also be called upon to greet guests.

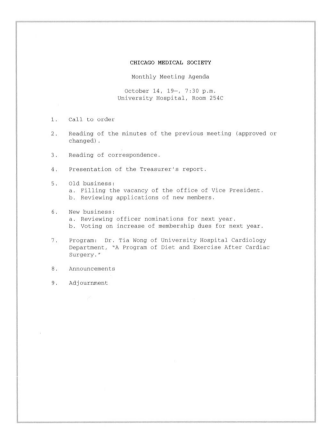

Figure 14-2 Meeting Agenda

Prepare an agenda for the staff meeting on November 10. This agenda should be posted in various locations throughout the office. Dr. Newman is going to discuss the following issues at the meeting: the National Medical Society meeting he will be attending in Phoenix from November 16 through 19; upcoming changes in office hours; additions to the office staff; medical students scheduled for family practice rotations in the practice; and updating charge slips to include additional common disease conditions.

File the agenda in your Miscellaneous folder.

Recording the Minutes

The official record of the proceedings of a meeting is called the **minutes**. The recording secretary is responsible for taking these notes and may ask the assistant to key them after the meeting. Meetings are conducted according to parliamentary procedure. Minutes may be formatted, as shown in Figure 14-3, in *(a)* formal style or in *(b)* informal style.

In special situations, verbatim minutes are recorded and later transcribed. If you are asked to record the minutes, be sure to familiarize yourself with the agenda, review names of attendees, sit next to the chairperson, and concentrate on the meeting. Read and refer to the

CHICAGO MEDICAL SOCIETY MINUTES

University Hospital, Room 254C

October 14, 19--

CALL TO ORDER	The monthly meeting of the Chicago Medical Society was held on October 14, 19--, in Room 254C at University Hospital. The meeting was called to order at 7:30 p.m. by President Dr. Lee Wentworth.
ATTENDANCE	The following members were present: Dr. Ernest Dodd, Dr. Brian Frieze, Dr. Rose Garcia, Dr. Marvin Kaser, Dr. Carol Mason, Dr. Jane Meyer, Dr. Mark Newman, Dr. Peter Schmidt, Dr. Yan Tuo, Dr. Lisa Twen, and Dr. Lee Wentworth.
MINUTES READING	Upon motion made, seconded, and unanimously passed, the reading of the minutes from the last meeting was waived.
TREASURER'S REPORT	The Treasurer reported that the society's bank balance as of October 12, 19--, was $1,254.72. There is one outstanding bill of $162.50 to the University Hospital Catering Service. A motion was made, seconded, and unanimously made to pay the bill.
VICE PRESIDENT VACANCY	The next matter of business was obtaining nominations for the office of Vice President. After discussion concerning the elections to be held in December for officers for next year, it was decided that the Treasurer would assume the duties of Vice President until the elections are held.
MEMBERSHIP APPLICANTS	Dr. Ernest Dodd of the Membership Committee reported on three physicians who made application for membership. These included Dr. Galen Becker, Dr. Monica Hover, and Dr. Mia Song. Their credentials were presented. A motion was made, seconded, and unanimously carried to admit the three applicants to the society. Dr. Dodd will notify the applicants in writing.
OFFICER ELECTIONS	A Nomination Committee was formed to meet in two weeks to review the officer nominations. Doctors Kaser, Tuo, and Wentworth volunteered for the committee.
MEMBERSHIP DUES	A motion was made to increase membership dues by $100 for the next year. This was seconded and unanimously carried to apply the increase for next year.
ADJOURNMENT	Upon motion, the meeting was adjourned at 8:45 p.m.

_____   _____
Recording Secretary   President

(a)

CHICAGO MEDICAL SOCIETY MINUTES

University Hospital, Room 254C

October 14, 19--

The monthly meeting of the Chicago Medical Society was held on October 14, 19--, in Room 254C at University Hospital. The meeting was called to order at 7:30 p.m. by President Dr. Lee Wentworth.

The following members were present: Dr. Ernest Dodd, Dr. Brian Frieze, Dr. Rose Garcia, Dr. Marvin Kaser, Dr. Carol Mason, Dr. Jane Meyer, Dr. Mark Newman, Dr. Peter Schmidt, Dr. Yan Tuo, Dr. Lisa Twen, and Dr. Lee Wentworth.

The reading of the minutes from the last meeting was waived.

The Treasurer reported that the society's bank balance as of October 12, 19--, was $1,254.72. There is one outstanding bill of $162.50 to the University Hospital Catering Service. A motion was made, seconded, and unanimously made to pay the bill.

The next matter of business was obtaining nominations for the office of Vice President. After discussion concerning the elections to be held in December for officers for next year, it was decided that the Treasurer would assume the duties of Vice President until the elections are held.

Dr. Ernest Dodd of the Membership Committee reported on three physicians who made application for membership. These included Dr. Galen Becker, Dr. Monica Hover, and Dr. Mia Song. Their credentials were presented. A motion was made, seconded, and unanimously carried to admit the three applicants to the society. Dr. Dodd will notify the applicants in writing.

A Nomination Committee was formed to meet in two weeks to review the officer nominations. Doctors Kaser, Tuo, and Wentworth volunteered for the committee.

A motion was made to increase membership dues by $100 for the next year. This was seconded and unanimously carried to apply the increase for next year.

Upon motion, the meeting was adjourned at 8:45 p.m.

_____   _____
Recording Secretary   President

(b)

Figure 14-3   Examples of *(a)* Formal and *(b)* Informal Minutes

minutes of previous meetings. Do not hesitate to ask for clarification of a certain point if you are unsure of what was said.

In verbatim minutes, it is not necessary to write down every word said at the meeting, but the pertinent discussion must be recorded word for word. A tape recorder is often used to record verbatim minutes, which can later be transcribed.

The following facts about the meeting should be noted:

- Date, location, time, and purpose of the meeting.
- Name of the presiding officer.
- Names of members in attendance.
- Order of business from the agenda.
- Motions made, whether approved or rejected (some organizations state the names of people who motioned and seconded).
- Summaries of discussions.

Minutes are signed by the recording secretary. They are kept in an official book of minutes and are taken to every meeting. Often, copies of the minutes are sent to each member after the meeting or are attached to the agenda before the next meeting.

PROJECT 51   **Recording Minutes of a Meeting**

Dr. Newman asks you to record the minutes of the staff meeting on November 10. Prepare the minutes in an informal style for distribution.

The proceedings of the staff meeting include the following items:

Attendance: Greg from the laboratory, Sharon from X ray, Karia from the nurses' station, Dr. Newman, and yourself.

Dr. and Mrs. Newman will be on vacation November 15 through 29. Dr. Newman will be attending the National Medical Society meeting in Phoenix from November 16 to 19.

Dr. Wanda Norberg will be the family practice resident for the first three-month rotation, starting December 3. Her hours have not yet been determined. Dr. Newman will issue a memorandum when the hours are set. All new patients, walk-ins, and emergencies will be assigned to Dr. Norberg, and Dr. Newman may assign other patients to her as well. Dr. Newman may also lengthen his office hours.

The practice will hire a new laboratory person capable of taking X rays, to work from 1 to 4 p.m. each day. A part-time receptionist also will be hired. Consideration will be given to hiring additional nursing staff in the near future.

Dr. Newman and you will code common diseases for charge slips.

There will be one more staff meeting prior to Dr. Norberg's arrival on staff. You are to let Dr. Newman know any issues that should be discussed at the meeting.

File the completed minutes in your Miscellaneous folder.

■ **PROGRAM PARTICIPATION**

A doctor may be asked to participate as a program speaker by invitation, as a result of offering to report some new developments or research, or after responding to a call for papers by the society sponsoring the program. The title of the lecture and an outline or a summary usually must be submitted to the program committee by a specified date.

Preparing for the Lecture

After the doctor has accepted a speaking engagement, various tasks must be completed by the assistant. A folder for the speaking engagement should be prepared; it will contain all notes and correspondence pertaining to the lecture. If handouts are needed for the presentation, they must be created and an adequate number of copies must be made for distribution. Audiovisual material must be assembled, checked against the manuscript of the presentation, and arranged in proper order.

As soon as possible, the following information about the presentation should be given to the program chairperson:

- Exact title of the lecture.
- Approximate length of the lecture.
- Audiovisual equipment that will be needed.
- Biographical credentials of the speaker.

The chairperson needs a curriculum vitae in order to introduce the speaker, to print excerpts in the program, and to use for publicity purposes. A **curriculum vitae**, like the one shown in Figure 14-4, is biographical information about a person's education, experience, and professional and community activities.

CURRICULUM VITAE

KAREN LARSEN, M.D.
Board Certified in Family Practice
2785 South Ridgeway Avenue
Chicago, IL 60647-2700
312-555-2700

EDUCATION:		
Resident:	University Medical School Chicago, Illinois Family Practice	1990–1992
Internships:	Western Family Practice Beltsville, Maryland	1989–1990
	University Family Clinic Chicago, Illinois	1988–1989
Medical School:	University Medical School Chicago, Illinois M.D. Degree	1988
Undergraduate:	University of Minnesota Minneapolis, Minnesota	
EXPERIENCE:	Medical Director, Family Practice Ridgeway Family Practice Chicago, Illinois	1995–present
	Associate Professor of Family Practice University Medical School, Chicago, Illinois	1993–1995
PROFESSIONAL ACTIVITIES:	American Board of Family Practice University Medical School Alumni American Medical Association Chicago Medical Society	
COMMUNITY ACTIVITIES:	Chicago Chamber of Commerce University Faculty Association Girl Scouts of America	

Figure 14-4   Curriculum Vitae

Keying the Lecture

The length of time allowed for reading a paper varies at different meetings. A paper should be carefully planned to conform to the time limitation. As a rule, a printed page of 250 words takes about two minutes to read at medium speed. If the author speaks freely or uses only notes, care should be taken to watch the time while lecturing. If the paper is read, the print should be clear and dark. Some speakers may prefer to have the notes printed in large type.

The draft of any speech or report is typed in standard manuscript style: double-spaced with 1-inch side margins. The final copy of the speech may be triple-spaced with even wider margins. This extra space allows easy reading and space for the doctor to make notes and indicate where audiovisual materials are to be used.

PROJECT 52   Confirming Speaking Arrangements

Dr. Newman has been asked to give a lecture to the local American Legion post at its January 12 meeting. Write a letter to Paul Berman, Commander of Post 211, 7431 West 82 Place, Chicago, IL 60652-1134.

Indicate that Dr. Newman is pleased to accept the invitation, that the speech is entitled "Caffeine Intoxication," and that it is about 30 minutes in length. Dr. Newman would like to use a chalkboard, if one is available.

Enclose a biographical sketch of Dr. Newman on a separate sheet of paper including the following information: Place of birth—Reno, Nevada; medical degree—University of Minnesota; internship—Cook County Hospital in Chicago; residency—Family Medicine, University of Minnesota Hospital; board certified in Family Medicine; currently on teaching staff at the University Medical School, Chicago, specializing in family practice; memberships—AMA, Illinois Medical Association, Chicago Medical Society; office address.

Date the letter and the biography November 10, and file the items in your Miscellaneous folder.

■ PREPARATIONS FOR A TRIP

When the doctor travels for professional or personal reasons, the medical assistant will be involved in preparing for the trip and will have many obligations while the doctor is away. In preparing for the doctor's trip, the assistant must consult with the doctor, carefully noting the date and time of departure, destinations, length of stay at each destination, and times of arrival at and departure from each destination.

A folder should be kept for any information about the trip. After the doctor returns, some of this material can be discarded, and the rest filed in the usual manner.

Travel Arrangements

The best resource for travel information is a skilled agent at a reputable travel agency. The travel agent is trained to assist in almost every aspect of travel plans—making travel and hotel reservations, issuing tickets for travel, renting cars, helping to get documentation for foreign travel, and obtaining tickets for entertainment.

Reservations should be made at the earliest possible time to allow the travel agent an opportunity to secure economical rates for the best means of travel available and to research alternative arrangements. The travel agent can provide information about luggage limitations, car rental plans, and international travel.

Foreign countries have various requirements regarding immunizations, passports, and **visas** (temporary visitation permits). In order to travel abroad, a traveler must obtain a **passport** in advance by submitting a passport picture and an application to a passport agent's office. Once issued, the passport is good for five years.

If travel reservations are made by telephone, tickets may be sent to the office or may have to be picked up at a certain location. After receiving the tickets, carefully check them to be sure all information is correct.

Hotel Reservations

As soon as possible, hotel accommodations should be made and a room reserved. Most resort hotels and hotel chains have toll-free telephone numbers for reservations. Some hotels require a deposit for a room reservation or a credit card number to hold a room for late arrival. Request confirmation of reservations in writing if time permits, and give the confirmation number to the doctor before departure.

Itinerary

If the doctor plans to visit several places, an itinerary must be prepared. Travel agencies provide itineraries as part of their service. An **itinerary** is a list that specifies each place the traveler will visit, the name and address of the hotel, and the date and time of arrival and departure. In addition to the doctor's copy, the assistant must keep a copy for reference in contacting the doctor. Itineraries may include a person's schedule at a convention. See Figure 14-5 for a sample itinerary format.

Travel Funds

One of the most practical methods of carrying money while traveling is **traveler's checks**. These can be purchased at most banks for a small charge. The purchaser signs each check at the time of purchase and then countersigns the check in the presence of the person cashing it. Thus, the doctor must obtain traveler's checks in person. If the traveler's checks are lost, the money is refunded.

Another popular method of payment during travel is the use of credit cards. People who travel can charge purchases, hotels, meals, and transportation. Some cards are universally accepted and provide the user with a quick method of payment for any necessary purchases or services.

```
                              ITINERARY
     Mark Newman, M.D.                                    April 19--
                       (Chicago, New York City, Boston)

     Friday, April 10
     (Chicago--New York City)
          5:00 p.m., CST     Depart Chicago, O'Hare International, American
                             Airlines, nonstop flight 104, 727.  Dinner.

          8:00 p.m., EST     Arrive New York, Kennedy International Airport.

                             Accommodations:  Americana Hotel, 52d Street and
                             Seventh Avenue, New York, NY  10019.

     Sunday, April 12
     (New York City--Boston)
          7:00 p.m., EST     Depart New York, La Guardia Airport, American
                             Airlines, nonstop flight 526, 727.

          8:01 p.m., EST     Arrive Boston, Logan International Airport.

                             Accommodation:  Sheraton-Boston Hotel, Prudential
                             Center, Boston, MA  02199.

     Monday, April 13
          Reminder           Make dinner reservations.

          7:30 p.m., EST     Dinner with Dr. and Mrs. Charles Whitfield.

     Tuesday, April 14
     (Boston--Chicago)
          6:45 p.m., EST     Depart Boston, Logan International Airport, American
                             Airlines, nonstop flight 157, DC10.  Dinner.

          8:12 p.m., CST     Arrive Chicago, O'Hare International.
```

Figure 14-5   Travel Itinerary

If the trip is connected with the doctor's practice, travel expenses may be deductible for income tax purposes. It is necessary, however, to retain receipts for every expenditure. The doctor will need to keep an accurate and detailed record of expenses. After the doctor's return, expenses can be tabulated and entered in the appropriate accounting records, and the receipts can be filed.

PROJECT 53   Keying An Itinerary

Dr. and Mrs. Newman will be leaving November 15 for the National Medical Society convention in Phoenix, Arizona. Dr. Newman hands you the convention itinerary (WPs 102 through 103) on which he checked the sessions he registered to attend. Also, he gives you the handwritten itinerary, WP 104, which includes addresses and telephone numbers of the hotels where he and his wife will be staying. Key a new itinerary for Dr. and Mrs. Newman by combining the checked sessions on the convention schedule with the handwritten itinerary. Place a copy of the new itinerary in the Travel folder after you photocopy it for the office file.

■ DUTIES DURING THE DOCTOR'S ABSENCE

The assistant has a double responsibility when left to run the office in the doctor's absence. In addition to regular duties, there are a variety of office management tasks that must be attended to, and the doctor must be kept informed of any new developments.

Financial Duties

Arrangements for paying bills during the doctor's absence must be made before the doctor leaves. If the doctor is away for an extended period of time, a lawyer or bank may be designated to take care of any expenses that the assistant forwards.

Appointments

As soon as dates for the doctor's trip are known, the appointment book must be marked accordingly so that no patients will be scheduled at that time. Patients who have regular appointments may have to be notified that the doctor will be away. A new appointment should be scheduled if necessary, and the patient should be told that another physician is on call if needed.

The name, address, and telephone number of the covering doctor should be placed by the telephone so that the information is readily available if a patient calls and needs to speak or meet with a physician.

Telephone Calls

Telephone calls are handled in the same way as they are when the doctor is in the office. The important point is to follow through on as many calls as possible so that only a few matters are left pending. A telephone log should be kept of all calls, noting the action taken. If a patient calls for an appointment and needs to be seen before the doctor returns, the patient should be referred to the doctor on call.

Mail and Reports

Whether or not to forward letters and status reports depends on the length of time the doctor is away from the office and the urgency of the matter. If a reply to a letter must wait until the doctor returns, acknowledge receipt of the letter and state the circumstances and when the physician will return.

If the doctor is absent for a month or more, the doctor may request that the assistant forward a written office status report or that the assistant check in periodically and make a verbal report over the telephone. Keep a daily log of phone calls, correspondence, and important matters that should be included in your report. Reports on other routine matters should be kept in a separate folder to await the doctor's return.

Spare Time

While the doctor is away, the assistant may have free time in the office. This is a good time to do many things for which there is little opportunity when the doctor has a busy appointment schedule. Here are a few suggestions:

- Clean out files and replace worn folders.
- Make new labels for all types of containers.
- Straighten out supply cabinets.
- Update procedures manual.
- Have curtains, rugs, and draperies cleaned.

Discuss this aspect of your responsibilities with the doctor. Perhaps other more extensive work can be done at this time, such as sending apparatus or furniture for repair, having the offices and examination rooms painted, or having floors waxed.

PROJECT 54 Changing the Schedule

Dr. Newman has helped you cancel patients' appointments scheduled for the days he will be away on vacation. The appointments have been rescheduled for earlier dates. Update your appointment book to reflect the following changes:

November 17: Change the Mitchell family appointments to November 12, with Erin Mitchell at 10:00 and Donald Mitchell at 10:15 (David Kramer does not need a separate appointment for his immunizations). Change Sarah Morton's appointment to 11:15 on November 12.

November 18: Change Clarence Rogers' consultation from November 12 to 11:30 on November 11, and change his vasectomy to 11:30 on November 12.

November 19: Change the November 19 appointments to the following times on November 11: Florence Sherman, 10:30; Theresa Dayton, 10:45; and Charles Jonathan III, 11:15.

Key Terms

The following terms appear in **boldface** type in this chapter. Do you recall what they mean? Refer to the chapter for definitions you need to review.

agenda	minutes
curriculum vitae	passport
itinerary	traveler's checks
Journal of the American Medical Association (JAMA)	visas

Topics for Discussion

1. It is your day to cover the switchboard. Dr. Newman asks you to attend a meeting and take minutes because he has an emergency and cannot attend the meeting. Discuss how will you handle this situation.

2. The office where you work has scheduled monthly staff meetings. At the meetings, each staff member is asked in turn if he or she has any concerns to be discussed. Lunch is provided during these meetings, since they take up the entire lunch period, but the meetings often seem unproductive. Discuss what suggestions might you offer.

Role-Playing

1. You have never taken minutes at a meeting before, and now you have been asked to do this task. Explain this situation to your supervisor.

2. During a meeting, one of the participants requests information that you know Dr. Newman has on a folder on his desk. Dr. Newman is not attending this meeting and is out of the office. How will you respond?

SIMULATION 4-A

Today you will begin your final simulation in Dr. Newman's office. The days will be Tuesday, November 11, and Wednesday, November 12.

PROCEDURES

Review the "General Procedures" in Simulation 1 for handling simulations. Follow the same instructions—under "Specific Procedures"—for Day 1 and 2 as in Simulation 1.

MATERIALS

The materials you will need are generally the same as those listed for Simulation 1. Each day, pull the patients' charts and ledgers according to the appointment calendar and put them in your To-Do folder.

Materials	Source

Appointment calendar

Card file

Supplies folder

Miscellaneous folder

Procedures Manual pages (5 items)	Project 47
"Caffeine Intoxication" manuscript	Project 48
Staff meeting announcement	Project 49
Agenda	Project 50
Staff minutes	Project 51
Letter to American Legion Post 211	Project 52
Dr. Newman's curriculum vitae	Project 52

Travel folder

Itinerary	Project 53

To-Do folder

Day 1
Patients' charts for November 3–11

Telephone Log	WP 105
To-do list	WP 106
Incoming letter	WP 107
Charge slips for November 11	WP 108
Rough draft FAX form	WP 109
Incoming checks	WP 110
Daily journal 11/3–10	WP 111
Daily journal 11/11	WP 112
Registration form for Ellen Stevens	WP 113
Insurance form for Florence Sherman	WP 114

Day 2
Patient's charts for November 11

Lab slips: Babcock and Armstrong	WP 115
Note concerning Sarah Morton	WP 116
Charge Slips	WP 116–117
Incoming checks	WP 118
Insurance form for Erin Mitchell	WP 119
Insurance form for Gary Robertson	WP 120
Daily journal 11/12	WP 121

Patients' folders
Patient charts and ledger cards for all current patients.

If you have not completed all the projects and do not have all these records set up in advance, talk with your instructor.

MEDICAL VOCABULARY

The following medical terms are used in Simulation 4. Review each term and its meaning.

clown–slapped appearance: pattern of erythema on cheeks.
dyschezia: pain during a bowel movement.
Fifth's disease: a disease whose symptoms include rash with characteristic cheek redness.
fulgurated: cauterized or burned.
omentum: one of several folds of the peritoneum lining the abdominal cavity.
otitis externa: inflammation of the external ear.
retro–ocular: located behind the eyeball.
rhomboideus muscle: a muscle located in the midupper back near the neck.
Saulter II fracture: a hand fracture with specific criteria.
Waters view of X ray: an X–ray technique used to demonstrate the sinuses.

SIMULATION 4-B

Simulation 4B is similar to Simulation 4A. However, the activities for Simulation 4B are meant to be done on the computer using MediSoft and the Student Data Disk. If you have not done exercises in this text in Medisoft earlier, read Appendix A of this textbook before proceeding.

The days of this simulation are Tuesday, November 11, and Wednesday, November 12, 1997.

Print Tuesday's schedule for Dr. Newman:

1. Put the Student Data Disk in drive A:.
2. At the prompt: c:\MEDISOFT> (with the Student Data Disk in drive A:), key *hours*.
3. Press Enter.
4. Press Spacebar. At Go to date on the screen, key *111197*.
5. Press F2 to print. Select *N* at Include empty time slots? (Y/N/Esc).
6. Select *S* at Print Detail or Summary list? (D/S/Esc).
7. Press ESC to exit.

Establish Dr. Norberg in the practice.

1. At the prompt: C:\MEDISOFT> (with the Student Data Disk in drive A:), key *ME*.
2. Press Enter. Key in a date or press Enter.
3. Select (1) for Set–Up Office and (2) for Provider Information.
4. Enter Dr. Norberg's information as follows:
   Same address and phone number as Dr. Newman.
   Social Security Number: 672–43–4576 (Key in number without hyphens.)
   License number is 1–78987
   Medicare PIN is WN–82732
   Medicaid PIN is 904323.
   CHAMPUS PIN is 678549.
5. Press F3 to save.

Go to the Office Hours Scheduler. (If you have questions, review Appendix A at this point.) Go to December 03, 1997 and block off everything except hours 2:00 to 4:00 on Dr. Norberg's schedule and make sure to save this information. Print a copy of the 12/03/97 schedule. Do the same for December 10, 1997. Print a copy of that schedule also.

Establish an appointment in the Entry Operations section of MediSoft for Florence Sherman with Dr. Norberg at 2:00 p.m. on December 10, for a Blood Pressure Check (takes 15 minutes) and save that information. (Refer to Appendix A if you have any questions.) Enter the patient information for Ellen Stevens on WP 113 into MediSoft. Check Appendix A if you have any questions. Make sure to save the information.

Enter the transactions shown on WP 111. Refer to Appendix A if you have any questions. Print a patient insurance form for each transaction. Print a Patient Day Sheet for 11/11/97.

Introduction to MediSoft

MediSoft is a widely used patient accounting program for medical and dental offices. In this text you are studying the administrative tasks of the medical assistant. When you work as an administrative medical assistant, it is likely that you will encounter some sort of patient accounting software. The MediSoft program includes the basic operations of all patient accounting software programs. Familiarizing yourself with MediSoft will enable you to learn almost any similar software in a very brief period of time.

For training purposes, a Student Data Disk accompanies this text. This disk allows you to work in MediSoft without anyone else putting information onto your disk. Before you start MediSoft on the school's computer, you must insert your own Student Data Disk. If you do not, the MediSoft on the school's computer will not work properly. Make sure to read the next section, "Handling Your Student Data Disk," before you actually start MediSoft.

Later on in this appendix, you will find specific instructions for the exercises in the text that are marked with the icon ▣. These instructions contain helpful hints for completion of the exercises.

■ HANDLING YOUR STUDENT DATA DISK

The Student Data Disk that you received with this textbook is where you will store data in MediSoft. Used in conjunction with the MediSoft software on your school's computer, you will work on patient accounting scheduling almost in the same way as in a medical office.

The first step before you actually use the Student Data Disk should be to make a copy. Some of the computers in your school will have special procedures or ways to copy disks. Consult your instructor. If you can get to the command prompt c:\>, follow the instructions below.

If you have DOS 3.3 or above and a single floppy drive, insert your Student Data Disk into drive A. At the command prompt C:\>, key *diskcopy a: a:* and then press Enter. After the machine reads your Student Data Disk, it will tell you to insert a new (blank) formatted disk. After you do so, the computer will tell you to press Enter. The computer will then copy the data back onto the blank disk.

If you have difficulty copying your disk, ask your instructor for help. Remember to always have your Student Data Disk in the machine when you go into and exit MediSoft.

■ STARTING MEDISOFT

The computer in your school may have several ways of accessing MediSoft software. There may be an icon which you double-click with a mouse, or you may have a prompt C:\MEDISOFT> on the screen. There are other alternatives depending on the setup at your particular school.

However you start MediSoft, the most important single thing to re-member is **to put the Student Data Disk into the floppy drive (usu-ally Drive A:) before** opening MediSoft. In the school situation, the data you input will go only to the Student Data Disk. Opening MediSoft without the disk will mean that you will not send data onto your disk and the program will not work properly.

If the school's computer opens to C:\MEDISOFT>, make sure the Student Data Disk is in Drive A: and key *me*. The opening screen (Figure A-1) will have the field: Enter Today's Date highlighted. Follow the date instructions for each exercise at the end of this appendix. See below for instructions on how to enter a date.

The MediSoft software in your school may be on a network. If so, you must specify the filename provided by your instructor to access MediSoft. Ask your instructor for specific directions.

> Always insert your Student Data Disk before starting MediSoft.

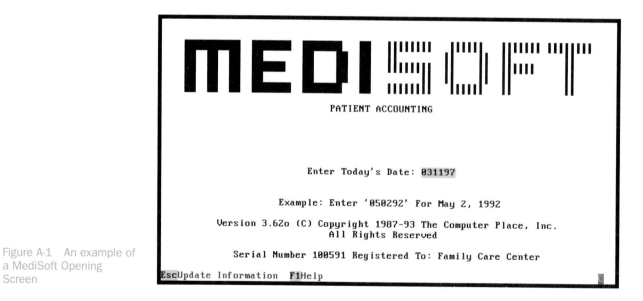

PATIENT ACCOUNTING

Enter Today's Date: `031197`

Example: Enter '050292' For May 2, 1992

Version 3.62o (C) Copyright 1987-93 The Computer Place, Inc.
All Rights Reserved

Serial Number 100591 Registered To: Family Care Center

`Esc`Update Information `F1`Help

Figure A-1 An example of a MediSoft Opening Screen

Entering a Date

To enter a date, enter the numbers in the MMDDYY format. MM stands for the month (for example, January is 01 and October is 10). DD stands for the day (for example, the ninth day of the month is 09). YY stands for the year (for example, 1997 is 97).

After entering the date, press Enter.

■ MEDISOFT MENUS

The screen following the opening screen is the MediSoft Operations Menu (Figure A-2). The Operations Menu has nine menu choices on the left. Each choice, when highlighted, changes the Sub-Menu Selection Window on the right. Press Enter to get into the Sub-Menu Selection Window.

The nine Operations Menu choices and their functions are as follows:

(1) **Set-Up Office** is used to enter all office information. In addition to the names of the doctors, important other names, addresses, and phone numbers, this is where all the data about the procedures performed in the office and the costs for those procedures are entered. Also, information about the insurance companies to which the office submits claims is entered here.

(2) **Patient Information** is the menu option that allows the medical assistant to enter all patient data. The information is first entered from the patient information forms that new patients fill out at their first visit. This information is updated whenever the patient changes address information, marital status, insurance companies, and so on.

(3) **Entry Operations** lets the medical assistant enter all financial transactions having to do with patient services. All charges and pay-

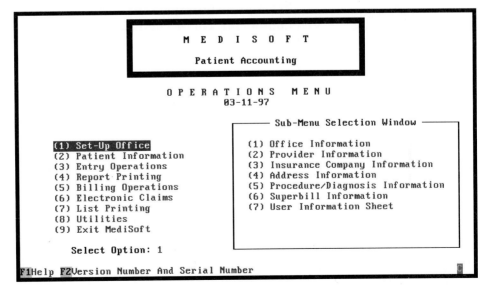

Figure A-2   An example of a MediSoft Operations Menu

ments are recorded here, as are patient appointments (other than those entered in the Office Hours Scheduler discussed later).

(4) **Report Printing** This option allows the printing of reports about the practice and about patients' accounts.

(5) **Billing Operations** This option is used to print insurance claim forms, patient statements, and various other insurance-related items.

(6) **Electronic Claims** Many medical practices submit claims electronically. This menu option is used to transmit insurance claims electronically either directly to insurance companies or indirectly through a clearing house that handles claims.

(7) **List Printing** This menu option is used to print a variety of lists having to do with the practice in general, such as patient lists, or with some specific item, such as lists of appointments by the day, week, or month.

(8) **Utilities** This group of sub-menu selections includes the housekeeping functions, such as backing up data, restoring files, month-end processing, and so on. Data in MediSoft is backed up onto the C:\ drive and the data is condensed automatically. (The Utilities menu will not be used in your school setting. If you were to back up data, you would not be able to reuse your Student Data Disk.)

> Never try to back up data when using the Student Data Disk.

(9) **Exit MediSoft** This menu option takes you out of the MediSoft Operations Menu and brings you to a flashing screen that recommends you make a backup of your MediSoft data every day. **DO NOT DO THIS**. In an office setting, you would do this every day. However, in this version, just press Enter to get to the C:\MEDISOFT> prompt.

■ SETTING UP THE OFFICE

In the previous section, you learned how to get to the MediSoft Operations Menu. This section discusses the first Sub-Menu Selection Window. Figure A-2 shows this sub-menu in the box on the right. When you press Enter, eight items appear in the sub-menu. Each will be described here. To get to the sub-menu, press Enter when the Set-Up Office choice is highlighted.

Office Information

The section on Office Information is automatically highlighted first. Press Enter. The screen shows Data Path: A:\ and asks Do You Want to Change The Current Data File Path? Select [N] for No. The next screen shows the office information for Dr. Mark Newman. He is the primary doctor in the office. (This information has already been set up on the Student Data Disk.)

name, the first two letters of the first name, and the digit 0, which represents head of household in the MediSoft software. If the last name has less than five letters, use more letters of the first name and even of the middle name if necessary. To find a patient who is already entered, you key in the appropriate chart number and press Enter. To enter a new patient, you enter the chart number and then add all the information you have into the various fields in the primary screen and the secondary screen of the Patient Information section.

If you do not know whether or not a patient is entered, press F6 to search and key the first letter of the patient's last name. Try to find the chart for Thomas Baab. You could either search the letter B, or you could put BAABTHOO in the Chart Number field. *Hint:* At the end of a search, press ESC to get back to the Chart Number field. Once you enter the chart number, press Enter to proceed.

Patient Data

Look at Thomas Baab's chart in MediSoft. The next fields under Chart Number are **Patient Name, Street, City Line, Phone, Social Security, Birth Date,** and **Sex**. These can usually be entered from a new Patient Information Form, if they are not already present. The Phone field is a ten-digit field, so enter only the numbers without any parentheses or hyphens. The Social Security Number field is nine digits, so do not enter any hyphens even though they will show up automatically on the chart.

Some of the fields are optional. When you come to 2nd phone, press Enter and proceed unless you know that the patient has a work number. If so, you can enter it there. Listed below are the other fields in the Patient Information section with instructions for entering data.

Billing Code: The billing code is set up for each individual office. For example, patients with billing code A are billed on the 15th of each month. For purposes of this text, key *X* in this field.

Indicator: Indicator is an optional code used to classify patients as a group. For instance, all diabetics might be given the Indicator D, so that a particular office would be sure to send out any appropriate newsletters or other mailings. For this text, press Enter and skip this field.

Assigned Provider: Enter *1* for Dr. Newman and *2* for Dr. Norberg. Press Enter.

Medicare?: Answer *Y* or *N*. Press Enter.

Employer: If patient is employed, enter the appropriate Employer name in this field and phone in the next.

Location: Location is an optional field if the patient works for an employer with several locations. Skip this field for this text.

Primary Insured Medisoft will automatically enter the patient's chart number in once you press Enter. In some situations, such as in a family practitioner's office, you may have a child as the patient and one of the parents as the primary insured. In other cases, only one spouse will have the primary insurance, and that spouse should be entered instead of the patient. When entering someone other than the patient into this field, key in the other person's chart number.

Rel. is short for relation. Enter one of the following codes in this field:

1 The patient is the insured.
2 The patient is the spouse of the insured.
3 The patient is the child of the insured.
4 Other.

Insurance Company,% covered, and **Policy Number** can usually be obtained from the new patient's information form. Enter a number for the insurance company. (***Hint:*** Get the number from the Insurance Company Information in the Set-Up Office section of the Operations Menu if you do not know it.) Most policies cover 80%, and that should be entered if it is the case.

Group is the Insurance group number; enter it if you know it. Otherwise, press Enter.

Secondary Insured is for additional insurance, such as when two members of a family carry insurance. The software will enter the patient unless otherwise instructed.

Accept Assignment?: is the field where you enter either *Y* (yes, the doctor accepts the insurance as payment) or *N* (no, the doctor does not accept it; the patient must pay and be reimbursed by the insurance company).

Signature on Ins.?: is the field in which you key *Y* to print the insured's name on the signature part of the insurance form or *N* to leave the signature line blank. Key *N* for patients in this text.

Balances will come up automatically if you have entered any transactions for a patient.

Patient Information—Supplement Screen

To move to the next page of Patient Information (Figure A-4), press F4. All the fields are optional and relate to particular accidents or illnesses for each patient. The bottom of the screen usually gives you the options for each field, such as *Y* for Yes or *N* for No. Several abbreviations that you may not be familiar with are EPSDT, which is the Medicaid well-baby program (*Y* if the patient qualifies, *N* if not), and LMP, which stands for *last menstrual period* (put a date in—use the MMDDYY format). Once you have entered all the patient information and checked your work, press F3 to save. Press ESC twice to exit to the Operations Menu.

Editing Patient Information

To change patient information, go to the patient's chart, use the up

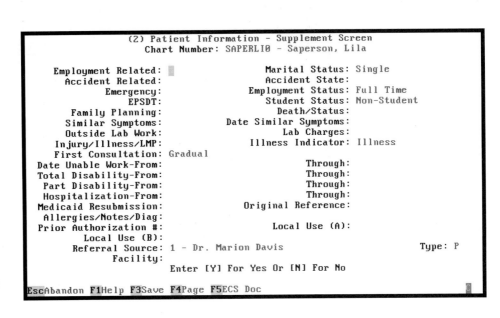

Figure A-4   Patient Information Supplemental Screen

and down arrows to move the cursor to the field you want changed, and key in the new information. When the field has been corrected, move the cursor to the end of the page (if you do not go all the way to the end, it will not save the changes), and press F3 to save.

■ ENTRY OPERATIONS

The sub-menu for Entry Operations has three choices: **Transaction Entry, Appointment Entry,** and **Exit to Medisoft Menu.** The first is used to record any charges, payments, procedures, and diagnoses given to patients on a particular date. The Appointment Entry option is usually used for callback appointments, and the Exit option is used to return to the main menu.

Transaction Entry—Recording Charges

Highlight the Transaction Entry option and press Enter (see Figure A-5). You will find the cursor at Chart Number. Key in the patient's chart number. If you do not know it, press F6 to search by the first letter of the patient's last name. Press ESC to close the search box.

Enter the patient's chart number and the cursor will move to the **Document.** The document number is the date of the transaction entry done as YYMMDD. Each patient may have a number of documents for transactions on different days but usually will have only one number on any given day.

Press Enter, and the date is automatically put under the date column. Next, the **Procedure** column is used to key in the procedure performed at a visit. If there are multiple procedures, enter the number of each procedure on a separate line. To find procedure numbers,

The document number for November 12, 1998 = 981112

```
Chart Number:                                    Document:
 DATE         PROCEDURE        LOC     DIAGNOSIS      CHARGE UNITS PROV




















 Perm. Diag:                                        Total:
 Med:   Pri:
        Sec:
      Balance:          Last Pay Amount:          Last Pay Date:


EscMenu F1Help F5Recall F6Search F8Add F9Change
```

Figure A-5 Transaction
Entry Screen

press F6 to search. For example, if the procedure is a hospital visit, either search for the letter h or the letter v to find out the procedure number. Press ESC to exit the search once you have the number. Key the number in the procedure column.

The next column is **LOC.**, short for Location. Most offices have a series of codes indicating whether the visit took place at the hospital, a clinic, in the office, and so on. For this text, press Enter to leave this column blank.

The cursor then moves to the **Diagnosis** column. Again, if you know the diagnosis code, key it in the column; if not, press F6 to search any letter in the diagnosis. You can also leave this column blank if you do not know the diagnosis. The software will automatically repeat the patient's diagnosis for each procedure once you have entered it. If you do not want it, you must use the delete key on the keyboard to remove it character by character.

Next, the charge will be entered automatically, or you can key it in manually. Then the cursor moves to **Units.** This is usually 1 but can be more. For example, if a patient has had three hospital visits at $70.00 per visit, key 3, and the amount will be changed. The cursor goes to the **PROV** column, which is where you key the provider number. Check your work and press F3 to total the amounts and then press Enter to save.

Transaction Entry—Recording Payments

Payments are recorded in the same area as charges. In the Entry Operations Sub-Menu, highlight Transaction Entry and press Enter. Key in the patient's Chart Number. The Document number is the date in YYMMDD format. Press Enter to move to the Date field. Enter the date of the payment if it is not the same as the date shown.

Go to the procedure field. Most offices will set up a coding system for the type of payment received. For the purposes of this text, choose the appropriate code from the following list:

01 Patient payment, cash
02 Patient payment, check
03 Insurance carrier payment
04 Adjustment, insurance company
05 Adjustment, patient

Enter all payments without a dollar sign. You only need to include a decimal point for amounts that include cents. For example, a payment of $27.50 is keyed as –27.50.

Skip the Location field. In Diagnosis, enter a check number or other note about the payment.

In Charge, enter the amount of the payment or adjustment. Always show the payment or adjustment as a negative, since this reduces the amount the patient owes.

In Units, key *1*. In Prov, key the number of the patient's provider. Check all the data, press Enter until you get to **Last Pay Date**, and press F3 to save.

NOTE: Remember that some payments may cover a number of charges. This is particularly true for insurance payments that may cover many charges. Make sure to enter each portion of the payment that applies to a specific charge separately so that the amounts will be applied to the correct charge. In **Charge,** key in only the portion of the payment applicable to a specific charge.

Appointment Entry

The next sub-menu item is **Appointment Entry**. This section is generally used for recall appointments. For example, the doctor writes a note about having the patient return in two weeks for a specific text. You find out what time is convenient for the patient, go to the sub-menu item, and press Enter (Figure A-6).

The first field is **Patient.** Enter the appropriate chart number. (You can use F6 search if you are not sure.) The next field is **Provider.** Key in the appropriate provider number.

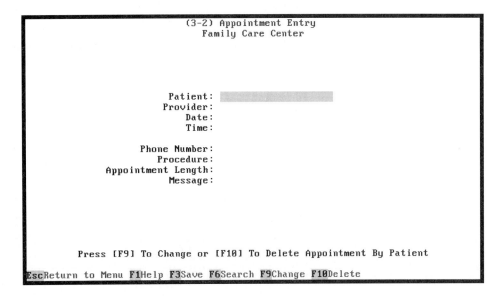

```
                    (3-2) Appointment Entry
                       Family Care Center




                Patient:  ▒▒▒▒▒▒▒▒▒▒▒▒▒▒▒▒
               Provider:
                   Date:
                   Time:

           Phone Number:
              Procedure:
      Appointment Length:
                Message:




        Press [F9] To Change or [F10] To Delete Appointment By Patient
EscReturn to Menu F1Help F3Save F6Search F9Change F10Delete
```

Figure A-6 Appointment Entry Screen

The next two fields call for a **Date** and **Time** of the appointment. Then key in the patient's phone number in the next field if it does not appear automatically. The **Procedure** field calls for a code to be entered. Press F6 to search if you need to. You may also leave this field blank.

The last two fields are for **Appointment Length** and **Message.** Both of these fields can be left blank by pressing Enter. If you know the length of the appointment or if it does not appear automatically, key in the number of minutes. The message field is for any notes the doctor may have about the appointment, up to 30 characters.

Press F3 to save the appointment or ESC if you do not want to save it. To delete an appointment once the appointment is displayed, press F10. (To display an appointment, press F9 in the patient field. Once you have entered the patient's Chart Number, all appointments will be displayed by pressing F9. Choose the appointment you wish to delete.)

NOTE: All appointments made in Appointment entry are also stored in the Office Hours Scheduler and vice versa.

The third sub-menu option returns you to the MediSoft Operations Menu.

■ REPORT PRINTING

Highlight the **Report Printing** option and press Enter. The sub-menu has six choices for types of reports. Reports are needed to analyze cash flow in a practice, to verify a daily total, to look at patients' accounts, and so on.

Transaction Entries

The first option, **Transaction Entries,** gives you lists of transactions (charges, adjustments, or payments) that have taken place over a specific period of time and for a specific provider or all providers. Highlight this option and press Enter (Figure A-7).

The **Date of Report** field should be the date on which you are printing the report. The **Range of Procedure Codes** should be all (which is the default for this field) if you wish to see all transactions for a period of time. A report could, however, list only deliveries or x-rays performed if that is what is specified.

The next field is **Range of Dates.** Key the dates for which you want transactions given. This could be a day, all (the default), or a week, a month, and so on. Use the MMDDYY-MMDDYY format to key in the range or just one date (MMDDYY) for one day.

Range of Entries is a field either to limit the number of transactions you wish to print or to print all (the default). The bottom of the screen tells you how many entries are available to print. These numbers represent the number of transactions entered (a number is given to each transaction).

```
                    (4-1) Print Transaction Entries
                           Family Care Center




                     Date of Report: ▒▒▒▒▒
              Range of Procedure Codes:
                        Range of Dates:
                       Range of Entries:
                     Range of Providers:
```

EscReturn to Menu F1Help

Figure A-7   Sample Print Screen Options

Range of Providers allows you to print each provider's transactions separately or all together. Enter the provider numbers you want.

When you press Enter at the end of the last field, the field **Enter Print Option** will be displayed. Key in *P* to print the report, *D* to display the report on the screen, and *F* to save the report to a file for later printing or use. Figure A-8 shows a sample transaction journal report.

Print Patient Ledgers

The next sub-menu choice, **Print Patient Ledgers,** allows you to print a record of a patient's account, including all charges, payments, and adjustments. If a patient has a question about an account, it is useful

```
                          Family Care Center
                          TRANSACTIONS JOURNAL              Page 1
                              07-31-95

Entry  Date   Pat #    Document  Location-Diagnosis     Code    Prov   Amount

1     101497 ARMSTMO0  971014   OF-627.0 menopausal bleedi99212   1    30.00
2     101497 ARMSTMO0  971014   OF-                      85022    1    20.00
3     101497 ARMSTMO0  971014   OF-                      80012    1    30.00
4     101497 ARMSTMO0  971014   OF-                      81000    1    10.00
5     101497 ARMSTMO0  971014   OF-                      82270    1    15.00
6     101697 ARMSTMO0  971014   OF-V70.0 health maintenanc76091   1    80.00
7     101497 KRAMEAN1  971014   OF-382.9 unspecified otiti99212   1    30.00
8     101497 LUNDLAW1  971014   OF-625.3 dysmenorrhea    99214    1    75.00
9     101497 LUNDLAW1  971014   OF-                      88156    1    35.00
10    101497 MITCHAL1  971014   OF-V22.1 supervision of ot99203   1    50.00

                       Total Charges                           $375.00
                       Total Standard Receipts                   $0.00
                       Total Insurance Receipts                  $0.00
                       Total Standard Debit Adjustments          $0.00
                       Total Standard Credit Adjustments         $0.00
                       Total Insurance Debit Adjustments         $0.00
                       Total Insurance Credit Adjustments        $0.00
                       Total of Entries                        $375.00
```

Figure A-8   Sample Transaction Journal Report

to view the account while investigating the question. Highlight **Print Patient Ledgers** and press Enter.

Key the Date that you want at the top of the report. Then in the **Sort By Document Number** field, key *Y* if you want the transactions sorted by document number or press Enter to accept the default, which is *N*. The *N* means that the transactions will be in the order in which they were entered.

Summarize Document Detail is a field that asks if you want to print all details for each entry. For this text, accept the default by pressing Enter.

The rest of the fields on the screen ask which patients you want and how you want the report printed. At the end of this screen, press Enter, and you will have a Print Option choice just as you do for all reports. When you are finished, press ESC to return to the menu.

Aging Reports

The next two sub-menu choices are for aging reports. The **Patient Aging** option shows which patients have overdue balances of a specific length of time, such as 60 days or 90 days, or for a variety of periods. The **Insurance Aging** report does the same for payments due from insurers. Such reports help when doing collections for an office. They also help keep track of how many receivables are due the office.

Print Patient Day Sheet

A patient day sheet is a summary of the activity of patients on any given day. It includes the procedures for each patient and a summary of all moneys received that day. This summary can be used to check the day's bank deposit. Select the **Print Patient Day Sheet** option and press Enter.

The fields for this report are the same as the other reports discussed earlier until you reach Print a Patient Day Sheet. Key *Y* to print the patient day sheet portion; key *N* to print the procedure day sheet and payment day sheet portions.

The last three fields ask if you want all details printed. Press Enter to accept the default, *Y*.

Practice Analysis Report

A practice analysis report shows the practice's revenue for a period of time. Such a report is used as a basis for financial statements and profit analysis.

■ BILLING OPERATIONS

This option allows you to format and print patient statements and patient insurance forms. It also has a selection for printing insurance mailing labels and insurance carrier analysis. All of these billing options make it easy to send out bills and statements. Using the formatting choices can result in having various types of messages put on bills automatically. For example, every bill 90 days overdue can include a note such as, "Fast payment will avoid further action."

Printing Superbills

The Print Superbills selection is used for the day's patients who have scheduled appointments. Highlight this choice and press Enter (Figure A-9).

First enter the **Superbill Date** and the **Range of Providers.** For **Range of Appointment Times,** press Enter for all. If you want the superbill to preprint the charges for procedures, key *Y*. If not press Enter to accept *N*. The last field is **Number of Blank Superbills.** You generally want to print a few blanks for each day for patients who arrive unexpectedly. After you have completed all the fields, press Enter to get to the **Enter Print Option** field. Press *P* for printing.

■ ELECTRONIC CLAIMS

The next Operations Menu option is for **Electronic Claims.** Many medical offices are filing insurance claims electronically to save time. If you are in an office that files electronically, you will most likely work in MediSoft or a similar software already connected to the electronic processor to which you will send claims. The procedure is similar to billing by mail. You set up the bill electronically and then send it.

■ LIST PRINTING

MediSoft prints a variety of valuable lists. Patient lists can be used for everything from marketing a practice to sending out birthday cards. Other lists help in financial analysis.

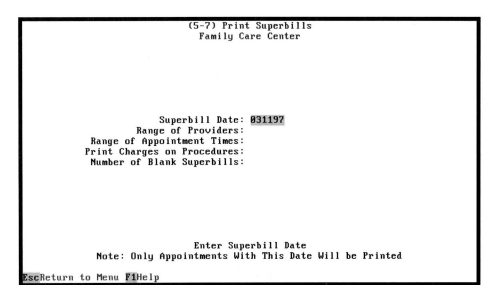

```
                    (5-7) Print Superbills
                      Family Care Center






                      Superbill Date: 031197
                      Range of Providers:
             Range of Appointment Times:
            Print Charges on Procedures:
           Number of Blank Superbills:






                    Enter Superbill Date
         Note: Only Appointments With This Date Will be Printed
EscReturn to Menu F1Help
```

Figure A-9 Example of a Superbill Options Screen

To print a patient list, press Enter at List Printing to get to the Sub-Menu Selection Window. The option, Print Patient Lists, is highlighted, press Enter. The next screen has the cursor at Select Patient List Format. Key *A* for List of Patients. At the next screen, select Print Patient list and press Enter to accept the default for all fields. This will result in a list of all patients in the practice. You can limit the list by changing any of the fields, such as provider number. Next, at Enter Print Option, key either *D* for display to see the list on the screen or *P* for print to actually print the list. (Note: the list will be long so check with your instructor before printing the entire list.)

The procedure code lists and diagnosis code lists are items that are set up for a particular office. The procedures are entered along with charges that will show up when a procedure is entered into the transaction entry option of the Entry Operations Sub-Menu. The diagnosis codes are used in billing insurance companies. The codes are generally accepted in the insurance industry and can be easily understood.

The List Printing option also allows the printing of appointment lists as by the week or month so that a provider can look at his or her calendar. Such a calendar is also useful for the office staff.

■ UTILITIES

The Utilities option is the area where the storing and handling of data takes place in an office. Most files are backed up daily and a disk is often taken from the premises in case of fire. In the school situation, you will not use the Utilities options because the student data disk will be harmed if you try to perform backup and restore functions.

■ EXIT MEDISOFT

Select option (9) Exit to leave MediSoft. Press Enter, and you will see a flashing screen warning you to make a backup of your data every day. **DO NOT DO THIS IN THE SCHOOL SETTING.** Instead, press Enter and you will be at the C:\MEDISOFT> prompt. Remove your student disk if you are done.

■ USING THE OFFICE HOURS SCHEDULER

In addition to the Operations Menu, MediSoft has a scheduler option. You can schedule appointments electronically in MediSoft in two ways. Recall appointments are often scheduled in the **Appointment Entry Sub-Menu** section under **Entry Operations.** The more common way is to use the Office Hours Scheduler.

At the C:\MEDISOFT> prompt, key *hours10k*. Then press ALT + S. Do this when you first begin MediSoft. This will activate the scheduler. The scheduling screen is shown in Figure A-10. Most appointments made in MediSoft are recorded in the Office Hours Scheduler, which is

```
┌─O F F I C E──────┐  ┌─Appointment List───────────────────────────────┐
│────H O U R S─────│  │  6:00a                       1:30              │
│─September 1997───│  │  6:15                        1:45              │
│Su Mo Tu We Th Fr Sa│ │  6:30                        2:00p             │
│    1  2  3  4  5  6 │ │  6:45                        2:15              │
│ 7  8  9 10 11 12 13 │ │  7:00a                       2:30              │
│14 15 16 17 18 19 20 │ │  7:15                        2:45              │
│21 22 23 24 25 26 27 │ │  7:30                        3:00p             │
│28 29 30          │  │  7:45                        3:15              │
│                  │  │  8:00a                       3:30              │
│                  │  │  8:15                        3:45              │
│                  │  │  8:30                        4:00p             │
│─Staff────────────│  │  8:45                        4:15              │
│Dr. Katherine Van │  │  9:00a                       4:30              │
│Dr. John Rudner   │  │  9:15                        4:45              │
│Dr. Jessica Rudner│  │  9:30                        5:00p             │
│                  │  │  9:45                        5:15              │
│                  │  │ 10:00a                       5:30              │
│                  │  │ 10:15                        5:45              │
│                  │  │ 10:30                        6:00p             │
│                  │  │ 10:45                        6:15              │
│                  │  │ 11:00a                       6:30              │
│                  │  │ 11:15                        6:45              │
└──────────────────┘  └────────────────────────────────────────────────┘
 F1-Help F2-Print F4-Purge F5-Staff F6-Find SPACE-Goto PgDn/Up-Next/Prev ESC-Exit
```

Figure A-10 Office Hours Schedule Screen

a separate MediSoft program accessible from any of the Operations Menu areas by pressing ALT + S.

In the first section of the scheduler, you will find the monthly calendar. Use the page up and page down keys to move by month. Use the four arrow keys to move by day or week.

After you find the date that you want, make sure that the provider you want is highlighted under **Staff**. If not, press F5 to change the provider and use the up and down arrow keys to move the highlight. Press ESC when finished. This returns you to the monthly calendar.

Press Tab to move to the **Appointment List** or hourly schedule. Use the up and down arrow keys to move to a specific time slot. When you are ready to key in an appointment, press Enter and the Appointment Entry window appears (see Figure A-11).

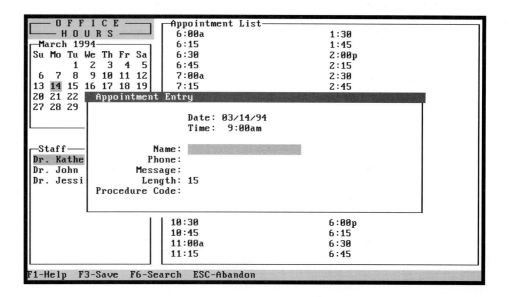

Figure A-11 Example of an Appointment Entry Window

To move around the scheduler, you press Tab, F5, Shift + Tab, or ESC depending on where you are:

In the calendar, press Enter or Tab to move to the Appointment List. Press F5 to go to **Staff.** If you press ESC in the calendar, you will exit the scheduler and go back to MediSoft.

In **Staff,** press Tab to move to the monthly calendar or press Shift + Tab to move to the Appointment List or hourly calendar. Press Tab or ESC to move back to the monthly calendar.

In **Appointment List,** press Tab or F5 to move to Staff. Shift + Tab or ESC moves back to the monthly calendar.

In Appointment List, press Enter and the cursor will be at **Name.** Enter the patient's Chart Number or a task (for example, Hospital Rounds). If you do not know the number, press F6 to search. If the patient's phone number does not come up automatically, find it, and key it in. The message field is for any message up to 30 characters long. The next field is length (of appointment). Key in the minutes scheduled for the appointment if you know it. Then enter the procedure code if you know it. (You can use F6 to search for a code.) Once you are finished, press F3 to save.

To change an appointment, use the same procedure as entering an appointment. When you get to the **Appointment Entry** window, change the appointment and save the changes by pressing F3.

To delete an appointment, highlight the appointment in the hourly calendar (Appointment List) and press F10. The screen will ask: Delete this appointment? (Y/N/ESC). Select Y to delete.

Printing the Calendar

To print a daily calendar, press F2. The bottom of the screen will ask you whether you want to display empty slots and then whether you want a detailed or a summary schedule. Once you answer these questions, the schedule will be printed.

■ MEDISOFT ASSIGNMENTS IN TEXT CHAPTERS 5–14

An icon precedes certain projects and simulations throughout this textbook. The icon indicates that all or part of a practice task can also be done in MediSoft using the Student Data Disk you received with this package. Make sure to read Appendix A up to this point before you start. Listed below are the specific MediSoft exercises that may be assigned by your instructor. (Note: Remember not every part of every project can be done in MediSoft. Follow instructions below.)

Project 19 (page 92)

Dr. Newman's practice is already set up on the Student Data Disk. After inserting the disk, enter October 13, 1997 as the starting date and use the Office Hours Scheduler to enter, cancel, and reschedule the appointments on the calendar pages referred to in Project 19.

Project 20 (page 95)

Using the Office Hours Scheduler in MediSoft, enter the appointments in Project 20.

Project 21 (page 99)

Using the Office Hours Scheduler in MediSoft, cancel and reschedule the appointments in Project 21.

Project 23 (page 113)

Print a list in MediSoft of all patients. Check the information for each patient shown on WP 40 and 41.

Project 26 (page 128)

Enter all the names and addresses shown on WP 43 into the Address Information part of MediSoft. Abbreviate North, South, East, West, Avenue, Street, and Drive. Put Suite number on address lines and put other comments on c/o line.

Simulation 1 (pages 135–137)

Print Doctor Newman's schedule for October 14 and 15. (**Hint:** Use Alt + S to get to the scheduler.)

Project 35 (page 158)

Enter all the transactions into the Transaction Entry section of MediSoft and prepare superbills (insurance claim forms) for all the charges in Project 35. (**Hints:** Use a new Document number, for each patient for each date. To edit transactions, press F9.)

Simulation 2 (pages 170–171)

Enter all transactions that you have not already entered. Print Doctor Newman's schedules from the Office Hours Scheduler for October 21 and 22. Prepare a superbill for all patients to be seen on October 21 and 22.

Project 38 (page 188)

Prepare a Patient Insurance form for Florence Sherman in MediSoft. (**Hints:** Choose A for Insurance Form Format and make sure to change default N at Rebill Insurance Companies to Y.)

Project 39 (page 189)

Prepare a Patient Insurance form for Cheng Sun in MediSoft.

Project 40 (page 196)

Enter all the charges and payments shown for October 27. Print a patient statement for any patient who made a payment.

Project 43 (page 201)

Enter the transactions shown and prepare patient statements for all patients seen on October 28. Print a Day Sheet for October 28.

Simulation 3 (pages 209–210)

Enter any transactions that you have not already entered. Prepare superbills for all patients with appointments on October 29, 30, and 31. Print Patient Insurance Forms as needed. Print Day sheets for all three days.

Project 54 (page 247)

Make the appointment changes in MediSoft for the days shown in Project 54.

Simulation 4B (page 251)

Follow the instructions to do the entire simulation in MediSoft.

Index

Job advancement, certification and, 13
Journal of the American Medical Association (JAMA), 229, 233, 236
Journals, medical, 11, 113–114, 120, 227–234, 236
Judgment, 20

Labels, file folder, 106
Laboratories
  appointments with, 99–100
  career opportunities in, 12, 13
  findings from, 147–148
  X ray. *See* X rays
Language, 30–31
Lateral files, 104
Laundry, 223
Lectures, preparation of, 242–243
Ledgers
  general, 195
  patients', 103, 155–157, 160, 182, 195
Legal issues. *See* Medical law
Letters, 124–132
  background materials for, 120
  collection, 162, 164, 166
  concerning fees, 154
  confidentiality of, 28–29
  copies of, 121, 127, 132
  for the doctor's signature, 125–129
  equipment for writing, 124. *See also* Word processing software
  filing of, 113–114
  follow-up, 130
  formatting of, 125
  general and medical correspondence, 103
  incoming, 119–121
  from the medical assistant, 130
  outgoing, 121–124
  professional courtesy, 162, 163
  referral, 127–129
  reprints and, 233
  style of, 125–127
  transcription equipment and, 130–131
  withdrawal or termination, 50
Libel, 48–49
Libraries, use of, 227–229
Licenses, 222
  medical, 37
  narcotic, 37
  records retention for, 117
  renewal of, 37
Litigation, 51–54
  court appearances, 54–56
  safeguards against, 53–54
Living wills, 34
Lunch breaks, 20, 21

Mail, 119–124
  absence of doctor and, 120–121, 246
  billing by, 161
  classifications, 122
  equipment and supplies, 121–122

incoming, 119–121
outgoing, 121–124
postal services, 50, 122–123
samples received by, 120
Maintenance, of office, 222–224
Major medical insurance, 175, 177–178
Malpractice, 48
  court appearances and, 54–55
  insurance for, 52, 223–224
  safeguards against litigation and, 53–54
Manuals
  office procedures, 215–220, 234
  personnel, 214
Maturity, 23–24
Medicaid, 10, 188
Medical assistants, 2–15
  administrative tasks of, 2–3, 5, 6, 13
  career opportunities for, 7–12
  career qualifications of. *See* Career qualifications
  clinical tasks of, 2–3, 6, 13
  daily routine of, 5–7, 217
  desk area, 221
  ethical responsibilities of, 35–36
  functions of, 5, 14–15
  interpersonal skills of, 4, 16–19, 25–32
  letters written by, 130
  negligence of, 19, 42, 48–49
  professional status of, 13–15, 23–24
  skills of, 3–4, 14–15
Medical editorial assistants, 11
Medical ethics, 33–36, 38
  assistant's responsibility in, 35–36
  bioethics, 34–35
  confidentiality and, 27–29, 36, 39–45, 48–49, 75–76, 92
  etiquette in, 33–34, 62–64, 162, 163
  Hippocratic oath, 34
  principles of, 34, 35
  violation of, 51
Medical history
  court cases and, 55–56
  databases, 146
  procedure for taking, 141–144
Medical insurance, 175, 187
Medical law, 33, 36–56
  confidentiality and, 27–29, 36, 39–45, 48–49, 75–76, 92
  consent, 45–47
  court appearances, 54–56
  licensing, 37, 117
  litigation, 51–54
  Medical Practice Acts, 36–37
  narcotic registration, 37
  negligence. *See* Negligence
  physician-patient relationship, 27–29, 38–39, 49–50, 168
  privileged communications, 39–45
  professional liability and, 48–54, 117, 223–224
  specialization, 37
  workers' compensation and,

189–190
Medical management consultants, 212–213
Medical Practice Acts, 36–37
Medical records, 103, 138–150
  canceled appointments in, 97
  contents of, 102–103, 138–145, 219
  court cases and, 55–56
  discharge and, 139, 150
  durable power of attorney in, 34–35
  errors in, 140, 141
  facsimile transmittal, 75–76
  forms, 145
  insurance information in, 117, 162, 179
  medical reports in, 147–148
  obtaining clinical data, 139–144
  ownership of, 149
  patient access to, 29, 42
  preparation of, 95
  problem-oriented, 146–147
  professional liability and, 48–51, 139, 149–150
  quality assurance in, 37, 150
  recording transactions in, 155–158
  referrals and, 100, 127–129
  release of information from, 39–45, 107, 127–129, 179, 180, 217
  retention of, 116–117, 149
  telephone messages in, 70, 72
  transferring, 217
  workers' compensation claims and, 189–190
Medical reports, 219
  fees for preparing, 44–45, 149
  statutory, 41
  types of, 147–148
Medical societies, 236–243
  meetings of, 236–243
  program participation and, 241–243
  types and functions of, 236–237
  See also specific societies
Medicare, 10, 186–187
Medication records, 148
MediSoft, 92, 253–272
Memorandums, interoffice, 130, 131
Microfiche, 106
Micrographics, 106, 149
Minors, consent and, 45–46
Minutes, of meetings, 240–241
Missing files, location of, 117
Mobile-aisle files, 105
Modems, 123–124
Monitors, computer, 124
Monthly summary, 199–200
Mouse, computer, 124

Narcotics, 37
National Board of Medical Examiners, 13, 37
National Library of Medicine, 229
Negligence
  court appearances and, 54–55
  damage suits and, 56

Working Papers

MEDICAL SPECIALISTS

Directions: Match the specialist from Column 2 with its definition in Column 1.

COLUMN 1

____ 1. Specializes in treating diseases of the nervous system.

____ 2. Diagnoses and treats diseases of the skin.

____ 3. Diagnoses and treats illness in children.

____ 4. Specializes in diagnosing and treating conditions of the eye.

____ 5. Performs surgery to repair and reconstruct body structures.

____ 6. Diagnoses and treats disease through the use of X rays.

____ 7. Treats diseases of the endocrine glands, such as diabetes.

____ 8. Relieves pain and maintains a patient in stable condition during surgery and diagnostic procedures.

____ 9. Studies laboratory specimens to diagnose disease.

____ 10. Studies and treats disorders of the kidney.

____ 11. Diagnoses and treats mental and behavioral disorders.

____ 12. Studies and treats conditions of the heart and blood vessels.

____ 13. Specializes in the treatment of the ear, nose, and throat.

____ 14. Performs chest surgery.

____ 15. Gives immediate care to trauma victims.

____ 16. Uses physical means such as heat, cold, water, and exercise to restore physical function.

____ 17. Diagnoses and treats disorders of the musculoskeletal system.

____ 18. Diagnoses and treats conditions affecting the urinary system.

____ 19. Provides care during pregnancy and childbirth.

____ 20. Diagnoses and treats cancer.

COLUMN 2

a. Anesthesiologist
b. Cardiologist
c. Dermatologist
d. Emergency physician
e. Endocrinologist
f. Nephrologist
g. Neurologist
h. Obstetrician
i. Oncologist
j. Ophthalmologist
k. Orthopedist
l. Otorhinolaryngologist
m. Pathologist
n. Pediatrician
o. Physiatrist
p. Plastic surgeon
q. Psychiatrist
r. Radiologist
s. Thoracic surgeon
t. Urologist

PROFESSIONAL CONDUCT

Directions: Match the term from Column 2 with the correct definition in Column 1.

COLUMN 1

____ 1. Able to adapt to new situations.

____ 2. Able to achieve a purpose without offending.

____ 3. Free of errors.

____ 4. Able to endure with calmness.

____ 5. Able to identify oneself with the situation of another.

____ 6. Marked by truth and integrity.

____ 7. Able to do what is expected.

____ 8. Able to come to a decision by evaluating a situation.

____ 9. On time, ready to work.

____ 10. Careful to complete all aspects of a task.

____ 11. Able to produce results with minimal effort.

____ 12. Able to express an idea with confidence.

COLUMN 2

a. Accurate

b. Assertive

c. Dependable

d. Efficient

e. Empathetic

f. Flexible

g. Honest

h. Having good judgment

i. Patient

j. Punctual

k. Tactful

l. Thorough

QUALITIES FOR A MEDICAL ASSISTANT

Directions: Rate yourself by checking Column 1 under the appropriate category for each quality. Your instructor will rate you in Column 2. You will rate yourself again at the end of the course using Column 3.

Qualities	Frequently			Sometimes			Seldom		
	1	2	3	1	2	3	1	2	3
Accurate									
Ambitious									
Assertive									
Cheerful									
Dependable									
Efficient									
Empathic									
Flexible									
Helpful									
Honest									
Independent									
Logical									
Mature									
Patient									
Poised									
Punctual									
Tactful									
Thorough									
Understanding									

INTERACTIONS WITH PATIENTS AND COWORKERS

Directions: Circle the best answer for each of the following situations.

1. Your office staff is friendly. Everyone, including the doctor, is on a first-name basis at office functions and parties. When the doctor arrives at the office after hospital rounds, you would say:
   a. "Good morning, Dr. Newman."
   b. "Good morning, Mark."
   c. "Good morning, Sir."
   d. "Good morning, Doctor."

2. A patient stops at your desk and quietly says, "My goodness, that patient next to me has an awful rash. What is it?"
   You would say:
   a. "I suggest you ask the doctor."
   b. "Just a minute, I'll check the chart."
   c. "I am sorry, but that information is confidential."
   d. "I think it is psoriasis."

3. Ellen Bronsky, who has been a patient at the clinic for several years, stops at the front desk after her appointment. You would say:
   a. "Good-bye."
   b. "I'm glad you came in today."
   c. "Hope to see you soon, Ellen."
   d. "Good-bye, Ellen."

4. George Ruiz has terminal cancer. When greeting him, you would say:
   a. "Good afternoon, Mr. Ruiz."
   b. "Mr. Ruiz, you look good. Evidently the medication hasn't made you sick."
   c. "You are looking good today after being so sick, Mr. Ruiz."
   d. "How are the radiation treatments going?"

5. Three children have been waiting half an hour for their mother, who is being treated by the doctor. They have been fairly quiet to this point, but now they have started chasing each other. The assistant would:
   a. Expect other patients to say something to the children.
   b. Give them time to work off their energy.
   c. Talk quietly to the children, showing them some books to read.
   d. Tell them to be quiet or they will have to leave.

6. At an outside office function, Leslie, who works in the office cafeteria, asks why Mrs. Jean Schmidt is a patient in your office. You would:
   a. Reply that she is going to have her gallbladder removed.
   b. Reply that the information is confidential.
   c. Reply that you have not read Mrs. Schmidt's chart yet.
   d. Reply that Leslie should ask the doctor.

7. A patient stops to chat at the front desk. A safe topic for conversation would be:
   a. Dr. Newman's new home.
   b. The local political convention.
   c. The patient's illness.
   d. The current sunny weather.

8. Mr. Di Angelo, a patient with pneumonia, tells the assistant about a new medication that is being used for pneumonia on elderly patients. The assistant would:
   a. Suggest that Mr. Di Angelo discuss the medication with the doctor.
   b. Tell Mr. Di Angelo that the new medication is too expensive.
   c. Tell Mr. Di Angelo that he is not elderly.
   d. Say that Dr. Newman will probably prescribe the medication for Mr. Di Angelo.

(Continued on next page.)

9. Harriet Wong, a salesperson for a surgical supply company, arrives at the office during a busy time. Dr. Newman has previously told you that he is not interested in purchasing any new surgical supplies at this time. You would:
   a. Tell Harriet that Dr. Newman sees all the salespeople on the first Wednesday of the month from 11 a.m. to noon.
   b. Take Harriet's business card, and tell her that someone will get back to her.
   c. Tell Harriet that Dr. Newman is not purchasing any surgical supplies at this time.
   d. Send Harriet in to see the head nurse, who handles all the surgical supplies.

10. John Walters, a patient, stops at the front desk. You notice that John is trying to read the papers that are on the desk. You would:
    a. Tell John that everything on the desk is confidential.
    b. Calmly cover the papers that are on the desk.
    c. Tell the other assistant that John is trying to read the items on the desk.
    d. Tell the doctor that John is trying to read the items on the desk.

OBLIGATIONS OF THE PHYSICIAN AND PATIENT

Directions: The following numbered items refer to the obligations of the physician and of the patient. Mark each statement completion either "T" for *true* or "F" for *false.*

1. The AMA Principles of Medical Ethics:
   ___ State the length of time to keep the medical record.
   ___ State that the doctor may refuse to accept a new patient.
   ___ Give the doctor permission to charge a fee for referring a patient to a specialist.
   ___ Allow the assistant to perform emergency measures.
   ___ Require the doctor to obtain a consultation in a complex case.

2. The patient has the right to:
   ___ Refuse treatment.
   ___ Delay payment of charges until the patient is recovered from a specific illness.
   ___ Obtain a second opinion.
   ___ Select another physician within the practice.
   ___ Refuse before-and-after photographing of treatment in plastic surgery cases for advertising purposes.

3. The doctor is legally obligated to:
   ___ Inform a patient of all possible reactions to drug treatment.
   ___ Accept an indigent patient.
   ___ Refuse to perform an unapproved procedure.
   ___ Prescribe the medication requested by the patient.
   ___ Suggest a referral when complications beyond the physician's scope of knowledge occur during hospitalization.

4. A license to practice medicine:
   ___ Is issued by the individual states.
   ___ Is granted after application by a university graduate.
   ___ Is good for the life of the doctor.
   ___ May be obtained after passing an examination from the National Board of Examiners.
   ___ May be obtained by reciprocity.
   ___ May be revoked.
   ___ Is available to the nurse after completion of a master's degree in science.
   ___ Is on display in the doctor's office.

AUTHORIZATION FOR RELEASE OF INFORMATION

Directions: The following numbered items refer to the release of information. Mark each statement completion either "T" for *true* or "F" for *false.*

1. The authorization form for release of information:
   ___ Is signed by the patient.
   ___ Is necessary when filling out a registration form for a new patient.
   ___ Gives office employees permission to give family members information from the patient's medical record.
   ___ Is necessary for the forwarding of records from the patient's previous doctor.
   ___ Is cosigned by the doctor.
   ___ Releases the doctor from malpractice suits.
   ___ Can be accomplished over the telephone.
   ___ Needs to be signed before information can be given to a patient's employer.
   ___ Gives permission for the doctor to perform mole excision.
   ___ Should be sent to the patient's attorney.
   ___ Should be sent to the doctor's attorney.
   ___ Is retained in the patient's medical file.

2. Harriet Lewis has moved from Chicago to Belleville. She used to be Dr. Newman's patient and would like to have her medical records transferred to her new physician in Belleville. Dr. Newman's assistant would:
   ___ Send the records with her.
   ___ Send the records to one of the clinics in Belleville.
   ___ Ask Harriet to sign a release form.
   ___ Ask Dr. Newman to sign a release form.
   ___ Write to the clinic to ask whether it wants the records.
   ___ File the original request in the chart and send a photocopy of the release with the records.
   ___ Telephone the clinic to ask whether it wants the records.
   ___ Hold the release form Harriet signed until Harriet moves and a request is forwarded from the new doctor.

3. An authorization for release of information must be signed:
   ___ Before minor surgery.
   ___ When sending a patient's chest X rays along with a patient to a specialist.
   ___ When a doctor writes a referral letter to another doctor.
   ___ At the time a patient has an X ray so the radiologist can send the radiology report to the patient's family doctor.
   ___ Before information can be given to a minor regarding his or her parent's illness.
   ___ By a child so his or her parent can get information from the child's medical chart.

CONSENT

Directions: The following numbered items refer to a patient's consent for treatment in the medical office. Mark each statement completion either "T" for *true* or "F" for *false.*

1. A written consent for treatment is necessary:

    ___ To prescribe experimental medications.

    ___ Before a patient takes part in a medical research project.

    ___ When the patient requests lab results.

    ___ For minor office surgery.

    ___ When the doctor discusses a child's disease with his or her parents.

    ___ In emergency situations.

    ___ At the time an office appointment is made.

    ___ When sending the surgeon an X-ray report.

    ___ Before treating a child that has been brought to the office from a day care facility while the child's parents are at work.

2. Dr. Newman plans to perform a lymph node biopsy on a patient. The patient:

    ___ May refuse.

    ___ Will be asked to sign a consent.

    ___ May go to another doctor for a second opinion.

    ___ Does not have to sign a consent because the procedure is part of a study Dr. Newman is doing and the patient will not be charged.

    ___ Should receive a copy of the consent form, if signed.

    ___ Gives Dr. Newman permission to have pictures taken of the procedure by signing a consent form.

    ___ Is giving expressed consent by signing a consent form.

    ___ Must ask the doctor to sign the consent form.

    ___ Must ask to have a copy of the consent form sent to his or her attorney.

MALPRACTICE AND THE ASSISTANT'S RESPONSIBILITY

Directions: In each of the following numbered items, the decisions of the medical assistant will play a part in preventing possible malpractice claims. Mark each statement completion "T" for *true* or "F" for *false.*

1. Marie, one of Dr. Newman's patients, calls to say that she feels much better and asks you whether she should continue her medication. As Dr. Newman's assistant, you should:
   ___ Tell her to take the medication until it is gone.
   ___ Tell her to cut back to half the dosage.
   ___ Take a message for Dr. Newman.
   ___ Record the call in the medical record.
   ___ Suggest that she call the pharmacist.
   ___ Tell her to hold while you check with Dr. Newman.

2. Dr. Newman is attending a convention out of town. Henry, a patient Dr. Newman saw last week, calls to describe a rash. You should:
   ___ Tell Henry to discontinue any medication.
   ___ Recognize this as a possible drug reaction.
   ___ Tell Henry to go to the emergency room.
   ___ Ask Henry to come in so that you can see the rash.
   ___ Make an appointment for Henry for the first available time after Dr. Newman returns.
   ___ Give the patient the name and telephone number of the doctor taking Dr. Newman's calls.
   ___ Record the call in Henry's chart.
   ___ Suggest that Henry see another doctor.

3. A person identifying herself as an insurance clerk phones requesting information about a patient. You should:
   ___ Give her the information because the insurance company is responsible for the bill.
   ___ Suggest that she write a letter specifying the requested information.
   ___ Check the chart for the patient's signed release.
   ___ Refer the caller to the hospital's billing department.
   ___ Take a message.
   ___ Verify the caller's identity by returning the call.
   ___ Suggest that the caller get the information from the patient.
   ___ Photocopy the patient's chart and send it to the insurance company.

LEGAL TERMS

Directions: Match each legal term in Column 2 with the proper definition in Column 1.

COLUMN 1

_____ 1. Law protecting doctors from liability when treating an emergency case.

_____ 2. Legal age.

_____ 3. Written summons requiring presence in court.

_____ 4. Any court action or lawsuit.

_____ 5. Protection against financial liability when a doctor is sued.

_____ 6. Principles of right and wrong.

_____ 7. Legally binding agreement between doctor and patient.

_____ 8. Testimony under oath but not in court.

_____ 9. Agreement to receive care after discussion of treatment options.

_____ 10. Time limit within which a lawsuit can be started.

_____ 11. Law regulating doctor's professional behavior.

_____ 12. Mutual acceptance of licensing requirements.

_____ 13. Outlines of a patient's responsibility.

_____ 14. A doctor's leaving a case before patient is recovered.

_____ 15. The person claimed to be at fault in a lawsuit.

_____ 16. Permission granted by law to perform a special function.

_____ 17. Negligence, malpractice.

_____ 18. Patient's agreement to a procedure.

_____ 19. Not disclosing information without patient's permission.

_____ 20. Permission to send a patient's records.

_____ 21. Person filing a lawsuit.

_____ 22. Confidential reports sent to department of health.

_____ 23. Performance of surgery beyond what patient consented to.

_____ 24. False information given to injure someone's reputation.

_____ 25. Patient's verbal or written agreement to receive care.

_____ 26. The understood agreement to receive care when a patient comes to a doctor for treatment.

COLUMN 2

a. Abandonment
b. Battery
c. Confidentiality
d. Consent
e. Contract
f. Defendant
g. Deposition
h. Ethics
i. Expressed consent
j. Good samaritan act
k. Implied consent
l. Informed consent
m. Liability
n. License
o. Litigation
p. Majority
q. Malpractice insurance
r. Medical Practice Act
s. Patient's Bill of Rights
t. Plaintiff
u. Reciprocity
v. Release of information
w. Slander
x. Statute of limitations
y. Statutory reports
z. Subpoena

SCREENING CALLS

Directions: Dr. Newman is in the office seeing patients. Explain how you would respond to each of the calls described in Column 1. Indicate your response by choosing one of the answers shown in Column 2. You may use an answer from Column 2 for more than one item in Column 1.

COLUMN 1

____ 1. A pharmacist calls for a prescription refill.

____ 2 An emergency room nurse calls to talk with Dr. Newman about a patient in the emergency room.

____ 3. A nurse calls to ask for routine orders for a patient admitted to the hospital.

____ 4. A mother calls because her child has a temperature of 104 degrees.

____ 5. The auto insurance representative calls about a change in Dr. Newman's policy.

____ 6. A patient calls complaining of occasional chest pain.

____ 7. Dr. Martin calls for Dr. Newman.

____ 8. A patient calls with a rash; he is not on medication.

____ 9. A patient calls to ask for test results.

____ 10. Dr. Newman's daughter calls for Dr. Newman.

____ 11. A patient calls to ask whether it is OK to treat an eye injury with a hot pack.

____ 12. A laboratory technician calls with a report for Dr. Newman.

____ 13. A home health aide at a patient's house calls to ask about a patient's present treatment.

____ 14. A patient calls after having fallen off a ladder; she may have a fracture or dislocation.

____ 15. A patient calls with a temperature of 103 degrees; he has no transportation.

____ 16. A patient calls because she thinks she is in labor.

____ 17. A patient calls to ask what laboratory work needs to be done before a physical examination with Dr. Newman.

____ 18. An insurance clerk calls to ask about the diagnosis of a patient.

____ 19. A hospital administrator calls for Dr. Newman.

____ 20. A patient asks for Dr. Newman and wants to know when to go into the hospital for short-stay surgery.

COLUMN 2

a. Take a message.
b. Give information or advice.
c. Transfer caller to the appointment desk.
d. Transfer caller to the nurse.
e. Transfer caller to the doctor.

MESSAGE

TO _____

DATE _____ TIME _____

FROM _____

PHONE _____

☐ PLEASE CALL   ☐ RETURNED YOUR CALL   ☐ WILL CALL AGAIN

REGARDING _____

_____

_____

_____

TAKEN BY _____

MESSAGE

TO _____

DATE _____ TIME _____

FROM _____

PHONE _____

☐ PLEASE CALL   ☐ RETURNED YOUR CALL   ☐ WILL CALL AGAIN

REGARDING _____

_____

_____

_____

TAKEN BY _____

MESSAGE

TO _____

DATE _____ TIME _____

FROM _____

PHONE _____

☐ PLEASE CALL   ☐ RETURNED YOUR CALL   ☐ WILL CALL AGAIN

REGARDING _____

_____

_____

_____

TAKEN BY _____

MESSAGE

TO _____

DATE _____ TIME _____

FROM _____

PHONE _____

☐ PLEASE CALL   ☐ RETURNED YOUR CALL   ☐ WILL CALL AGAIN

REGARDING _____

_____

_____

_____

TAKEN BY _____

MESSAGE

TO _____

DATE _____ TIME _____

FROM _____

PHONE _____

☐ PLEASE CALL ☐ RETURNED YOUR CALL ☐ WILL CALL AGAIN

REGARDING _____

_____

_____

_____

TAKEN BY _____

MESSAGE

TO _____

DATE _____ TIME _____

FROM _____

PHONE _____

☐ PLEASE CALL ☐ RETURNED YOUR CALL ☐ WILL CALL AGAIN

REGARDING _____

_____

_____

_____

TAKEN BY _____

MESSAGE

TO _____

DATE _____ TIME _____

FROM _____

PHONE _____

☐ PLEASE CALL ☐ RETURNED YOUR CALL ☐ WILL CALL AGAIN

REGARDING _____

_____

_____

_____

TAKEN BY _____

MESSAGE

TO _____

DATE _____ TIME _____

FROM _____

PHONE _____

☐ PLEASE CALL ☐ RETURNED YOUR CALL ☐ WILL CALL AGAIN

REGARDING _____

_____

_____

_____

TAKEN BY _____

MESSAGE

TO _____ DATE _____ TIME _____

FROM _____

PHONE _____

☐ PLEASE CALL ☐ RETURNED YOUR CALL ☐ WILL CALL AGAIN

REGARDING _____

_____

_____

_____

TAKEN BY _____

MESSAGE

TO _____ DATE _____ TIME _____

FROM _____

PHONE _____

☐ PLEASE CALL ☐ RETURNED YOUR CALL ☐ WILL CALL AGAIN

REGARDING _____

_____

_____

_____

TAKEN BY _____

MESSAGE

TO _____ DATE _____ TIME _____

FROM _____

PHONE _____

☐ PLEASE CALL ☐ RETURNED YOUR CALL ☐ WILL CALL AGAIN

REGARDING _____

_____

_____

_____

TAKEN BY _____

MESSAGE

TO _____ DATE _____ TIME _____

FROM _____

PHONE _____

☐ PLEASE CALL ☐ RETURNED YOUR CALL ☐ WILL CALL AGAIN

REGARDING _____

_____

_____

_____

TAKEN BY _____

MESSAGE

TO _____

DATE _____ TIME _____

FROM _____

PHONE _____

☐ PLEASE CALL   ☐ RETURNED YOUR CALL   ☐ WILL CALL AGAIN

REGARDING _____

_____

_____

TAKEN BY _____

MESSAGE

TO _____

DATE _____ TIME _____

FROM _____

PHONE _____

☐ PLEASE CALL   ☐ RETURNED YOUR CALL   ☐ WILL CALL AGAIN

REGARDING _____

_____

_____

TAKEN BY _____

MESSAGE

TO _____

DATE _____ TIME _____

FROM _____

PHONE _____

☐ PLEASE CALL   ☐ RETURNED YOUR CALL   ☐ WILL CALL AGAIN

REGARDING _____

_____

_____

TAKEN BY _____

MESSAGE

TO _____

DATE _____ TIME _____

FROM _____

PHONE _____

☐ PLEASE CALL   ☐ RETURNED YOUR CALL   ☐ WILL CALL AGAIN

REGARDING _____

_____

_____

TAKEN BY _____

MESSAGE

TO _____

DATE _____ TIME _____

FROM _____

PHONE _____

☐ PLEASE CALL ☐ RETURNED YOUR CALL ☐ WILL CALL AGAIN

REGARDING _____
_____
_____
_____

TAKEN BY _____

MESSAGE

TO _____

DATE _____ TIME _____

FROM _____

PHONE _____

☐ PLEASE CALL ☐ RETURNED YOUR CALL ☐ WILL CALL AGAIN

REGARDING _____
_____
_____
_____

TAKEN BY _____

MESSAGE

TO _____

DATE _____ TIME _____

FROM _____

PHONE _____

☐ PLEASE CALL ☐ RETURNED YOUR CALL ☐ WILL CALL AGAIN

REGARDING _____
_____
_____
_____

TAKEN BY _____

MESSAGE

TO _____

DATE _____ TIME _____

FROM _____

PHONE _____

☐ PLEASE CALL ☐ RETURNED YOUR CALL ☐ WILL CALL AGAIN

REGARDING _____
_____
_____
_____

TAKEN BY _____

MESSAGE

TO _____
DATE _____ TIME _____
FROM _____
PHONE _____
☐ PLEASE CALL   ☐ RETURNED YOUR CALL   ☐ WILL CALL AGAIN
REGARDING _____
_____
_____
_____
TAKEN BY _____

MESSAGE

TO _____
DATE _____ TIME _____
FROM _____
PHONE _____
☐ PLEASE CALL   ☐ RETURNED YOUR CALL   ☐ WILL CALL AGAIN
REGARDING _____
_____
_____
_____
TAKEN BY _____

MESSAGE

TO _____
DATE _____ TIME _____
FROM _____
PHONE _____
☐ PLEASE CALL   ☐ RETURNED YOUR CALL   ☐ WILL CALL AGAIN
REGARDING _____
_____
_____
_____
TAKEN BY _____

MESSAGE

TO _____
DATE _____ TIME _____
FROM _____
PHONE _____
☐ PLEASE CALL   ☐ RETURNED YOUR CALL   ☐ WILL CALL AGAIN
REGARDING _____
_____
_____
_____
TAKEN BY _____

MESSAGE

TO _____

DATE _____ TIME _____

FROM _____

PHONE _____

☐ PLEASE CALL ☐ RETURNED YOUR CALL ☐ WILL CALL AGAIN

REGARDING _____

_____

_____

_____

TAKEN BY _____

MESSAGE

TO _____

DATE _____ TIME _____

FROM _____

PHONE _____

☐ PLEASE CALL ☐ RETURNED YOUR CALL ☐ WILL CALL AGAIN

REGARDING _____

_____

_____

_____

TAKEN BY _____

MESSAGE

TO _____

DATE _____ TIME _____

FROM _____

PHONE _____

☐ PLEASE CALL ☐ RETURNED YOUR CALL ☐ WILL CALL AGAIN

REGARDING _____

_____

_____

_____

TAKEN BY _____

MESSAGE

TO _____

DATE _____ TIME _____

FROM _____

PHONE _____

☐ PLEASE CALL ☐ RETURNED YOUR CALL ☐ WILL CALL AGAIN

REGARDING _____

_____

_____

_____

TAKEN BY _____

MESSAGE

TO _____

DATE _____ TIME _____

FROM _____

PHONE _____

☐ PLEASE CALL   ☐ RETURNED YOUR CALL   ☐ WILL CALL AGAIN

REGARDING _____

_____

_____

_____

TAKEN BY _____

MESSAGE

TO _____

DATE _____ TIME _____

FROM _____

PHONE _____

☐ PLEASE CALL   ☐ RETURNED YOUR CALL   ☐ WILL CALL AGAIN

REGARDING _____

_____

_____

_____

TAKEN BY _____

MESSAGE

TO _____

DATE _____ TIME _____

FROM _____

PHONE _____

☐ PLEASE CALL   ☐ RETURNED YOUR CALL   ☐ WILL CALL AGAIN

REGARDING _____

_____

_____

_____

TAKEN BY _____

MESSAGE

TO _____

DATE _____ TIME _____

FROM _____

PHONE _____

☐ PLEASE CALL   ☐ RETURNED YOUR CALL   ☐ WILL CALL AGAIN

REGARDING _____

_____

_____

_____

TAKEN BY _____

TELEPHONE SKILLS

Directions: Circle the best answer for each of the following telephone situations.

1. Telephone calls that the assistant should handle include all of the following *except:*
   a. Prescription refills.
   b. Routine reports from hospitals (histories, physicals, discharge summaries, etc.).
   c. Patients who will not reveal symptoms.
   d. X-ray and lab reports.
   e. Return appointments.

2. In answering the telephone, all of the following would be acceptable on your part as the assistant *except:*
   a. Answering on the second ring.
   b. Identifying the office first and then yourself.
   c. Answering, "Doctors Jones and Smith." (These are the only two doctors in the office.)
   d. Saying, "Good morning" first, then identifying the office and yourself.
   e. Answering by saying, "Doctor's office, please hold."

3. The minimum information required when taking a telephone message includes all of the following *except:*
   a. The caller's name.
   b. The caller's telephone number.
   c. The reason for the call.
   d. The full name of the person taking the message.
   e. The action to be taken.

4. Which of the following calls would the assistant not be able to answer or handle without a return call from the doctor:
   a. An appointment for a new patient.
   b. A request for assistance with an insurance form.
   c. A satisfactory progress report from a patient.
   d. An inquiry about a bill.
   e. A patient's questions about lab results and their meaning.

5. If a telephone caller insists on talking to the doctor but refuses to give a name or state the nature of the call, the assistant should:
   a. Put the call through to the doctor.
   b. Tell the caller to try again at the end of the day when the office is less busy.
   c. Tell the caller to leave a telephone number and that the doctor will return the call.
   d. Suggest to the caller that a letter be written to the doctor concerning the nature of the caller's request.
   e. Suggest to the caller that the doctor be called at home that evening.

6. The first way to communicate courtesy to the telephone caller is to:
   a. Answer promptly.
   b. Identify yourself and the office.
   c. Use the caller's name frequently.
   d. Take a message.
   e. Excuse yourself if you must put the caller on hold.

7. As soon as you identify the office and yourself, you should:
   a. Put the caller on hold.
   b. Put the call right through to the doctor.
   c. Obtain the name of the caller.
   d. Take a message.
   e. Find out the reason for the call.

(Continued on next page.)

8. When an emergency call comes in and you are in the office alone, you should:
   a. Obtain the caller's name and the nature of the emergency.
   b. Give the patient simple first aid directions.
   c. Tell the patient to go to the hospital emergency room.
   d. Tell the patient that the doctor will return the call as soon as possible.
   e. Do a, b, and c.
   f. Do a, b, and d.

9. When two phone lines ring at the same time, the assistant should:
   a. Answer Line 1 with, "Dr. Newman's office, could you hold please?" and then complete the call on Line 2.
   b. Answer Line 1 with, "Dr. Newman's office, could you hold please?"; then answer Line 2 with the same message, and return to Line 1.
   c. Answer Line 1, determine the nature of the call, ask whether the caller can hold, and then answer Line 2 to complete that call.
   d. Answer Line 1, determine the nature of the call, and ask whether the caller can hold; then answer Line 2, determine the nature of the call, and return to Line 1 to complete that call; and finally return to Line 2.

10. When returning to a call that has been on hold, the assistant should say:
    a. "Thank you for holding."
    b. "I can help you now."
    c. "This is Linda Jenson; sorry for the interruption."
    d. "This has been such a busy day; could I help you now?"

TELEPHONE SITUATIONS

Directions: Circle the best answer for each of the following telephone situations.

1. On Tuesday, an assistant needs to make a number of calls to cancel Thursday's appointments. The assistant would:
   a. Ask someone else to make the calls since there have been so many incoming calls.
   b. Make all of the calls early in the day.
   c. Make all of the calls at the end of the day.
   d. Make all of the calls during the lunch hour.
   e. Allow an interval of about five minutes between each call.
   f. Send the patients postcards telling of the cancellation.

2. When taking a telephone call from a patient who insists on speaking with the doctor, the best response the assistant can give would be:
   a. "The doctor is busy now."
   b. "The doctor is with a patient. Could I take a message?"
   c. "The doctor is not in."
   d. "I cannot interrupt the doctor now. Could I help you?"

3. When the assistant is talking with one patient on the telephone and another call comes in, the assistant should:
   a. Answer the other call by asking "Could you hold?"
   b. Answer the other call, identify the office, and ask the caller to hold.
   c. Answer the other call by identifying the office, asking the nature of the call, and then determining whether that caller can hold.
   d. Ignore the other call because someone else in the office will answer it.

4. The assistant has two lines on hold and has forgotten which patient is on which line. The assistant should return to one line by saying:
   a. "Thank you for holding. May I help you?"
   b. "Dr. Newman's office, Linda speaking. May I help you?"
   c. "Is this John Edison?"
   d. "I'm sorry for the interruption. Could I help you?"

5. A patient calls and asks to speak to the doctor, who is out of the office. The assistant should say:
   a. "I'm sorry, the doctor is not in right now."
   b. "The doctor is at the hospital. You could try calling there."
   c. "I will contact the doctor for you."
   d. "The doctor is not available right now. Could I help you?"

SCHEDULING WORKSHEET

Directions: For each of the following medical problems, indicate whether the patient should be scheduled (a) stat, (b) today, (c) tomorrow, or (d) when available. Also indicate with an asterisk (*) which problems would require more than one time slot in the appointment book.

____ 1. Earache

____ 2. Wart removal

____ 3. Pap smear

____ 4. College physical

____ 5. Recheck of cast

____ 6. Sore throat

____ 7. Postoperative check

____ 8. Athletic physical

____ 9. Lump in breast

____ 10 Suture removal

____ 11. Abdominal pain

____ 12. Presurgical exam

____ 13. Six-week postpartum

____ 14. Laryngitis

____ 15. Something in the eye

____ 16. Pain when urinating

____ 17. Diabetic recheck

____ 18. Laceration

____ 19. Postoperative bleeding

____ 20. Croup

____ 21. First OB physical exam

____ 22. Blood in urine

____ 23. Cyst on the back

____ 24. Cast repair

____ 25. Fatigue

____ 26. Cough

____ 27. Routine OB checkup

____ 28. Rash

____ 29. Dressing change

____ 30. Migraine

____ 31. Plantar wart

____ 32. Routine adult physical

____ 33. Congestion

____ 34. Infected hangnail

____ 35. Vaginal discharge

____ 36. Nosebleed

____ 37. Blurry vision

____ 38. Vomiting

____ 39. Preschool physical

____ 40. Diarrhea

DR. MARK NEWMAN'S OFFICE SCHEDULE
2235 South Ridgeway Avenue
Chicago, IL 60623-2240
312-555-6022

MONDAY, TUESDAY, AND WEDNESDAY

Hospital rounds	8	– 10
Appointments with patients	10:30	– 12
Lunch	12	– 1
University Hospital	1	– 5

THURSDAY

University Hospital	All day

FRIDAY

Hospital rounds	8	– 10
Office for dictation, messages, writing, and course preparation	10:30	– 12
Afternoon off		

Physical examination	1 hour
Routine check	15 minutes

Allow 1/2 hour transportation time to office after hospital rounds.

APPOINTMENT ABBREVIATIONS

abd	abdominal
bldg	bleeding
BP	blood pressure
✓	checkup
Dx	diagnosis
drsg	dressing
EKG	electrocardiogram
F/U	follow-up visit
FX	fracture
GI	gastrointestinal
inf	infection
N & V	nausea and vomiting
NP	new patient
NS	no-show (for appointment)
CP, CPE, PE	physical examination
poss	possible
preop	preoperative
postop	postoperative
pg	pregnancy
OB	prenatal visit
pp	postpartum
prob	problem

Monday, October 13	Tuesday, October 14	Wednesday, October 15

Monday, October 13

8:00
8:15
8:30
8:45
9:00   Hospital
9:15   Rounds
9:30
9:45
10:00   Travel
10:15   ↓
10:30
10:45
11:00
11:15
11:30
11:45
12:00
12:15
12:30   Lunch
12:45
1:00
1:15
1:30
1:45
2:00
2:15
2:30   University
2:45   Hospital
3:00
3:15
3:30
3:45
4:00
4:15
4:30
4:45
5:00
5:15
5:30
5:45

Tuesday, October 14

8:00
8:15
8:30
8:45
9:00   Hospital
9:15   Rounds
9:30
9:45
10:00   Travel
10:15   ↓
10:30
10:45
11:00
11:15
11:30
11:45
12:00
12:15
12:30   Lunch
12:45
1:00
1:15
1:30
1:45
2:00
2:15
2:30   University
2:45   Hospital
3:00
3:15
3:30
3:45
4:00
4:15
4:30
4:45
5:00
5:15
5:30
5:45

8:00 Chicago Medical Society

Wednesday, October 15

8:00
8:15
8:30
8:45
9:00   Hospital
9:15   Rounds
9:30
9:45
10:00   Travel
10:15   ↓
10:30
10:45
11:00
11:15
11:30
11:45
12:00
12:15
12:30   Lunch
12:45
1:00
1:15
1:30
1:45
2:00
2:15
2:30   University
2:45   Hospital
3:00
3:15
3:30
3:45
4:00
4:15
4:30
4:45
5:00
5:15
5:30
5:45

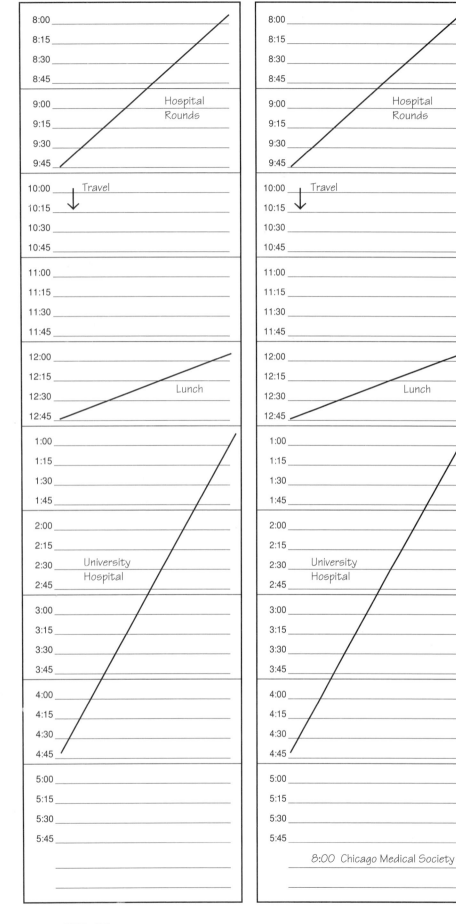
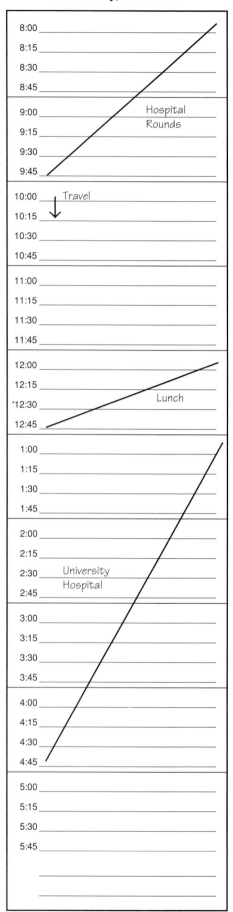

Thursday, October 16

8:00	
8:15	
8:30	
8:45	
9:00	
9:15	
9:30	
9:45	
10:00	
10:15	
10:30	
10:45	
11:00	
11:15	
11:30	
11:45	
12:00	
12:15	
12:30	
12:45	
1:00	
1:15	
1:30	
1:45	
2:00	
2:15	
2:30	
2:45	
3:00	
3:15	
3:30	
3:45	
4:00	
4:15	
4:30	
4:45	
5:00	
5:15	
5:30	
5:45	

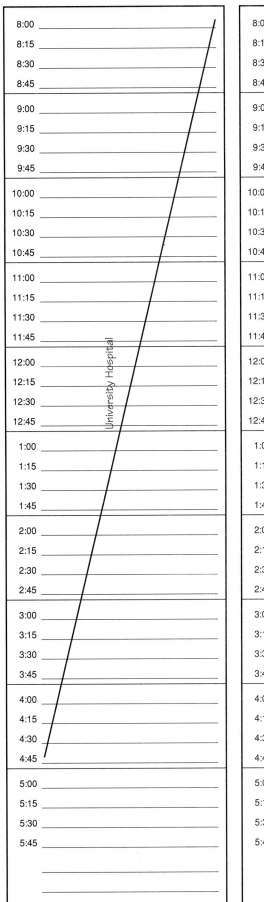

University Hospital

Friday, October 17

8:00	
8:15	
8:30	
8:45	
9:00	
9:15	
9:30	
9:45	
10:00	
10:15	
10:30	
10:45	
11:00	
11:15	
11:30	
11:45	
12:00	
12:15	
12:30	
12:45	
1:00	
1:15	
1:30	
1:45	
2:00	
2:15	
2:30	
2:45	
3:00	
3:15	
3:30	
3:45	
4:00	
4:15	
4:30	
4:45	
5:00	
5:15	
5:30	
5:45	

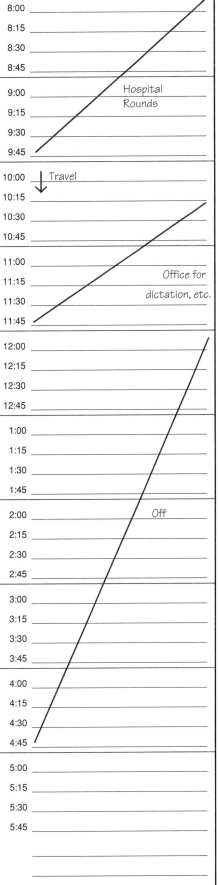

Hospital Rounds

↓ *Travel*

Office for dictation, etc.

Off

Saturday, October 18

8:00	
8:15	
8:30	
8:45	
9:00	
9:15	
9:30	
9:45	
10:00	
10:15	
10:30	
10:45	
11:00	
11:15	
11:30	
11:45	
12:00	
12:15	
12:30	
12:45	

October

S	M	T	W	T	F	S
			1	2	3	4
5	6	7	8	9	10	11
12	13	14	15	16	17	18
19	20	21	22	23	24	25
26	27	28	29	30	31	

November

S	M	T	W	T	F	S
						1
2	3	4	5	6	7	8
9	10	11	12	13	14	15
16	17	18	19	20	21	22
23	24	25	26	27	28	29
30						

December

S	M	T	W	T	F	S
	1	2	3	4	5	6
7	8	9	10	11	12	13
14	15	16	17	18	19	20
21	22	23	24	25	26	27
28	29	30	31			

Monday, October 20

8:00 _____
8:15 _____
8:30 _____
8:45 _____

9:00 _____
9:15 _____
9:30 _____
9:45 _____

10:00 _____
10:15 _____
10:30 _____
10:45 _____

11:00 _____
11:15 _____
11:30 _____
11:45 _____

12:00 _____
12:15 _____
12:30 _____
12:45 _____

1:00 _____
1:15 _____
1:30 _____
1:45 _____

2:00 _____
2:15 _____
2:30 _____
2:45 _____

3:00 _____
3:15 _____
3:30 _____
3:45 _____

4:00 _____
4:15 _____
4:30 _____
4:45 _____

5:00 _____
5:15 _____
5:30 _____
5:45 _____

_____
_____

Tuesday, October 21

8:00 _____
8:15 _____
8:30 _____
8:45 _____

9:00 _____
9:15 _____
9:30 _____
9:45 _____

10:00 _____
10:15 _____
10:30 _____
10:45 _____

11:00 _____
11:15 _____
11:30 _____
11:45 _____

12:00 _____
12:15 _____
12:30 _____
12:45 _____

1:00 _____
1:15 _____
1:30 _____
1:45 _____

2:00 _____
2:15 _____
2:30 _____
2:45 _____

3:00 _____
3:15 _____
3:30 _____
3:45 _____

4:00 _____
4:15 _____
4:30 _____
4:45 _____

5:00 _____
5:15 _____
5:30 _____
5:45 _____

_____
_____

Wednesday, October 22

8:00 _____
8:15 _____
8:30 _____
8:45 _____

9:00 _____
9:15 _____
9:30 _____
9:45 _____

10:00 _____
10:15 _____
10:30 _____
10:45 _____

11:00 _____
11:15 *Marc Phan - cough 555-3344*
11:30 _____
11:45 _____

12:00 _____
12:15 _____
12:30 _____
12:45 _____

1:00 _____
1:15 _____
1:30 _____
1:45 _____

2:00 _____
2:15 _____
2:30 _____
2:45 _____

3:00 _____
3:15 _____
3:30 _____
3:45 _____

4:00 _____
4:15 _____
4:30 _____
4:45 _____

5:00 _____
5:15 _____
5:30 _____
5:45 _____

_____
_____

Thursday, October 23

8:00 _____
8:15 _____
8:30 _____
8:45 _____

9:00 _____
9:15 _____
9:30 _____
9:45 _____

10:00 _____
10:15 _____
10:30 _____
10:45 _____

11:00 _____
11:15 _____
11:30 _____
11:45 _____

12:00 _____
12:15 _____
12:30 _____
12:45 _____

1:00 _____
1:15 _____
1:30 _____
1:45 _____

2:00 _____
2:15 _____
2:30 _____
2:45 _____

3:00 _____
3:15 _____
3:30 _____
3:45 _____

4:00 _____
4:15 _____
4:30 _____
4:45 _____

5:00 _____
5:15 _____
5:30 _____
5:45 _____

_____
_____

Friday, October 24

8:00 _____
8:15 _____
8:30 _____
8:45 _____

9:00 _____
9:15 _____
9:30 _____
9:45 _____

10:00 _____
10:15 _____
10:30 _____
10:45 _____

11:00 _____
11:15 _____
11:30 _____
11:45 _____

12:00 _____
12:15 _____
12:30 _____
12:45 _____

1:00 _____
1:15 _____
1:30 _____
1:45 _____

2:00 _____
2:15 _____
2:30 _____
2:45 _____

3:00 _____
3:15 _____
3:30 _____
3:45 _____

4:00 _____
4:15 _____
4:30 _____
4:45 _____

5:00 _____
5:15 _____
5:30 _____
5:45 _____

_____
_____

Saturday, October 25

8:00 _____
8:15 _____
8:30 _____
8:45 _____

9:00 _____
9:15 _____
9:30 _____
9:45 _____

10:00 _____
10:15 _____
10:30 _____
10:45 _____

11:00 _____
11:15 _____
11:30 _____
11:45 _____

12:00 _____
12:15 _____
12:30 _____
12:45 _____

October

S	M	T	W	T	F	S
			1	2	3	4
5	6	7	8	9	10	11
12	13	14	15	16	17	18
19	20	21	22	23	24	25
26	27	28	29	30	31	

November

S	M	T	W	T	F	S
						1
2	3	4	5	6	7	8
9	10	11	12	13	14	15
16	17	18	19	20	21	22
23	24	25	26	27	28	29
30						

December

S	M	T	W	T	F	S
	1	2	3	4	5	6
7	8	9	10	11	12	13
14	15	16	17	18	19	20
21	22	23	24	25	26	27
28	29	30	31			

Monday, October 27

8:00 _____
8:15 _____
8:30 _____
8:45 _____

9:00 _____ Hospital
9:15 _____ Rounds
9:30 _____
9:45 _____

10:00 ____ Travel
10:15 ↓
10:30 _____
10:45 _____

11:00 _____
11:15 Marc Phan - cough 555-3344
11:30 _____
11:45 _____

12:00 _____
12:15 _____
12:30 _____ Lunch
12:45 _____

1:00 _____
1:15 _____
1:30 _____
1:45 _____

2:00 _____
2:15 _____
2:30 ____ University
2:45 ____ Hospital

3:00 _____
3:15 _____
3:30 _____
3:45 _____

4:00 _____
4:15 _____
4:30 _____
4:45 _____

5:00 _____
5:15 _____
5:30 _____
5:45 _____

_____

Tuesday, October 28

8:00 _____
8:15 _____
8:30 _____
8:45 _____

9:00 _____ Hospital
9:15 _____ Rounds
9:30 _____
9:45 _____

10:00 ____ Travel
10:15 ↓
10:30 _____
10:45 _____

11:00 _____
11:15 _____
11:30 _____
11:45 _____

12:00 _____
12:15 _____
12:30 _____ Lunch
12:45 _____

1:00 _____
1:15 _____
1:30 _____
1:45 _____

2:00 _____
2:15 _____
2:30 ____ University
2:45 ____ Hospital

3:00 _____
3:15 _____
3:30 _____
3:45 _____

4:00 _____
4:15 _____
4:30 _____
4:45 _____

5:00 _____
5:15 _____
5:30 _____
5:45 _____

_____

Wednesday, October 29

8:00 _____
8:15 _____
8:30 _____
8:45 _____

9:00 _____ Hospital
9:15 _____ Rounds
9:30 _____
9:45 _____

10:00 ____ Travel
10:15 ↓
10:30 _____
10:45 _____

11:00 _____
11:15 _____
11:30 _____
11:45 _____

12:00 _____
12:15 _____
12:30 _____ Lunch
12:45 _____

1:00 _____
1:15 _____
1:30 _____
1:45 _____

2:00 _____
2:15 _____
2:30 ____ University
2:45 ____ Hospital

3:00 _____
3:15 _____
3:30 _____
3:45 _____

4:00 _____
4:15 _____
4:30 _____
4:45 _____

5:00 _____
5:15 _____
5:30 _____
5:45 _____

_____

Thursday, October 30

8:00	
8:15	
8:30	
8:45	
9:00	
9:15	
9:30	
9:45	
10:00	
10:15	
10:30	
10:45	
11:00	
11:15	
11:30	
11:45	
12:00	
12:15	
12:30	
12:45	
1:00	
1:15	
1:30	
1:45	
2:00	
2:15	
2:30	
2:45	
3:00	
3:15	
3:30	
3:45	
4:00	
4:15	
4:30	
4:45	
5:00	
5:15	
5:30	
5:45	

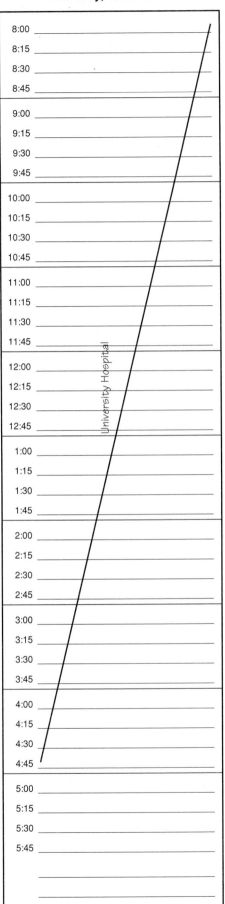

University Hospital

Friday, October 31

8:00	
8:15	
8:30	
8:45	
9:00	
9:15	
9:30	
9:45	
10:00	
10:15	
10:30	
10:45	
11:00	
11:15	
11:30	
11:45	
12:00	
12:15	
12:30	
12:45	
1:00	
1:15	
1:30	
1:45	
2:00	
2:15	
2:30	
2:45	
3:00	
3:15	
3:30	
3:45	
4:00	
4:15	
4:30	
4:45	
5:00	
5:15	
5:30	
5:45	

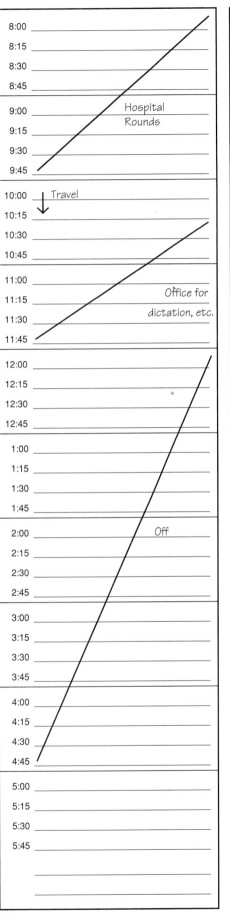

Hospital Rounds

↓ *Travel*

Office for dictation, etc.

Off

Saturday, November 1

8:00	
8:15	
8:30	
8:45	
9:00	
9:15	
9:30	
9:45	
10:00	
10:15	
10:30	
10:45	
11:00	
11:15	
11:30	
11:45	
12:00	
12:15	
12:30	
12:45	

October

S	M	T	W	T	F	S
			1	2	3	4
5	6	7	8	9	10	11
12	13	14	15	16	17	18
19	20	21	22	23	24	25
26	27	28	29	30	31	

November

S	M	T	W	T	F	S
						1
2	3	4	5	6	7	8
9	10	11	12	13	14	15
16	17	18	19	20	21	22
23	24	25	26	27	28	29
30						

December

S	M	T	W	T	F	S
	1	2	3	4	5	6
7	8	9	10	11	12	13
14	15	16	17	18	19	20
21	22	23	24	25	26	27
28	29	30	31			

Monday, November 3	Tuesday, November 4	Wednesday, November 5
8:00	8:00	8:00
8:15	8:15	8:15
8:30	8:30	8:30
8:45	8:45	8:45
9:00 _Hospital_	9:00 _Hospital_	9:00 _Hospital_
9:15 _Rounds_	9:15 _Rounds_	9:15 _Rounds_
9:30	9:30	9:30
9:45	9:45	9:45
10:00 _Travel_	10:00 _Travel_	10:00 _Travel_
10:15 ↓	10:15 ↓	10:15 ↓
10:30	10:30	10:30
10:45 _Ana Mendez - Sinus 555-3606_	10:45	10:45
11:00 _Stephen Villano - Rash 555-3493_	11:00	11:00
11:15	11:15	11:15
11:30	11:30	11:30
11:45	11:45	11:45
12:00	12:00	12:00
12:15	12:15	12:15
12:30 _Lunch_	12:30 _Lunch_	12:30 _Lunch_
12:45	12:45	12:45
1:00	1:00	1:00
1:15	1:15	1:15
1:30	1:30	1:30
1:45	1:45	1:45
2:00	2:00	2:00
2:15	2:15	2:15
2:30 _University_	2:30 _University_	2:30 _University_
2:45 _Hospital_	2:45 _Hospital_	2:45 _Hospital_
3:00	3:00	3:00
3:15	3:15	3:15
3:30	3:30	3:30
3:45	3:45	3:45
4:00	4:00	4:00
4:15	4:15	4:15
4:30	4:30	4:30
4:45	4:45	4:45
5:00	5:00	5:00
5:15	5:15	5:15
5:30	5:30	5:30
5:45	5:45	5:45

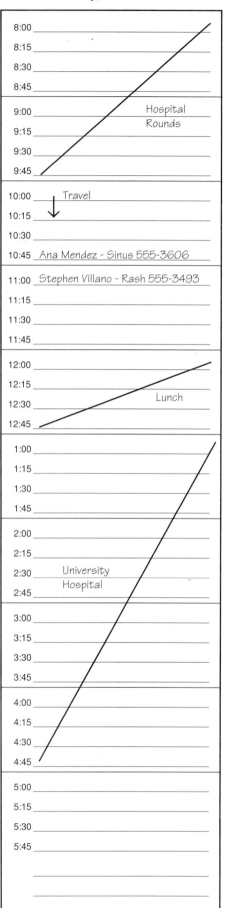
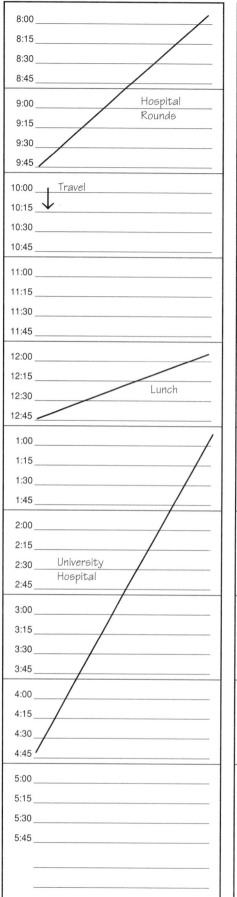
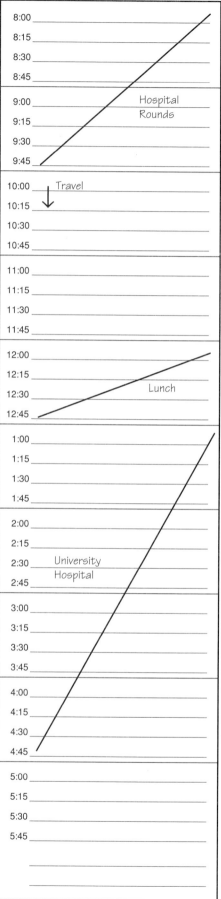

Thursday, November 6	Friday, November 7	Saturday, November 8

Thursday, November 6

8:00 ___
8:15 ___
8:30 ___
8:45 ___

9:00 ___
9:15 ___
9:30 ___
9:45 ___

10:00 ___
10:15 ___
10:30 ___
10:45 ___

11:00 ___
11:15 ___
11:30 ___
11:45 ___

University Hospital

12:00 ___
12:15 ___
12:30 ___
12:45 ___

1:00 ___
1:15 ___
1:30 ___
1:45 ___

2:00 ___
2:15 ___
2:30 ___
2:45 ___

3:00 ___
3:15 ___
3:30 ___
3:45 ___

4:00 ___
4:15 ___
4:30 ___
4:45 ___

5:00 ___
5:15 ___
5:30 ___
5:45 ___

_____
_____

Friday, November 7

8:00 ___
8:15 ___
8:30 ___
8:45 ___

9:00 ___ *Hospital*
9:15 ___ *Rounds*
9:30 ___
9:45 ___

10:00 ___ ↓ *Travel*
10:15 ___
10:30 ___
10:45 ___

11:00 ___
11:15 ___ *Office for*
11:30 ___ *dictation, etc.*
11:45 ___

12:00 ___
12:15 ___
12:30 ___
12:45 ___

1:00 ___
1:15 ___
1:30 ___
1:45 ___

2:00 ___ *Off*
2:15 ___
2:30 ___
2:45 ___

3:00 ___
3:15 ___
3:30 ___
3:45 ___

4:00 ___
4:15 ___
4:30 ___
4:45 ___

5:00 ___
5:15 ___
5:30 ___
5:45 ___

_____
_____

Saturday, November 8

8:00 ___
8:15 ___
8:30 ___
8:45 ___

9:00 ___
9:15 ___
9:30 ___
9:45 ___

10:00 ___
10:15 ___
10:30 ___
10:45 ___

11:00 ___
11:15 ___
11:30 ___
11:45 ___

12:00 ___
12:15 ___
12:30 ___
12:45 ___

October

S	M	T	W	T	F	S
			1	2	3	4
5	6	7	8	9	10	11
12	13	14	15	16	17	18
19	20	21	22	23	24	25
26	27	28	29	30	31	

November

S	M	T	W	T	F	S
						1
2	3	4	5	6	7	8
9	10	11	12	13	14	15
16	17	18	19	20	21	22
23	24	25	26	27	28	29
30						

December

S	M	T	W	T	F	S
	1	2	3	4	5	6
7	8	9	10	11	12	13
14	15	16	17	18	19	20
21	22	23	24	25	26	27
28	29	30	31			

Monday, November 10	Tuesday, November 11	Wednesday, November 12

Tuesday subheader: **VETERANS DAY**

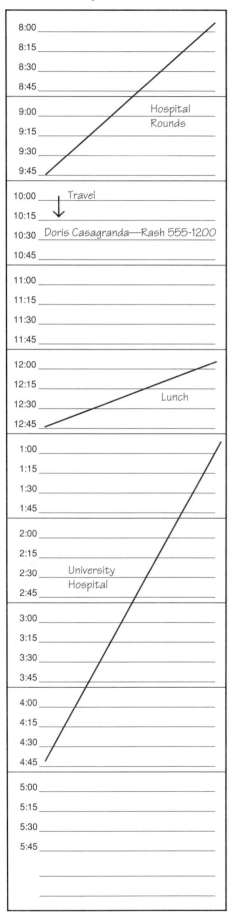

Monday, November 10

- 8:00
- 8:15
- 8:30
- 8:45
- 9:00 — Hospital Rounds
- 9:15
- 9:30
- 9:45
- 10:00 — Travel
- 10:15
- 10:30 — Doris Casagranda—Rash 555-1200
- 10:45
- 11:00
- 11:15
- 11:30
- 11:45
- 12:00
- 12:15
- 12:30 — Lunch
- 12:45
- 1:00
- 1:15
- 1:30
- 1:45
- 2:00
- 2:15
- 2:30 — University Hospital
- 2:45
- 3:00
- 3:15
- 3:30
- 3:45
- 4:00
- 4:15
- 4:30
- 4:45
- 5:00
- 5:15
- 5:30
- 5:45

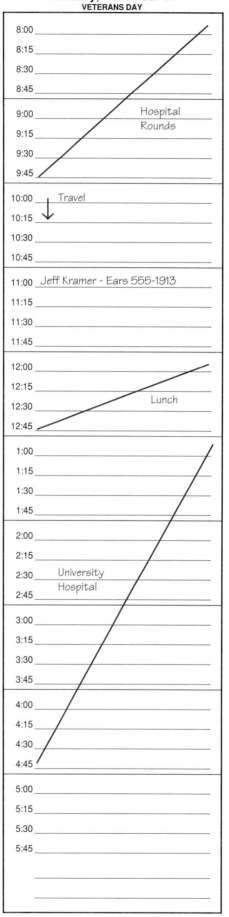

Tuesday, November 11

- 8:00
- 8:15
- 8:30
- 8:45
- 9:00 — Hospital Rounds
- 9:15
- 9:30
- 9:45
- 10:00 — Travel
- 10:15
- 10:30
- 10:45
- 11:00 — Jeff Kramer - Ears 555-1913
- 11:15
- 11:30
- 11:45
- 12:00
- 12:15
- 12:30 — Lunch
- 12:45
- 1:00
- 1:15
- 1:30
- 1:45
- 2:00
- 2:15
- 2:30 — University Hospital
- 2:45
- 3:00
- 3:15
- 3:30
- 3:45
- 4:00
- 4:15
- 4:30
- 4:45
- 5:00
- 5:15
- 5:30
- 5:45

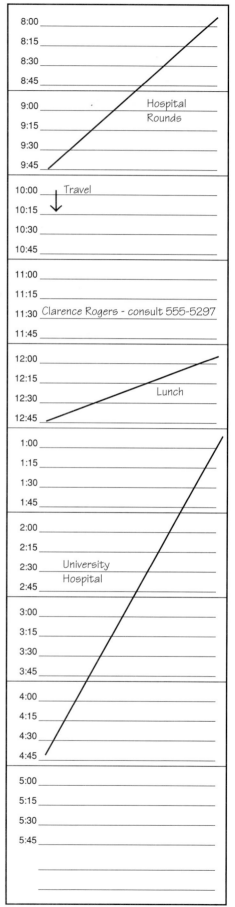

Wednesday, November 12

- 8:00
- 8:15
- 8:30
- 8:45
- 9:00 — Hospital Rounds
- 9:15
- 9:30
- 9:45
- 10:00 — Travel
- 10:15
- 10:30
- 10:45
- 11:00
- 11:15
- 11:30 — Clarence Rogers - consult 555-5297
- 11:45
- 12:00
- 12:15
- 12:30 — Lunch
- 12:45
- 1:00
- 1:15
- 1:30
- 1:45
- 2:00
- 2:15
- 2:30 — University Hospital
- 2:45
- 3:00
- 3:15
- 3:30
- 3:45
- 4:00
- 4:15
- 4:30
- 4:45
- 5:00
- 5:15
- 5:30
- 5:45

Thursday, November 13

8:00 ___
8:15 ___
8:30 ___
8:45 ___

9:00 ___
9:15 ___
9:30 ___
9:45 ___

10:00 ___
10:15 ___
10:30 ___
10:45 ___

11:00 ___
11:15 ___
11:30 ___
11:45 ___

12:00 ___
12:15 ___
12:30 ___
12:45 ___

1:00 ___
1:15 ___
1:30 ___
1:45 ___

2:00 ___
2:15 ___
2:30 ___
2:45 ___

3:00 ___
3:15 ___
3:30 ___
3:45 ___

4:00 ___
4:15 ___
4:30 ___
4:45 ___

5:00 ___
5:15 ___
5:30 ___
5:45 ___

___

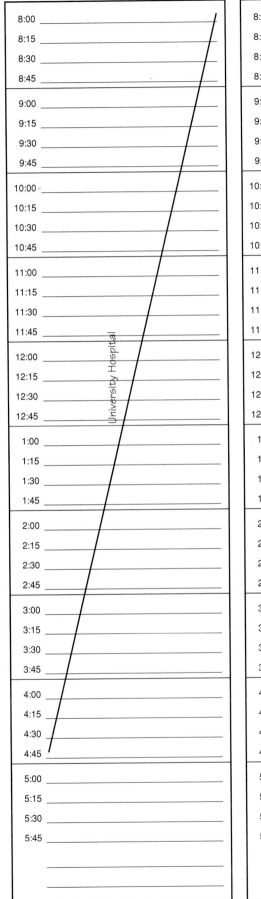

University Hospital

Friday, November 14

8:00 ___
8:15 ___
8:30 ___
8:45 ___

9:00 ___
9:15 ___
9:30 ___
9:45 ___

Hospital Rounds

10:00 ___
10:15 ___
10:30 ___
10:45 ___

Travel

11:00 ___
11:15 ___
11:30 ___
11:45 ___

Office for dictation, etc.

12:00 ___
12:15 ___
12:30 ___
12:45 ___

1:00 ___
1:15 ___
1:30 ___
1:45 ___

2:00 ___
2:15 ___
2:30 ___
2:45 ___

Off

3:00 ___
3:15 ___
3:30 ___
3:45 ___

4:00 ___
4:15 ___
4:30 ___
4:45 ___

5:00 ___
5:15 ___
5:30 ___
5:45 ___

___

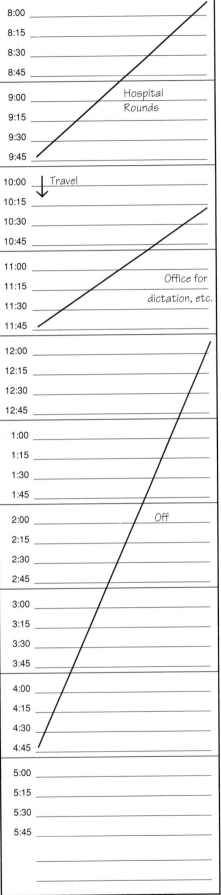

Saturday, November 15

8:00 ___
8:15 ___
8:30 ___
8:45 ___

9:00 ___
9:15 ___
9:30 ___
9:45 ___

10:00 ___
10:15 ___
10:30 ___
10:45 ___

11:00 ___
11:15 ___
11:30 ___
11:45 ___

12:00 ___
12:15 ___
12:30 ___
12:45 ___

October

S	M	T	W	T	F	S
			1	2	3	4
5	6	7	8	9	10	11
12	13	14	15	16	17	18
19	20	21	22	23	24	25
26	27	28	29	30	31	

November

S	M	T	W	T	F	S
						1
2	3	4	5	6	7	8
9	10	11	12	13	14	15
16	17	18	19	20	21	22
23	24	25	26	27	28	29
30						

December

S	M	T	W	T	F	S
	1	2	3	4	5	6
7	8	9	10	11	12	13
14	15	16	17	18	19	20
21	22	23	24	25	26	27
28	29	30	31			

Monday, November 17	**Tuesday, November 18**	**Wednesday, November 19**
8:00	8:00	8:00
8:15	8:15	8:15
8:30	8:30	8:30
8:45	8:45	8:45
9:00 Hospital	9:00 Hospital	9:00 Hospital
9:15 Rounds	9:15 Rounds	9:15 Rounds
9:30	9:30	9:30
9:45	9:45	9:45
10:00 Travel	10:00 Travel	10:00 Travel
10:15	10:15	10:15
10:30 Erin Mitchell - PP✔ 555-8153	10:30 Clarence Rogers - Vasectomy 555-5297	10:30
10:45 Donald Mitchell - 2-wk ✔ 555-8153	10:45	10:45 Theresa Dayton - Headache 555-2231
11:00 Sarah Morton - Hand injury 555-2324	11:00	11:00 Charles Jonathan III - Knee 555-3097
11:15	11:15	11:15
11:30	11:30	11:30
11:45	11:45	11:45
12:00	12:00	12:00
12:15	12:15	12:15
12:30 Lunch	12:30 Lunch	12:30 Lunch
12:45	12:45	12:45
1:00	1:00	1:00
1:15	1:15	1:15
1:30	1:30	1:30
1:45	1:45	1:45
2:00	2:00	2:00
2:15	2:15	2:15
2:30 University	2:30 University	2:30 University
2:45 Hospital	2:45 Hospital	2:45 Hospital
3:00	3:00	3:00
3:15	3:15	3:15
3:30	3:30	3:30
3:45	3:45	3:45
4:00	4:00	4:00
4:15	4:15	4:15
4:30	4:30	4:30
4:45	4:45	4:45
5:00	5:00	5:00
5:15	5:15	5:15
5:30	5:30	5:30
5:45	5:45	5:45

Thursday, November 20

8:00 _____
8:15 _____
8:30 _____
8:45 _____

9:00 _____
9:15 _____
9:30 _____
9:45 _____

10:00 _____
10:15 _____
10:30 _____
10:45 _____

11:00 _____
11:15 _____
11:30 _____
11:45 _____

12:00 _____
12:15 _____
12:30 _____
12:45 _____

1:00 _____
1:15 _____
1:30 _____
1:45 _____

2:00 _____
2:15 _____
2:30 _____
2:45 _____

3:00 _____
3:15 _____
3:30 _____
3:45 _____

4:00 _____
4:15 _____
4:30 _____
4:45 _____

5:00 _____
5:15 _____
5:30 _____
5:45 _____

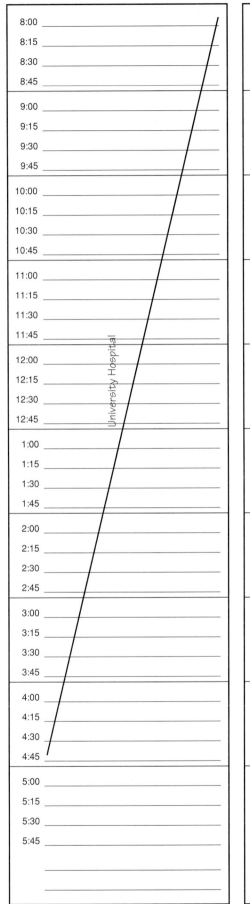

University Hospital

Friday, November 21

8:00 _____
8:15 _____
8:30 _____
8:45 _____

9:00 _____
9:15 _____
9:30 _____
9:45 _____

10:00 _____
10:15 _____
10:30 _____
10:45 _____

11:00 _____
11:15 _____
11:30 _____
11:45 _____

12:00 _____
12:15 _____
12:30 _____
12:45 _____

1:00 _____
1:15 _____
1:30 _____
1:45 _____

2:00 _____
2:15 _____
2:30 _____
2:45 _____

3:00 _____
3:15 _____
3:30 _____
3:45 _____

4:00 _____
4:15 _____
4:30 _____
4:45 _____

5:00 _____
5:15 _____
5:30 _____
5:45 _____

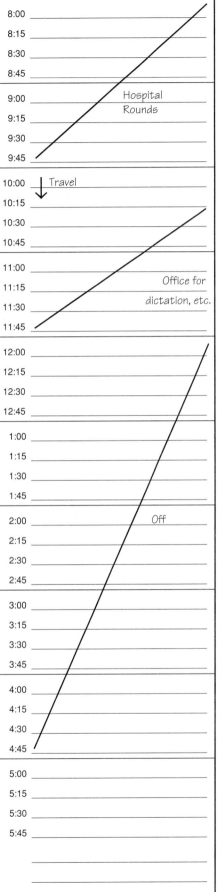

Hospital Rounds

↓ *Travel*

Office for dictation, etc.

Off

Saturday, November 22

8:00 _____
8:15 _____
8:30 _____
8:45 _____

9:00 _____
9:15 _____
9:30 _____
9:45 _____

10:00 _____
10:15 _____
10:30 _____
10:45 _____

11:00 _____
11:15 _____
11:30 _____
11:45 _____

12:00 _____
12:15 _____
12:30 _____
12:45 _____

October

S	M	T	W	T	F	S
			1	2	3	4
5	6	7	8	9	10	11
12	13	14	15	16	17	18
19	20	21	22	23	24	25
26	27	28	29	30	31	

November

S	M	T	W	T	F	S
						1
2	3	4	5	6	7	8
9	10	11	12	13	14	15
16	17	18	19	20	21	22
23	24	25	26	27	28	29
30						

December

S	M	T	W	T	F	S
	1	2	3	4	5	6
7	8	9	10	11	12	13
14	15	16	17	18	19	20
21	22	23	24	25	26	27
28	29	30	31			

Monday, November 24

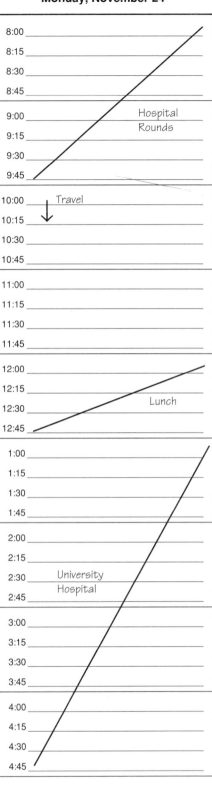

8:00 _____
8:15 _____
8:30 _____
8:45 _____

9:00 _____ Hospital
9:15 _____ Rounds
9:30 _____
9:45 _____

10:00 ____ ↓ Travel
10:15 ____
10:30 _____
10:45 _____

11:00 _____
11:15 _____
11:30 _____
11:45 _____

12:00 _____
12:15 _____
12:30 _____ Lunch
12:45 _____

1:00 _____
1:15 _____
1:30 _____
1:45 _____

2:00 _____
2:15 _____
2:30 _____ University
2:45 _____ Hospital

3:00 _____
3:15 _____
3:30 _____
3:45 _____

4:00 _____
4:15 _____
4:30 _____
4:45 _____

5:00 _____
5:15 _____
5:30 _____
5:45 _____

_____
_____

Tuesday, November 25

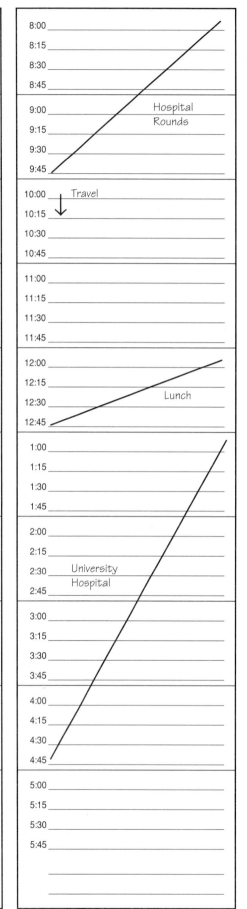

8:00 _____
8:15 _____
8:30 _____
8:45 _____

9:00 _____ Hospital
9:15 _____ Rounds
9:30 _____
9:45 _____

10:00 ____ ↓ Travel
10:15 ____
10:30 _____
10:45 _____

11:00 _____
11:15 _____
11:30 _____
11:45 _____

12:00 _____
12:15 _____
12:30 _____ Lunch
12:45 _____

1:00 _____
1:15 _____
1:30 _____
1:45 _____

2:00 _____
2:15 _____
2:30 _____ University
2:45 _____ Hospital

3:00 _____
3:15 _____
3:30 _____
3:45 _____

4:00 _____
4:15 _____
4:30 _____
4:45 _____

5:00 _____
5:15 _____
5:30 _____
5:45 _____

_____
_____

Wednesday, November 26

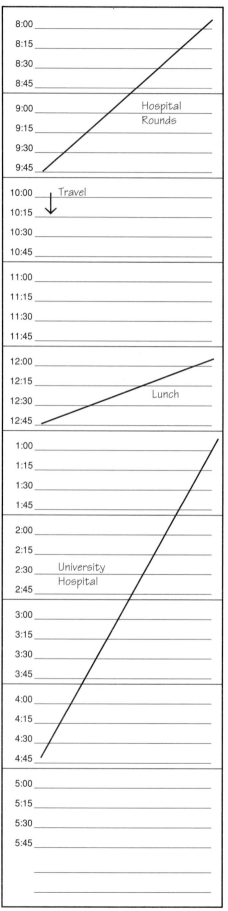

8:00 _____
8:15 _____
8:30 _____
8:45 _____

9:00 _____ Hospital
9:15 _____ Rounds
9:30 _____
9:45 _____

10:00 ____ ↓ Travel
10:15 ____
10:30 _____
10:45 _____

11:00 _____
11:15 _____
11:30 _____
11:45 _____

12:00 _____
12:15 _____
12:30 _____ Lunch
12:45 _____

1:00 _____
1:15 _____
1:30 _____
1:45 _____

2:00 _____
2:15 _____
2:30 _____ University
2:45 _____ Hospital

3:00 _____
3:15 _____
3:30 _____
3:45 _____

4:00 _____
4:15 _____
4:30 _____
4:45 _____

5:00 _____
5:15 _____
5:30 _____
5:45 _____

_____
_____

Thursday, November 27
THANKSGIVING DAY

8:00	
8:15	
8:30	
8:45	
9:00	
9:15	
9:30	
9:45	
10:00	
10:15	
10:30	
10:45	
11:00	
11:15	
11:30	
11:45	
12:00	University Hospital
12:15	
12:30	
12:45	
1:00	
1:15	
1:30	
1:45	
2:00	
2:15	
2:30	
2:45	
3:00	
3:15	
3:30	
3:45	
4:00	
4:15	
4:30	
4:45	
5:00	
5:15	
5:30	
5:45	

Friday, November 28

8:00	
8:15	
8:30	
8:45	
9:00	Hospital
9:15	Rounds
9:30	
9:45	
10:00	↓ Travel
10:15	
10:30	
10:45	
11:00	
11:15	Office for
11:30	dictation, etc.
11:45	
12:00	
12:15	
12:30	
12:45	
1:00	
1:15	
1:30	
1:45	
2:00	Off
2:15	
2:30	
2:45	
3:00	
3:15	
3:30	
3:45	
4:00	
4:15	
4:30	
4:45	
5:00	
5:15	
5:30	
5:45	

Saturday, November 29

8:00	
8:15	
8:30	
8:45	
9:00	
9:15	
9:30	
9:45	
10:00	
10:15	
10:30	
10:45	
11:00	
11:15	
11:30	
11:45	
12:00	
12:15	
12:30	
12:45	

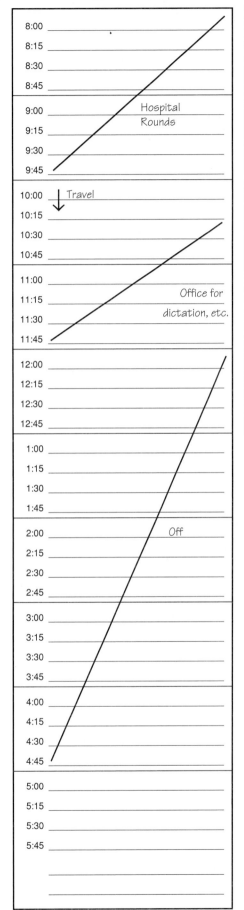

October

S	M	T	W	T	F	S
			1	2	3	4
5	6	7	8	9	10	11
12	13	14	15	16	17	18
19	20	21	22	23	24	25
26	27	28	29	30	31	

November

S	M	T	W	T	F	S
						1
2	3	4	5	6	7	8
9	10	11	12	13	14	15
16	17	18	19	20	21	22
23	24	25	26	27	28	29
30						

December

S	M	T	W	T	F	S
	1	2	3	4	5	6
7	8	9	10	11	12	13
14	15	16	17	18	19	20
21	22	23	24	25	26	27
28	29	30	31			

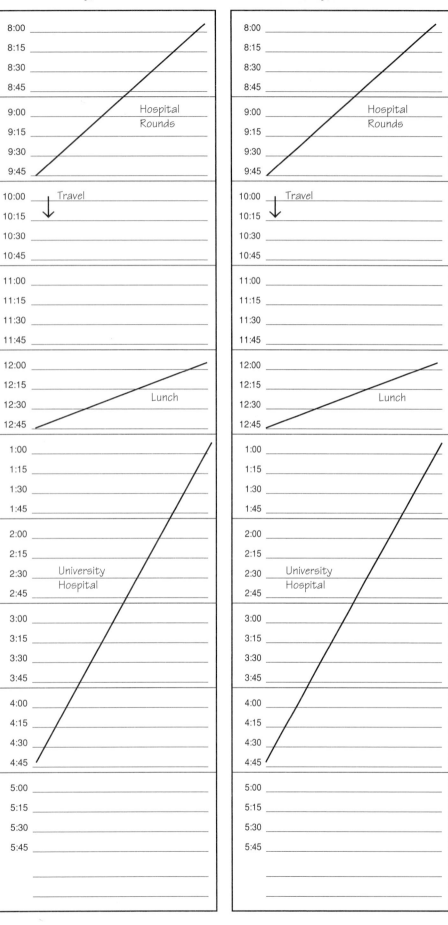
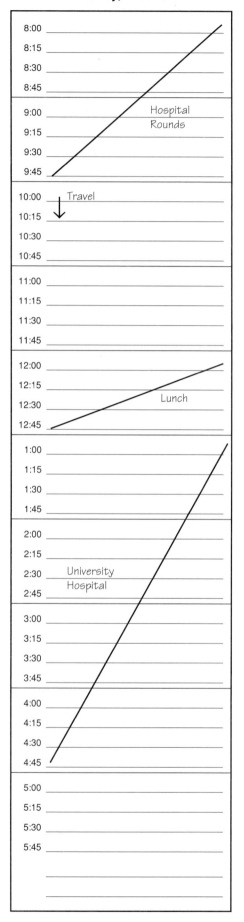

Monday, December 1

8:00	
8:15	
8:30	
8:45	
9:00	Hospital
9:15	Rounds
9:30	
9:45	
10:00	Travel
10:15	
10:30	
10:45	
11:00	
11:15	
11:30	
11:45	
12:00	
12:15	
12:30	Lunch
12:45	
1:00	
1:15	
1:30	
1:45	
2:00	
2:15	
2:30	University
2:45	Hospital
3:00	
3:15	
3:30	
3:45	
4:00	
4:15	
4:30	
4:45	
5:00	
5:15	
5:30	
5:45	

Tuesday, December 2

8:00	
8:15	
8:30	
8:45	
9:00	Hospital
9:15	Rounds
9:30	
9:45	
10:00	Travel
10:15	
10:30	
10:45	
11:00	
11:15	
11:30	
11:45	
12:00	
12:15	
12:30	Lunch
12:45	
1:00	
1:15	
1:30	
1:45	
2:00	
2:15	
2:30	University
2:45	Hospital
3:00	
3:15	
3:30	
3:45	
4:00	
4:15	
4:30	
4:45	
5:00	
5:15	
5:30	
5:45	

Wednesday, December 3

8:00	
8:15	
8:30	
8:45	
9:00	Hospital
9:15	Rounds
9:30	
9:45	
10:00	Travel
10:15	
10:30	
10:45	
11:00	
11:15	
11:30	
11:45	
12:00	
12:15	
12:30	Lunch
12:45	
1:00	
1:15	
1:30	
1:45	
2:00	
2:15	
2:30	University
2:45	Hospital
3:00	
3:15	
3:30	
3:45	
4:00	
4:15	
4:30	
4:45	
5:00	
5:15	
5:30	
5:45	

Monday, December 1 **Tuesday, December 2** **Wednesday, December 3**

YOUR APPOINTMENT IS:

_____ AT _____

SPECIAL INSTRUCTIONS:

MARK NEWMAN, M.D.
2235 South Ridgeway Avenue
Chicago, IL 60623-2240
312-555-6022

PLEASE CALL IF YOU CANNOT KEEP THIS APPOINTMENT.

YOUR APPOINTMENT IS:

_____ AT _____

SPECIAL INSTRUCTIONS:

MARK NEWMAN, M.D.
2235 South Ridgeway Avenue
Chicago, IL 60623-2240
312-555-6022

PLEASE CALL IF YOU CANNOT KEEP THIS APPOINTMENT.

YOUR APPOINTMENT IS:

_____ AT _____

SPECIAL INSTRUCTIONS:

MARK NEWMAN, M.D.
2235 South Ridgeway Avenue
Chicago, IL 60623-2240
312-555-6022

PLEASE CALL IF YOU CANNOT KEEP THIS APPOINTMENT.

YOUR APPOINTMENT IS:

_____ AT _____

SPECIAL INSTRUCTIONS:

MARK NEWMAN, M.D.
2235 South Ridgeway Avenue
Chicago, IL 60623-2240
312-555-6022

PLEASE CALL IF YOU CANNOT KEEP THIS APPOINTMENT.

YOUR APPOINTMENT IS:

_____ AT _____

SPECIAL INSTRUCTIONS:

MARK NEWMAN, M.D.
2235 South Ridgeway Avenue
Chicago, IL 60623-2240
312-555-6022

PLEASE CALL IF YOU CANNOT KEEP THIS APPOINTMENT.

YOUR APPOINTMENT IS:

_____ AT _____

SPECIAL INSTRUCTIONS:

MARK NEWMAN, M.D.
2235 South Ridgeway Avenue
Chicago, IL 60623-2240
312-555-6022

PLEASE CALL IF YOU CANNOT KEEP THIS APPOINTMENT.

YOUR APPOINTMENT IS:

_____ AT _____

SPECIAL INSTRUCTIONS:

MARK NEWMAN, M.D.
2235 South Ridgeway Avenue
Chicago, IL 60623-2240
312-555-6022

PLEASE CALL IF YOU CANNOT KEEP THIS APPOINTMENT.

YOUR APPOINTMENT IS:

_____ AT _____

SPECIAL INSTRUCTIONS:

MARK NEWMAN, M.D.
2235 South Ridgeway Avenue
Chicago, IL 60623-2240
312-555-6022

PLEASE CALL IF YOU CANNOT KEEP THIS APPOINTMENT.

YOUR APPOINTMENT IS:

_____ AT _____

SPECIAL INSTRUCTIONS:

MARK NEWMAN, M.D.
2235 South Ridgeway Avenue
Chicago, IL 60623-2240
312-555-6022

PLEASE CALL IF YOU CANNOT KEEP THIS APPOINTMENT.

YOUR APPOINTMENT IS:

_____ AT _____

SPECIAL INSTRUCTIONS:

MARK NEWMAN, M.D.
2235 South Ridgeway Avenue
Chicago, IL 60623-2240
312-555-6022

PLEASE CALL IF YOU CANNOT KEEP THIS APPOINTMENT.

YOUR APPOINTMENT IS:

_____ AT _____

SPECIAL INSTRUCTIONS:

MARK NEWMAN, M.D.
2235 South Ridgeway Avenue
Chicago, IL 60623-2240
312-555-6022

PLEASE CALL IF YOU CANNOT KEEP THIS APPOINTMENT.

YOUR APPOINTMENT IS:

_____ AT _____

SPECIAL INSTRUCTIONS:

MARK NEWMAN, M.D.
2235 South Ridgeway Avenue
Chicago, IL 60623-2240
312-555-6022

PLEASE CALL IF YOU CANNOT KEEP THIS APPOINTMENT.

YOUR APPOINTMENT IS:

_____ AT _____

SPECIAL INSTRUCTIONS:

MARK NEWMAN, M.D.
2235 South Ridgeway Avenue
Chicago, IL 60623-2240
312-555-6022

PLEASE CALL IF YOU CANNOT KEEP THIS APPOINTMENT.

YOUR APPOINTMENT IS:

_____ AT _____

SPECIAL INSTRUCTIONS:

MARK NEWMAN, M.D.
2235 South Ridgeway Avenue
Chicago, IL 60623-2240
312-555-6022

PLEASE CALL IF YOU CANNOT KEEP THIS APPOINTMENT.

YOUR APPOINTMENT IS:

_____ AT _____

SPECIAL INSTRUCTIONS:

MARK NEWMAN, M.D.
2235 South Ridgeway Avenue
Chicago, IL 60623-2240
312-555-6022

PLEASE CALL IF YOU CANNOT KEEP THIS APPOINTMENT.

10/12   Raymond Murray   House call

76-year-old with end-stage COPD. Home O_2. Increased respiratory distress x 2 d. yellow sputum. No fever, chill, sweat. Appetite, down. Increased wheezing; need O_2 24 h/d. Exam: BP, 115/70. Pulse, 110 and regular. Dyspneic. No JVD. Lungs, scattered medium inspiratory wheezes; no crackles. Cor, normal. 1+ pedal edema. Dx—acute exacerbation of COPD; bronchitis. Treatment—Erythromycin 250 mg q.i.d x 10 d. Call 2-3 days for progress report.

HOUSECALL SLIP   Date _____

Patient_____

Address_____ Phone _____

Bill to _____

****

Symptoms_____

_____

_____

_____

Exam_____

_____

_____

Diagnosis _____

Treatment _____

_____

OUT-OF-OFFICE CALL   Date _____

Patient_____

Address_____ Phone _____

Bill to _____

****

Symptoms_____

_____

_____

_____

Exam_____

_____

_____

Diagnosis _____

Treatment _____

_____

KRAMER, JEFFREY
5103 N. Marine Drive
Chicago, IL 60640-5607
312-555-1913
SSN: 990-22-3948
DOB: 04/22/ , Age 8
Employer: Western Travels
(father)
312-555-8820
Kramer, Andrew
Northstar Premium Insurance
747-22-3401-02 Group: 411

BABCOCK, SARA
131 N. Mason Avenue
Chicago, IL 60644-4455
312-555-5441
SSN: 987-87-3759
DOB: 12/20/ , Age 22
Employer: Kaiser Insurance
312-555-9966
Kaiser Insurance
987-87-3759

BAAB, THOMAS
5015 N. Ridgeway Avenue
Chicago, IL 60625-1220
312-555-3478
SSN: 581-57-0376
DOB: 10/06/ , Age 54
Employer: Sears Auto Parts
312-555-8830
University Health Plan
581-57-0376-59 Group: A87

DAYTON, THERESA
105 W. Chestnut Street
Chicago, IL 60610-2816
312-555-2231
SSN: 767-90-1128
03/13/ , Age 22
Employer: St. Anne Medical
Center
312-555-8832
University Health Plan
767-90-1128 Group: S357C

ARMSTRONG, MONICA
5518 W. Monroe Street
Chicago, IL 60644-5519
312-555-4413
SSN: 486-29-3789
DOB: 08/12/ , Age 50
Employer: Ostrom Electric
312-555-8825
Blue Cross/Blue Shield
486-29-3789-1

GRANT, TODD
1440 W. Olive Street
Chicago, IL 60660-3299
312-555-9825
SSN: 399-11-2939
DOB: 05/18/ , Age 32
Employer: University Hospital
312-555-2500
Prudential Plan
399-11-2939

CASAGRANDA, DORIS
3132 W. 42d Street
Chicago, IL 60632-1406
312-555-1200
SSN: 890-29-5649
DOB: 09/01/ , Age 16
Employer: Self-employed (father)
312-555-1200
National Insurance
497-27-3367-05

CASTRO, JOSEPH
4377 N. Oak Park Avenue
Chicago, IL 60634-3727
312-555-1020
SSN: 876-91-3629
DOB: 11/02/ , Age 19
Employer: University Hospital
312-555-2500
University Health Plan
876-91-3629 Group: A287-05

SHERMAN, FLORENCE
6111 N. Lincoln Avenue
Chicago, IL 60608-3173
312-555-1217
SSN: 669-35-2244
DOB: 05/22/ , Age 65
Employer: Retired
Medicare
669-35-2244B

ROBERTS, SUZANNE
133 N. Mason Avenue
Chicago, IL 60625-4433
312-555-2267
SSN: 340-20-1827
DOB: 07/07/ , Age 23
Employer: Rollins Club
312-555-8835
No insurance

SUN, CHENG
2235 W. School Street
Chicago, IL 60618-5785
312-555-3750
SSN: 285-90-2125
DOB: 08/11/ , Age 44
Employer: Billings, Inc.
312-555-8149
Metro State Plan
285-90-2125 Group: 35A

LUND, LAURA
13419 S. Buffalo Avenue
Chicago, IL 60633-2010
312-555-4106
SSN: 899-90-0072
DOB: 01/01/ , Age 17
Employer: North Auto Parts
(father)
312-555-8840
Lund, Lawrence
Employee Benefit
200-66-3986-01

BURTON, RANDY
4345 W. Grace Street
Chicago, IL 60641-6730
312-555-7292
SSN: ---
DOB: 01/16/ , Age 2
Employer: Unemployed (father)
Burton, Paul
No insurance

VILLANO, STEPHEN
3518 South 23d Street
Chicago, IL 60623-7355
312-555-3493
SSN: 880-29-0399
DOB: 02/27/ , Age 4
Employer: Metro Bus Service
(father)
312-555-8842
Villano, Juan
Employee Benefit Plan
200-97-4811-02 Group: 35A

RICHARDS, WARREN
7952 S. Springfield Avenue
Chicago, IL 60623-2579
312-555-3621
SSN: 902-55-3391
DOB: 04/09/ , Age 77
Employer: Retired
Medicare: 902-55-3391B
Blue Cross: 902-55-3391

MATTHEWS, ARDIS
4443 W. Monroe Street
Chicago, IL 60624-8966
312-555-3178
SSN: 340-99-6546
DOB: 09/10/ , Age 27
Employer: Arling Electronics
(Earl)
312-555-8848
Matthews, Earl--spouse
Arling Employee Plan
294-82-8099-02 Group: 33A

JONATHAN III, CHARLES
5708 W. 63d Place
Chicago, IL 60638-3391
312-555-3097
SSN: 444-02-4422
DOB: 11/29/ , Age 38
Employer: ISD #212
312-555-8850
Kaiser Insurance
444-02-4422 Group: 991A

ROGERS, CLARENCE
4713 W. 82d Place
Chicago, IL 60652-2111
312-555-5297
SSN: 463-71-3030
DOB: 09/25/ , Age 28
Employer: Websters' Restaurant
312-555-8852
Metro State Plan
463-71-3030 Group: 55A

MENDEZ, ANA
3457 W. 63d Place
Chicago, IL 60629-4270
312-555-3606
SSN: 295-99-3325
DOB: 03/24/ , Age 34
Employer: Lisle School District
#12
312-555-8852
Blue Cross and Blue Shield
295-99-3325 Group: 354

MURRAY, RAYMOND
3908 N. Central Avenue
Chicago, IL 60634-3276
312-555-6343
SSN: 555-88-3822
DOB: 11/05/ , Age 76
Employer: Retired
Medicare
555-88-3822B

ROBERTSON, GARY
3449 W. Foster Avenue
Chicago, IL 60625-2377
312-555-9565
SSN: 255-74-1021
DOB: 12/31/ , Age 43
Employer: Robertson's Fishing
Fleet
312-555-8857
Prudential Group Health
255-74-1021

PHAN, MARC
9340 S. Green Street
Chicago, IL 60620-8129
312-555-3344
SSN: 888-99-9228
DOB: 10/23/ , Age 2
Employer: University Hospital
(dad)
312-555-2500
Phan, Tam
University Health Plan
465-77-3821-01 Group: 77C

MORTON, SARAH
723 W. Sixth Street
Chicago, IL 60621-2314
312-555-2324
SSN: 899-34-2834
DOB: 01/27/ , Age 14
Employer: Universal Photo, Inc.
(mother)
312-555-8876
Morton, Esther
Northstar Insurance
300-29-1874 Group: 255-03

SINCLAIR, EUGENE
2721 W. 18th Street
Chicago, IL 60608-6260
312-555-4381
SSN: 322-91-7722
DOB: 11/19/ , Age 79
Employer: Retired
Medicare: 322-91-7722A
Blue Cross: 322-91-7722

Clinical Data Sheet

Name _____ **Telephone** _____

Date of Birth _____ **Age** _____

OUTSIDE SERVICES

University Hospital
5500 North Ridgeway Avenue
Chicago, IL 60625-1200
555-2500
Ms. Yates: Ext. 2950

Elizabeth Miller-Young, M.D.
Suite 205
2901 West Fifth Avenue
Chicago, IL 60612-9002
555-3500
OB/GYN

Hugh Arnolds, M.D.
Suite 440
2785 South Ridgeway Avenue
Chicago, IL 60647-2700
555-6800
Internist

Martinez Transcription Service
2200 South Ridgeway Avenue
Chicago, IL 60623-2000
555-2424
Betze Martinez

Margery Pierce, M.D.
Suite 209
6452 North Ridgeway Avenue
Chicago, IL 60626-5462
555-4880
Pediatrician

Karen Larsen, M.D.
2785 South Ridgeway Avenue
Chicago, IL 60647-2700
555-2700
On-call doctor

Jason Berger, M.D.
5000 North Oak Park Drive
Chicago, IL 60634-0005
555-7050
Personal friend

Richard Diangelis, M.D.
Suite 280
2785 South Ridgeway Avenue
Chicago, IL 60647-2700
555-1575
Ophthalmologist

Lynn Corbett, M.D.
Suite 300
Professional Building
8672 South Ridgeway Avenue
Chicago, IL 60623-2240
555-2300
Cardiologist

Theresa Townsend, M.D.
500 South Dearborn Street
Chicago, IL 60605-0005
555-2200
Chairperson
Chicago Medical Society

Consumer Pharmacy
555-1252

Greg Koski, M.D.
Suite 350
Professional Building
8672 South Ridgeway Avenue
Chicago, IL 60623-2240
555-4500
Orthopedic surgeon

Laura Sinn, M.D.
Suite 100
2901 West Fifth Avenue
Chicago, IL 60612-9002
555-7850
Urologist

MARK NEWMAN, M.D.

2235 South Ridgeway Avenue
Chicago, IL 60623-2240
312-555-6022
FAX: 312-555-0025

Board Certified in Family Medicine

Name Sherman, Florence   **Telephone** 555-1217

Date of Birth 5/22/--   **Age** 65

10/08/--

CHIEF COMPLAINT: Trouble with vision.

SUBJECTIVE: Patient is a 65-year-old female who had two episodes during the last week of jagged lights occurring in central visual field. These lasted 15-20 minutes; no other symptoms. Patient has long history of migraines.

OBJECTIVE: Within normal limits; specifically, no evidence of tear or hole of the retina.

ASSESSMENT: Migraine equivalent vs. posterior vitreous detachment.

PLAN:
1. Discussed with ophthalmologist, Dr. Richard Diangelis. Patient advised about signs and symptoms of detachment of the retina and told to seek immediate medical attention should any of these signs appear.
2. Trial of Inderal 40 mg b.i.d. for migraines.
3. Recheck in one to two months.
4. Patient requests referral to Dr. Diangelis.

            Mark Newman, M.D./tjo

Name Matthews, Ardis   **Telephone** 555-3178

Date of Birth 9/10/--   **Age** 27

9/24/--

SUBJECTIVE: Patient is a 27-year-old nulligravida female who was seen in April for condyloma acuminata of the perineum. She was treated with podophyllum, and they subsequently disappeared; however, over the past six weeks, she has noticed recurrence. They seem to be more profuse. She states that her consort was checked and noted to have no lesions.

She is a smoker. She has a history of IV drug abuse several years ago. She tested HIV negative one year ago; that was approximately six months post last IV usage. She also admits to having shared needles at that time.

OBJECTIVE: Perineum has large exophytic growth of the perineum, which is consistent with recurrent condyloma acuminata. Inspection of the introitus and vaginal vault shows excrescences over the lateral vaginal wall. The cervix appeared grossly normal; however, Pap smear was taken.

ASSESSMENT: Recurrent condyloma acuminata of the vulva and vagina, possibly the cervix.

PLAN:
1. Will await the Pap smear results. If this shows any evidence of dysplastic cells, the patient should undergo colposcopy to determine the lesion. If this is negative, will refer for possible laser ablation of these lesions of the vulva and vagina.
2. Discussed her discontinuing smoking.
3. Discussed using condom contraception.
4. She is willing to undergo HIV testing again because of the persistent and rapid recurrence of her condyloma acuminata.
5. Patient will call in two weeks for results of her Pap smear.
Mark Newman, M.D./tjo

10/01/--

Pap smear, negative. Refer to Dr. Elizabeth Miller-Young.
Mark Newman, M.D./tjo

PATIENT REGISTRATION

DATE _____

Patient Name			Birth Date
(Last)	(First)	(Initial)	

Address			
City		State	ZIP
Telephone	Social Security No.		
Bill To	Relationship		
Address	City	State	ZIP

Employer
Address	Work Phone
City	State	ZIP

NOTIFY IN CASE OF EMERGENCY

Name	Relationship
Address	Phone
City	State	ZIP

INSURANCE INFORMATION

INSURANCE COMPANY	POLICY NO.	SUBSCRIBER
(1)		
(2)		

PATIENT REGISTRATION

DATE _____

Patient Name			Birth Date	
(Last)	(First)	(Initial)		

Address			

City		State	ZIP

Telephone	Social Security No.

Bill To	Relationship

Address	City	State	ZIP

Employer		

Address	Work Phone

City	State	ZIP

NOTIFY IN CASE OF EMERGENCY

Name	Relationship

Address	Phone

City	State	ZIP

INSURANCE INFORMATION

INSURANCE COMPANY	POLICY NO.	SUBSCRIBER
(1)		
(2)		

RECORDS RELEASE

TO: _____ Health care provider
_____ Address
_____ City, State, ZIP

I hereby authorize the above-named health care provider to release the specified information below to

Mark Newman, M.D.
2235 South Ridgeway Avenue
Chicago, IL 60623-2240
FAX: 312-555-0025

PATIENT: _____
Address: _____
City, State, ZIP_____
Birth Date: _____

Please include
___   Specific Records _____

Signed _____   Date _____

RECORDS RELEASE

TO: _____ Health care provider
_____ Address
_____ City, State, ZIP

I hereby authorize the above-named health care provider to release the specified information below to

Mark Newman, M.D.
2235 South Ridgeway Avenue
Chicago, IL 60623-2240
FAX: 312-555-0025

PATIENT: _____
Address: _____
City, State, ZIP_____
Birth Date: _____

Please include
___   Specific Records _____

Signed _____   Date _____

TELEPHONE LOG

DATE _____

TIME	CALLER	TELEPHONE NUMBER	REASON	DONE

TO-DO LIST

DATE _____

RUSH	THINGS TO DO	DONE

Baab. 10/15 This 54-year-old male enters for health maintenance care. He is expressing some anxiety about the ability to tolerate the stresses that occur at work; otherwise, doing well. ROS: Has excellent exercise tolerance without any exertional chest discomfort or dyspnea. Has good energy level; sleeping well; no nausea, vomiting, abdominal pain, or diarrhea. No difficulties with urination. Has some itching groin rash past few weeks. Medications: Multivitamins and daily aspirin. Surgeries: S/P tonsillectomy. SH: Does not smoke or consume alcoholic beverages. Married, 3 children. Employed as construction worker. PE: Height, 70 inches. Weight, 210 #. BP, 110/82; pulse, 64. Patient is pleasant, mildly obese; in no acute distress. HEENT: TMs, within normal limits. Eyes, full EOM; PERRLA; disc margins, sharp. Mouth, not inflamed. Neck: Supple; thyroid, normal. No cervical or axillary adenopathy present. Chest: Clear to A & P. Cardiac: Normal S1 and S2 without click, rub, or gallop. All pulses, intact; no carotid or abdominal bruit noted. Abdomen: Normal bowel sounds without hepatosplenomegaly. Soft and nontender. No masses or scars. Extremities: No cyanosis, clubbing, or edema. GU: Testes, no masses or tenderness; no hernias present. Rash consistent with tinea cruris is present. Rectal: Normal prostate. Neurological: Intact. IMPRESSION: Normal physical exam with exception of tinea cruris. PLAN: Lotrimin cream for tinea cruris. Flex sig. Labs: UA, CBC, and SMA-12.

OBSTETRICAL CHART

Name _____

Age _____   Gravida ___II___   Para ___I___   Phone _____

HISTORY OF PRESENT PREGNANCY (Nausea, Vomiting, Bleeding, Edema, Headache)

LMP _2/15/--_   EDC _11/8/--_   Quickening _June_

PAST MEDICAL HISTORY (Include Use of Drugs and Alcohol) _____

_____ See Dr. Tai's record. _____

PAST SURGICAL HISTORY _See Dr. Tai's record._ _____

_____

FAMILY HISTORY _____ See Dr. Tai's record. _____

_____

MENSTRUAL HISTORY Onset _13_   Cycle _q28-30_   Duration _4 days_

Amount _moderate_ Pain _occasional_   Leucorrhea _Ø_

OBSTETRICAL HISTORY

Year	Length	Type of Delivery	Labor	Complications	Sex/Wt.

PRENATAL VISITS

DATE	WEIGHT	BP	HGB	ALBUMIN	SUGAR	FUNDUS	POS	FHT	EDEMA	REMARKS
10/14/--	145	112/70	11.6					Good	Trace	No problems UA, negative

OBSTETRICAL CHART

Name ___Erin Mitchell___

Age ___21___	Grav. ___II___	Para ___I___	

HISTORY OF PRESENT PREGNANCY: LMP ___2-15___ EDC ___11-8___ Quickening ___June___

ROS: Negative. Generally healthy.

PE: Essentially negative. Pap smear, 4/17 neg.

PAST MEDICAL HISTORY: UCHD. Denies use of drugs; occasional alcohol.

FAMILY HISTORY: Mother & father, living and well; 2 siblings, living and well.

PAST SURGICAL HISTORY: T & A age 5

MENSTRUAL HISTORY: Onset ___13___   Cycle ___q 28-30___

Duration ___4 days___

Amount ___Moderate___   Pain ___Occasional___   Leucorrhea ___—___

OBSTETRICAL HISTORY: Year ___(5 years ago)___   Length Pregnancy ___40 weeks___

Type of Delivery ___Spontaneous___

Length of Labor ___12 hours___

Complications ___Episiotomy___

Sex ___M___   Weight ___8 lb 7 oz___   Length ___21 in___

PRENATAL VISITS:

Date ___4/17___   Weight ___126___   Blood pressure ___122/64___   Hemoglobin ___12.5___
Albumin ___Neg.___   Sugar ___Neg.___   Fundus _____   POS _____
FHT ___—___   Edema ___—___   Titre results _____
Remarks and treatment ___Occasional N & V___

Date ___6/20___   Weight ___127___   Blood pressure ___124/64___   Hemoglobin ___12.3___
Albumin ___—___   Sugar ___—___   Fundus _____   POS _____
FHT ___+___   Edema ___—___   Titre results _____
Remarks and treatment _____

Date ___7/19___   Weight ___131___   Blood pressure ___120/68___   Hemoglobin ___11.9___
Albumin ___—___   Sugar ___—___   Fundus _____   POS _____
FHT ___+___   Edema ___—___   Titre results _____
Remarks and treatment ___Vitamins. No problems.___

Date ___8/22___   Weight ___134___   Blood pressure ___110/70___   Hemoglobin ___11.9___
Albumin ___—___   Sugar ___—___   Fundus _____   POS _____
FHT ___120+___   Edema _____   Titre results _____
Remarks and treatment ___No trouble___

Date ___9/22___   Weight ___137___   Blood pressure ___112/70___   Hemoglobin ___12.0___
Albumin ___—___   Sugar ___—___   Fundus _____   POS _____
FHT ___+___   Edema ___slight___   Titre results _____
Remarks and treatment ___Fetus active. Will be moving.___

10/15 - Records transferred to Mark Newman, M.D.

HEMATOLOGY—CHEMISTRY

Name _Thomas Baab_ • Doctor _Newman_

Test Results

5.2	WBC	124	Glucose
44.2	Hematocrit	420	Cholesterol
13.6	Hemoglobin	10	BUN
	Differential	9	Calcium
42	PMN	3	Phosphorous
2	Bands	1	Bilirubin
48	Lymphs	4	Uric acid
3	Mono	75	Alkaline phosphatase
5	Eos	4.2	Albumin
	Baso	7	Protein, total
242,000	Platelets	200	LDH
	Thyroid	30	SGOT

MN

Date _10/15_

URINE—Miscellaneous *MN*

Name _Thomas Baab_   Doctor _Newman_

Color _clear yellow_   Pap Smear _____

pH _6_   _____

Specific Gravity _1.020_   _____

Protein _O_   Vaginal Smear _____

Glucose _O_   _____

Ketone _____

WBCs/hpf _O-1_   Hemoccults _neg._

RBCs/hpf _O-1_   _____

Bacteria _____

_____

Culture _____

_____

Date _10/15_

HEMATOLOGY—CHEMISTRY

Name _Monica Armstrong_   Doctor _Newman_

Test Results

5.2	WBC	86	Glucose
43.0	Hematocrit	182	Cholesterol
13.6	Hemoglobin	15	BUN
	Differential	9	Calcium
50	PMN	3.1	Phosphorous
	Bands	0.5	Bilirubin
48	Lymphs	3.2	Uric acid
1	Mono		Alkaline phosphatase
1	Eos	4	Albumin
	Baso	6.9	Protein, total
247,000	Platelets	121	LDH
	Thyroid	15	SGOT

MN

Date _10/14_

URINE—Miscellaneous *MN*

Name _Monica Armstrong_   Doctor _Newman_

Color _clear yellow_   Pap Smear _____

pH _6_   _____

Specific Gravity _1.010_   _____

Protein _O_   Vaginal Smear _____

Glucose _O_   _____

Ketone _____

WBCs/hpf _O-1_   Hemoccults _neg._

RBCs/hpf _O-3_   _____

Bacteria _____

_____

Culture _____

_____

Date _10/14_

Name David Kramer   Doctor   Newman
Test Results Hemoglobin

____	WBC	____	Glucose
____	Hematocrit	____	Cholesterol
13.1	Hemoglobin	____	BUN
	Differential	____	Calcium
____	PMN	____	Phosphorous
____	Bands	____	Bilirubin
____	Lymphs	____	Uric acid
____	Mono	____	Alkaline phosphatase
____	Eos	____	Albumin
____	Baso	____	Protein, total
____	Platelets	____	LDH
____	Thyroid	____	SGOT

MN

HEMATOLOGY—CHEMISTRY

Date 10/14

Name David Kramer   Doctor Newman

Color _____   Pap Smear _____
pH _____   _____
Specific Gravity _____
Protein _____ Vaginal Smear _____
Glucose _____ _____
Ketone _____ neg.
WBCs/hpf _____ Hemoccults _____
RBCs/hpf _____ _____
Bacteria _____
_____

Culture _____   MN
_____

URINE—Miscellaneous

Date 10/14

Name Gary Robertson   Doctor Newman

Color yellow   Pap Smear _____
pH 5.6   _____
Specific Gravity _____
Protein neg. Vaginal Smear _____
Glucose neg. _____
Ketone neg.
WBCs/hpf 15-20 Hemoccults _____
RBCs/hpf 5-10 _____
Bacteria _____
_____

Culture urine culture pending
_____

URINE—Miscellaneous   MN

Date 10/14

Name _____   Doctor _____

Color _____   Pap Smear _____
pH _____   _____
Specific Gravity _____
Protein _____ Vaginal Smear _____
Glucose _____ _____
Ketone _____
WBCs/hpf _____ Hemoccults _____
RBCs/hpf _____ _____
Bacteria _____
_____

Culture _____
_____

URINE—Miscellaneous

Date _____

RE: Thomas Baab, 10/16/--

Flex sig: Indications — health care maintenance. Findings: Scope advanced to 21 cm, no further secondary to angulation of colon and spasms. No polyps, masses, or ulcers seen. Vascular pattern and mucosa are normal. No diverticula. Assessment: Negative flexible sigmoidoscopy to 21 cm.

MARK NEWMAN, M.D.

Board Certified in Family Medicine

2235 South Ridgeway Avenue
Chicago, IL 60623-2240
312-555-6022
FAX: 312-555-0025

FEE SCHEDULE

New Patients

99202	OV Focused (OVF)	40.00
99203	OV Expanded (OVE)	50.00

Established Patients

99212	OV Focused (OVF)	30.00
99213	OV Expanded (OVE)	40.00
99214	OV Detailed (OVD)	75.00
99215	OV Comprehensive	100.00

House Call

99352	HC	80.00

Hospital Visits

99221	Initial HV	100.00
99232	HV	70.00

Obstetrical/Genitourinary

99212	OVF (antepartum)	30.00
54150	Circumcision	75.00
59410	Delivery	650.00
99433	Newborn physical	35.00
99212	OVF (postpartum)	30.00
55250	Vasectomy	350.00

Miscellaneous

93000	EKG	65.00
45330	Flex sig	125.00
A4550	Sterile tray	20.00

X-rays

71020	Chest	70.00
73560	Knee films	75.00
76091	Mammogram	80.00
72090	Scoliosis Film	60.00
70210	Sinus	60.00

Laboratory

85022	CBC	20.00
82465	Cholesterol	10.00
85007	Differential	10.00
82270	Hemoccults x3	15.00
85018	Hemoglobin (Hgb)	10.00
86308	Mono test	20.00
88156	Pap Smear	35.00
89300	Semen Analysis	30.00
80012	SMA-12	30.00
86588	Strep Screen	20.00
89060	Synovial Fluid	20.00
81000	Urinalysis (UA)	10.00
87086	Urine Culture (UC)	10.00
85048	WBC	10.00
85009	WBC with Diff	15.50
87210	Wet Prep	15.00

Injections

J1030	DepoMedrol-40mg	15.00
J1040	DepoMedrol-80mg	15.00
90701	DPT	25.00
90702	DT	12.00
90724	Influenza	15.00
90707	MMR	40.00
90712	Oral Polio	20.00
90703	TT	13.00

Statement 1

STATEMENT

MARK NEWMAN, M.D.
2235 South Ridgeway Avenue
Chicago, IL 60623-2240
312-555-6022   Fax 312-555-0025

Family
1. Earl
2. Ardis
3.
4.
5.

Earl Matthews
2000 N. Lincoln Park West
Chicago, IL 60614-1411

NO.	DATE	DESCRIPTION	CHARGE	PAYMENT	ADJ.	CURRENT BALANCE
2	4/22	OVE (NP)/Pap	75.00	75.00		—
2	6/5	OVE	40.00			40.00
2	7/18	OVF/CBC/UA	60.00			100.00
2	8/12	OVE/Chest X ray	110.00			210.00
2	9/24	OVE/Pap	75.00			285.00
2	10/2	ROA		150.00		135.00

CBC—complete blood count
EKG—electrocardiogram
HC—house call
Hgb—hemoglobin
HV—hospital visit

INJ—injection
LAB—laboratory work
NP—new patient
OVD—office visit, detailed
OVE—office visit, expanded

OVF—office visit, focused
Pap—Pap smear
ROA—received on account
UA—urinalysis
UC—urine culture

Statement 2

STATEMENT

MARK NEWMAN, M.D.
2235 South Ridgeway Avenue
Chicago, IL 60623-2240
312-555-6022   Fax 312-555-0025

Family
1. Theresa
2.
3.
4.
5.

Theresa Dayton
105 W. Chestnut Street
Chicago, IL 60610-2816

NO.	DATE	DESCRIPTION	CHARGE	PAYMENT	ADJ.	CURRENT BALANCE
1	9/24	OV Comp/LAB/Pap	165.00	50.00		115.00
	10/3	ROA		115.00		—

CBC—complete blood count
EKG—electrocardiogram
HC—house call
Hgb—hemoglobin
HV—hospital visit

INJ—injection
LAB—laboratory work
NP—new patient
OVD—office visit, detailed
OVE—office visit, expanded

OVF—office visit, focused
Pap—Pap smear
ROA—received on account
UA—urinalysis
UC—urine culture

STATEMENT 1 (Warren)

STATEMENT

MARK NEWMAN, M.D.
2235 South Ridgeway Avenue
Chicago, IL 60623-2240
312-555-6022   Fax 312-555-0025

Family
1. Warren
2.
3.
4.
5.

Warren Richards
7952 S. Springfield Ave.
Chicago, IL 60623-2579

NO.	DATE	DESCRIPTION	CHARGE	CREDIT PAYMENT	CREDIT ADJ.	CURRENT BALANCE
1	9/6	Initial HV/4 HV 9/1-9/5	380.00			380.00
	10/6	ROA		300.00		80.00

CBC—complete blood count
EKG—electrocardiogram
HC—house call
Hgb—hemoglobin
HV—hospital visit

INJ—injection
LAB—laboratory work
NP—new patient
OVD—office visit, detailed
OVE—office visit, expanded

OVF—office visit, focused
Pap—Pap smear
ROA—received on account
UA—urinalysis
UC—urine culture

STATEMENT 2 (Ana)

STATEMENT

MARK NEWMAN, M.D.
2235 South Ridgeway Avenue
Chicago, IL 60623-2240
312-555-6022   Fax 312-555-0025

Family
1. Ana
2.
3.
4.
5.

Ana Mendez
3457 W. 63rd Place
Chicago, IL 60629-4270

NO.	DATE	DESCRIPTION	CHARGE	CREDIT PAYMENT	CREDIT ADJ.	CURRENT BALANCE
1	9/24	OV Comp/Pap/LAB/Mammogram	255.00			255.00
	10/1	ROA		100.00		155.00

CBC—complete blood count
EKG—electrocardiogram
HC—house call
Hgb—hemoglobin
HV—hospital visit

INJ—injection
LAB—laboratory work
NP—new patient
OVD—office visit, detailed
OVE—office visit, expanded

OVF—office visit, focused
Pap—Pap smear
ROA—received on account
UA—urinalysis
UC—urine culture

STATEMENT

MARK NEWMAN, M.D.
2235 South Ridgeway Avenue
Chicago, IL 60623-2240
312-555-6022   Fax 312-555-0025

	Family
1.	Clarence
2.	
3.	
4.	
5.	

Clarence Rogers
4713 W. 82d Place
Chicago, IL 60652-2111

NO.	DATE	DESCRIPTION	CHARGE	CREDIT PAYMENT	CREDIT ADJ.	CURRENT BALANCE
		Previous Balance				250.00
1	9/24	OVE/EKG/SMA-12	135.00			385.00
	10/7	ROA		150.00		235.00

CBC—complete blood count	INJ—injection	OVF—office visit, focused
EKG—electrocardiogram	LAB—laboratory work	Pap—Pap smear
HC—house call	NP—new patient	ROA—received on account
Hgb—hemoglobin	OVD—office visit, detailed	UA—urinalysis
HV—hospital visit	OVE—office visit, expanded	UC—urine culture

---

STATEMENT

MARK NEWMAN, M.D.
2235 South Ridgeway Avenue
Chicago, IL 60623-2240
312-555-6022   Fax 312-555-0025

	Family
1.	Suzanne
2.	
3.	
4.	
5.	

Suzanne Roberts
133 N. Mason Avenue
Chicago, IL 60625-4433

NO.	DATE	DESCRIPTION	CHARGE	CREDIT PAYMENT	CREDIT ADJ.	CURRENT BALANCE
1	7/25	OV Comp/UA/Pap/LAB	180.00			180.00
	9/30	Reminder note sent				
	10/10	Follow-up call				

CBC—complete blood count	INJ—injection	OVF—office visit, focused
EKG—electrocardiogram	LAB—laboratory work	Pap—Pap smear
HC—house call	NP—new patient	ROA—received on account
Hgb—hemoglobin	OVD—office visit, detailed	UA—urinalysis
HV—hospital visit	OVE—office visit, expanded	UC—urine culture

STATEMENT

MARK NEWMAN, M.D.
2235 South Ridgeway Avenue
Chicago, IL 60623-2240
312-555-6022   Fax 312-555-0025

Family
1.
2.
3.
4.
5.

NO.	DATE	DESCRIPTION	CHARGE	CREDIT PAYMENT	CREDIT ADJ.	CURRENT BALANCE

CBC—complete blood count
EKG—electrocardiogram
HC—house call
Hgb—hemoglobin
HV—hospital visit

INJ—injection
LAB—laboratory work
NP—new patient
OVD—office visit, detailed
OVE—office visit, expanded

OVF—office visit, focused
Pap—Pap smear
ROA—received on account
UA—urinalysis
UC—urine culture

STATEMENT

MARK NEWMAN, M.D.
2235 South Ridgeway Avenue
Chicago, IL 60623-2240
312-555-6022   Fax 312-555-0025

Family
1. Florence
2.
3.
4.
5.

Florence Sherman
6111 N. Lincoln Avenue
Chicago, IL 60608-3173

NO.	DATE	DESCRIPTION	CHARGE	CREDIT PAYMENT	CREDIT ADJ.	CURRENT BALANCE
		Previous Balance				375.00
1	10/8	OVE	40.00			415.00
		INS PAYMENT-Medicare		200.00	75.00	140.00

CBC—complete blood count
EKG—electrocardiogram
HC—house call
Hgb—hemoglobin
HV—hospital visit

INJ—injection
LAB—laboratory work
NP—new patient
OVD—office visit, detailed
OVE—office visit, expanded

OVF—office visit, focused
Pap—Pap smear
ROA—received on account
UA—urinalysis
UC—urine culture

STATEMENT

MARK NEWMAN, M.D.
2235 South Ridgeway Avenue
Chicago, IL 60623-2240
312-555-6022   Fax 312-555-0025

Family
1.
2.
3.
4.
5.

NO.	DATE	DESCRIPTION	CHARGE	CREDIT		CURRENT BALANCE
				PAYMENT	ADJ.	

CBC—complete blood count
EKG—electrocardiogram
HC—house call
Hgb—hemoglobin
HV—hospital visit

INJ—injection
LAB—laboratory work
NP—new patient
OVD—office visit, detailed
OVE—office visit, expanded

OVF—office visit, focused
Pap—Pap smear
ROA—received on account
UA—urinalysis
UC—urine culture

STATEMENT

MARK NEWMAN, M.D.
2235 South Ridgeway Avenue
Chicago, IL 60623-2240
312-555-6022   Fax 312-555-0025

Family
1.
2.
3.
4.
5.

NO.	DATE	DESCRIPTION	CHARGE	CREDIT		CURRENT BALANCE
				PAYMENT	ADJ.	

CBC—complete blood count
EKG—electrocardiogram
HC—house call
Hgb—hemoglobin
HV—hospital visit

INJ—injection
LAB—laboratory work
NP—new patient
OVD—office visit, detailed
OVE—office visit, expanded

OVF—office visit, focused
Pap—Pap smear
ROA—received on account
UA—urinalysis
UC—urine culture

TELEPHONE LOG

DATE _____

TIME	CALLER	TELEPHONE NUMBER	REASON	DONE

TO-DO LIST

DATE _____

RUSH	THINGS TO DO	DONE

Send a letter to Thomas Baab

This letter is to inform you of the results of your blood cholesterol level
from October 15. Your result was 420 — a cholesterol level around 200
is considered normal.

I suggest that you start taking measures to decrease your cholesterol
intake such as a low-fat diet and a low-cholesterol diet. If you need
such a
assistance in planning that diet, please call Linda at our clinic. She will
my office   can
send you a diet instruction sheet. You should also begin an exercise
program as we discussed at our last visit.

If you have other concerns or questions, please contact me.

October 17, 19--

Mark Newman, M.D.
2235 South Ridgeway Avenue
Chicago, IL 60623-2240

Dear Dr. Newman:

RE: David Kramer   DOB: 4/28/--

David is up to date on his immunizations. His immunization record
is as follows:

        DPT: 3 months (7/26/--)   Oral polio: 3 months (7/26/--)
                6 months (10/22/--)   6 months (10/22/--)
                9 months (1/29/--)   9 months (1/29/--)

        MMR: 2 years (5/2/--)

David is due for a booster DTP before starting kindergarten.

If you have any questions, please contact our office.

Sincerely,

Grace Tai, M.D.

Grace Tai, M.D.

jz

MN
Please file.

Ridgeway Radiology
2248 South Ridgeway Avenue
Chicago, IL 60623-224-
312-555-7357

PATIENT: Monica Armstrong
DOCTOR: Mark Newman, M.D.
DATE: 10/16/--

REPORT: Mammogram

Bilateral low-dose mammogram shows no dominant
mass or malignant calcium in either breast.

IMPRESSION: No radiologic evidence for
malignancy.

                                    HWC

H. Wilson Campbell, M.D./pa

Name _Stephen Villano_ Doctor _Newman_
Test Results _Strep screen—positive_

_____	WBC	_____	Glucose
_____	Hematocrit	_____	Cholesterol
_____	Hemoglobin	_____	BUN
	Differential	_____	Calcium
_____	PMN	_____	Phosphorous
_____	Bands	_____	Bilirubin
_____	Lymphs	_____	Uric acid
_____	Mono	_____	Alkaline phosphatase
_____	Eos	_____	Albumin
_____	Baso	_____	Protein, total
_____	Platelets	_____	LDH
_____	Thyroid	_____	SGOT

HEMATOLOGY—CHEMISTRY
Date _10/21_

Name _Gary Robertson_ Doctor _Newman_

Color _weak tea_   Pap Smear _____
pH _____   _____
Specific Gravity _____ _____
Protein _____   Vaginal Smear _____
Glucose _____   _____
Ketone _____
WBCs/hpf _20-25_   Hemoccults _____
RBCs/hpf _10-20_   _____
Bacteria _____
_____
Culture _____
_____

URINE—Miscellaneous
Date _10/22_

Name _Gary Robertson_ Doctor _Newman_
Test Results _____

13,400	WBC	_____	Glucose
_____	Hematocrit	_____	Cholesterol
_____	Hemoglobin	_____	BUN
	Differential	_____	Calcium
_____	PMN	_____	Phosphorous
_____	Bands	_____	Bilirubin
_____	Lymphs	_____	Uric acid
_____	Mono	_____	Alkaline phosphatase
_____	Eos	_____	Albumin
_____	Baso	_____	Protein, total
_____	Platelets	_____	LDH
_____	Thyroid	_____	SGOT

HEMATOLOGY—CHEMISTRY
Date _10/22_

NAME Jonathan III, Charles   **DATE** 10/21

Exam	Code	Charge
OVF	99212	
LAB:		
X RAY:		
OTHER:		
TOTAL		

Diagnosis: Tendinitis

NAME Sherman, Florence   **DATE** 10/21

Exam	Code	Charge
OVF	99212	
LAB: Hgb	85018	
X RAY:		
OTHER:		
TOTAL		

Diagnosis: Dizziness

NAME Dayton, Theresa   **DATE** 10/21

Exam	Code	Charge
OVE	99213	
LAB: Pap	88156	
X RAY: Mammogram	76091	
OTHER:		
TOTAL		

Diagnosis: Cyst right breast. Normal contraception. Female exam.

NAME Mitchell, Erin   **DATE** 10/21

Exam	Code	Charge
OVF	99212	
LAB: Hgb	85018	
UA	81000	
X RAY:		
OTHER:		
TOTAL		

Diagnosis: Pregnancy

NAME Villano, Stephen   **DATE** 10/21

Exam	Code	Charge
OVF	99212	
LAB: Strep screen	86588	
X RAY:		
OTHER:		
TOTAL		

Diagnosis: Strep pharyngitis

NAME Casagranda, Doris   **DATE** 10/20

Exam	Code	Charge
OVE	99212	
LAB:		
X RAY:		
OTHER:		
TOTAL		

Diagnosis: Hidradenitis, suppurative, mild

NAME Lund, Laura   **DATE** 10/21

Exam	Code	Charge
OVE	99213	
LAB:		
X RAY:		
OTHER:		
TOTAL		

Diagnosis: Acute cervical strain

NAME Sun, Cheng   **DATE** 10/21

Exam	Code	Charge
OVF	99212	
LAB:		
X RAY:		
OTHER: Sterile tray	A4550	
TOTAL		

Diagnosis: Removal of wooden splinter from underneath right 4th fingernail

NAME Castro, Joseph   **DATE** 10/22

Exam	Code	Charge
OVF	99212	
LAB:		
X RAY:		
OTHER: Sterile tray	A4550	
TOTAL		

Diagnosis: Foreign body, left eye ? tar

NAME Robertson, Gary   **DATE** 10/22

Exam	Code	Charge
OVD	99214	
LAB: UA	81000	
WBC	85048	
X RAY:		
OTHER:		
TOTAL		

Diagnosis: Pyelonephritis

NAME Mendez, Ana   **DATE** 10/22

Exam	Code	Charge
OVF	99212	
LAB:		
X RAY:		
OTHER:		
TOTAL		

Diagnosis: Acute tonsillitis with regional lymphadenitis

NAME Sherman, Florence   **DATE** 10/22

Exam	Code	Charge
OVD	99214	
LAB:		
X RAY:		
OTHER:		
TOTAL		

Diagnosis: Vestibular neuronitis

NAME Phan, Marc   **DATE** 10/22

Exam	Code	Charge
OVF	99212	
LAB:		
X RAY:		
OTHER:		
TOTAL		

Diagnosis: Bronchitis

NAME Sinclair, Eugene   **DATE** 10/22

Exam	Code	Charge
OVF	99212	
LAB:		
X RAY:		
OTHER:		
TOTAL		

Diagnosis: Nose lesion. R/O basal cell carcinoma

HEALTH INSURANCE TERMS

Directions: Match each health insurance term in Column 2 with the proper definition in Column 1.

COLUMN 1

____ 1. Insurance that covers large medical expenses

____ 2. The doctor who performs the health care

____ 3. Insurance that covers many subscribers under one master policy

____ 4. The rate charged for insurance coverage

____ 5. Insurance that covers physicians' fees

____ 6. The typical fee charged by comparable doctors in the same geographic area

____ 7. An amount the subscriber has to pay for each office visit

____ 8. A formal agreement between the subscriber and the carrier

____ 9. A provision that ensures nonduplication of health insurance coverage

____ 10. Insurance that covers the operating room charges for an inpatient

____ 11. The insurance company that provides insurance benefits

____ 12. The amount the subscriber must pay before the insurance company will pay

____ 13. Insurance protection against a specific accident or disease such as cancer

____ 14. A written agreement covering the subscriber, spouse, and the subscriber's unmarried and student-status dependents

____ 15. The way in which the dependents' primary carrier is determined

COLUMN 2

a. Birthday Rule
b. carrier
c. COB
d. contract
e. co-payment
f. customary fee
g. deductible
h. family contract
i. group insurance
j. hospital insurance
k. major medical insurance
l. medical insurance
m. premium
n. provider
o. special risk insurance

APPROVED OMB-0938-0008

CARRIER ▲

▼

PICA

HEALTH INSURANCE CLAIM FORM

PICA

1. MEDICARE	MEDICAID	CHAMPUS	CHAMPVA	GROUP HEALTH PLAN	FECA BLK LUNG	OTHER	1a. INSURED'S I.D. NUMBER	(FOR PROGRAM IN ITEM 1)
(Medicare #)	(Medicaid #)	(Sponsor's SSN)	(VA File #)	(SSN or ID)	(SSN)	(ID)		

2. PATIENT'S NAME (Last Name, First Name, Middle Initial)

3. PATIENT'S BIRTH DATE MM | DD | YY   SEX M ☐ F ☐

4. INSURED'S NAME (Last Name, First Name, Middle Initial)

5. PATIENT'S ADDRESS (No., Street)

6. PATIENT RELATIONSHIP TO INSURED

Self ☐ Spouse ☐ Child ☐ Other ☐

7. INSURED'S ADDRESS (No., Street)

CITY   STATE

8. PATIENT STATUS

Single ☐ Married ☐ Other ☐

Employed ☐ Full-Time Student ☐ Part-Time Student ☐

CITY   STATE

ZIP CODE   TELEPHONE (Include Area Code)

ZIP CODE   TELEPHONE (INCLUDE AREA CODE)

9. OTHER INSURED'S NAME (Last Name, First Name, Middle Initial)

10. IS PATIENT'S CONDITION RELATED TO:

11. INSURED'S POLICY GROUP OR FECA NUMBER

a. OTHER INSURED'S POLICY OR GROUP NUMBER

a. EMPLOYMENT? (CURRENT OR PREVIOUS)
☐ YES ☐ NO

a. INSURED'S DATE OF BIRTH MM | DD | YY   SEX M ☐ F ☐

b. OTHER INSURED'S DATE OF BIRTH MM | DD | YY   SEX M ☐ F ☐

b. AUTO ACCIDENT?   PLACE (State)
☐ YES ☐ NO

b. EMPLOYER'S NAME OR SCHOOL NAME

c. EMPLOYER'S NAME OR SCHOOL NAME

c. OTHER ACCIDENT?
☐ YES ☐ NO

c. INSURANCE PLAN NAME OR PROGRAM NAME

d. INSURANCE PLAN NAME OR PROGRAM NAME

10d. RESERVED FOR LOCAL USE

d. IS THERE ANOTHER HEALTH BENEFIT PLAN?
☐ YES ☐ NO *If yes*, return to and complete item 9 a-d.

READ BACK OF FORM BEFORE COMPLETING & SIGNING THIS FORM.

12. PATIENT'S OR AUTHORIZED PERSON'S SIGNATURE I authorize the release of any medical or other information necessary to process this claim. I also request payment of government benefits either to myself or to the party who accepts assignment below.

SIGNED   DATE

13. INSURED'S OR AUTHORIZED PERSON'S SIGNATURE I authorize payment of medical benefits to the undersigned physician or supplier for services described below.

SIGNED

PATIENT AND INSURED INFORMATION ▲ ▼

14. DATE OF CURRENT: MM | DD | YY ◄ ILLNESS (First symptom) OR INJURY (Accident) OR PREGNANCY(LMP)

15. IF PATIENT HAS HAD SAME OR SIMILAR ILLNESS. GIVE FIRST DATE MM | DD | YY

16. DATES PATIENT UNABLE TO WORK IN CURRENT OCCUPATION FROM MM | DD | YY TO MM | DD | YY

17. NAME OF REFERRING PHYSICIAN OR OTHER SOURCE

17a. I.D. NUMBER OF REFERRING PHYSICIAN

18. HOSPITALIZATION DATES RELATED TO CURRENT SERVICES FROM MM | DD | YY TO MM | DD | YY

19. RESERVED FOR LOCAL USE

20. OUTSIDE LAB? $ CHARGES
☐ YES ☐ NO

21. DIAGNOSIS OR NATURE OF ILLNESS OR INJURY. (RELATE ITEMS 1,2,3 OR 4 TO ITEM 24E BY LINE)

1. L___ . ___   3. L___ . ___

2. L___ . ___   4. L___ . ___

22. MEDICAID RESUBMISSION CODE   ORIGINAL REF. NO.

23. PRIOR AUTHORIZATION NUMBER

24. A DATE(S) OF SERVICE From MM DD YY	To MM DD YY	B Place of Service	C Type of Service	D PROCEDURES, SERVICES, OR SUPPLIES (Explain Unusual Circumstances) CPT/HCPCS | MODIFIER	E DIAGNOSIS CODE	F $ CHARGES	G DAYS OR UNITS	H EPSDT Family Plan	I EMG	J COB	K RESERVED FOR LOCAL USE
1											
2											
3											
4											
5											
6											

25. FEDERAL TAX I.D. NUMBER   SSN ☐ EIN ☐

26. PATIENT'S ACCOUNT NO.

27. ACCEPT ASSIGNMENT? (For govt. claims, see back) ☐ YES ☐ NO

28. TOTAL CHARGE $

29. AMOUNT PAID $

30. BALANCE DUE $

31. SIGNATURE OF PHYSICIAN OR SUPPLIER INCLUDING DEGREES OR CREDENTIALS (I certify that the statements on the reverse apply to this bill and are made a part thereof.)

SIGNED   DATE

32. NAME AND ADDRESS OF FACILITY WHERE SERVICES WERE RENDERED (If other than home or office)

33. PHYSICIAN'S, SUPPLIER'S BILLING NAME, ADDRESS, ZIP CODE & PHONE #

PIN#   GRP#

PHYSICIAN OR SUPPLIER INFORMATION ▲ ▼

(APPROVED BY AMA COUNCIL ON MEDICAL SERVICE 8/88)

PLEASE PRINT OR TYPE

FORM HCFA-1500 (12-90)
FORM OWCP-1500   FORM RRB-1500
FORM OP 050191

WORKER'S COMPENSATION BOARD

ATTENDING PHYSICIAN'S 48-HOUR REPORT

PLEASE PRINT OR TYPE — INCLUDE ZIP CODE IN ALL ADDRESSES — CLAIMANT'S SS # MUST BE ENTERED BELOW ↓

WCB CASE NO. (If known)	CARRIER CASE NO. (If Known)	DATE OF INJURY AND TIME	ADDRESS WHERE INJURY OCCURRED (City, Town or Village)	SOCIAL SECURITY NUMBER

INJURED PERSON	NAME	AGE	ADDRESS	APT. NO.
EMPLOYER				
INSURANCE CARRIER				

H I S T O R Y

1. State how injury occurred and give source of this information. (If claim is for *occupational disease*, include occupational history and date of onset or related symptoms).

2. Is there a history of unconsciousness? ☐ YES ☐ NO   If "Yes," for how long?   Were X-Rays taken? ☐ YES ☐ NO

3. Was patient hospitalized? ☐ YES ☐ NO   If "Yes," state name and address of hospital:

4. Was patient previously under the care of another physician for this injury? ☐ YES ☐ NO   If "Yes," enter his name and address, and reason for transfer under "Remarks" (Item 10).

D I A G N O S I S

5. Describe nature and extent of injury or disease and specify *all* parts of body involved:

T R E A T M E N T

6. Nature of treatment:

Date of your first treatment: If treatment is continuing, estimate its duration.

If treatment is not continuing, is this your final report? ☐ YES ☐ NO   If "Yes," state date of last treatment:

DISA-BILITY

7. May the injury result in permanent restriction, total or partial loss of function of a part or member, or permanent facial, head or neck disfigurement? ☐ YES ☐ NO

8. Is patient working? ☐ YES ☐ NO   Is patient disabled? ☐ YES ☐ NO   If "Yes," estimate duration of disability:

CAUSAL RELATION

9. In your opinion, was the occurrence described above the competent producing cause of the injury and disability (if any) sustained? ☐ YES ☐ NO

R E M A R K S

10. Enter here additional information of value, requests for authorization, etc.:

11. Medical testimony is occasionally required. If your testimony should be necessary in this case, please indicate the days of the week (and hours) most convenient to you for this purpose:

Dated:	Typed or printed name of Attending Physician:		Address
WCB Rating Code	WCB Authorization No.	Telephone No.	Written Signature of Attending Physician

C-48   ANSWER ALL QUESTIONS. AVOID USE OF INDEFINITE TERMS

DAILY JOURNAL

DATE _October 22, 19--_   SHEET NO. _80_

RECEIPT NUMBER	DATE	DESCRIPTION-CODE	CHARGE	PAYMENT	ADJUSTMENTS	BALANCE	PREVIOUS BALANCE	NAME
1	10/22	OVF/sterile tray	50 00			50 00	—	Joseph Castro
2		OVD/UA/WBC	95 00			145 00	50 00	Gary Robertson
3		OVF	30 00			30 00	—	Eugene Sinclair
4		OVD	75 00			265 00	190 00	Florence Sherman
5		OVF	30 00			30 00	—	Marc Phan
6		OVF	30 00			185 00	155 00	Ana Mendez
7								
8								
9								
10								
11								
12								
13								
14								
15								
16								
17								
31								
32								
33								
34								
TOTALS			Column A 310 00	Column B	Column C	Column D 705 00	Column E 395 00	

◄ ALL RECEIPTS MUST BE IN NUMERICAL ORDER

PROOF OF POSTING

COLUMN E TOTAL	$ _____
"PLUS" COLUMN A TOTAL	$ _____
SUB TOTAL	$ _____
"MINUS" COLUMN B TOTAL	$ _____
EQUALS COLUMN D TOTAL	$ _____

ACCOUNTS RECEIVABLE CONTROL

PREVIOUS BALANCE	$ _8,055.00_
"PLUS" COLUMN A	$ _____
SUB TOTAL	$ _____
"MINUS" COLUMN B TOTAL	$ _____
PRESENT ACCT'S REC. BALANCE	$ _____

DAILY CASH SUMMARY

OPENING CASH ON HAND AT BEGINNING OF DAY	$ _____
CASH RECEIVED DURING DAY	$ _____
TOTAL	$ _____

FORM NO. 210-1

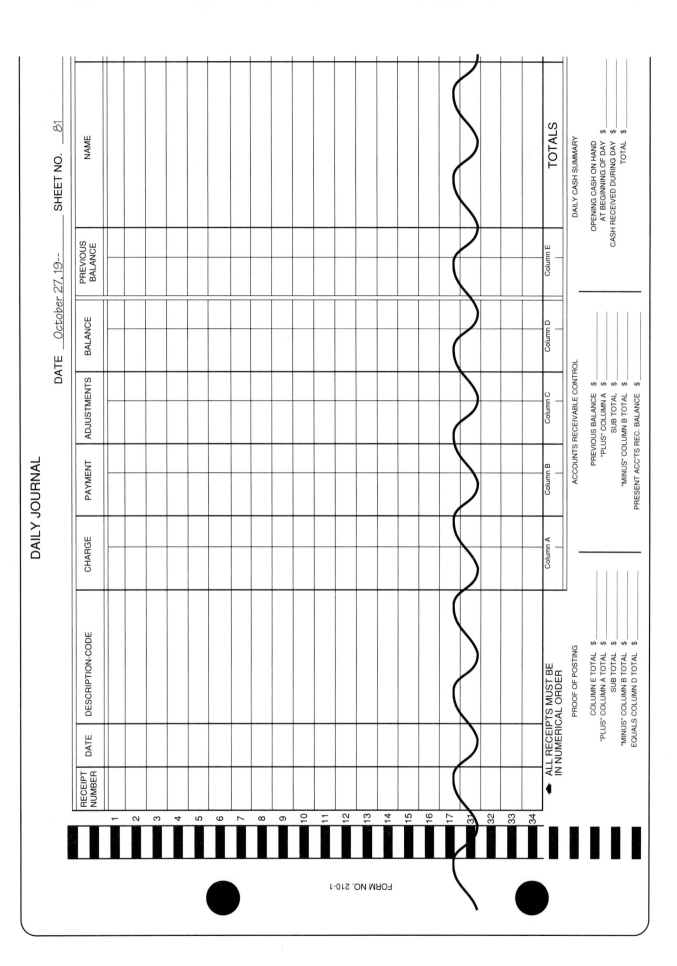

DAILY JOURNAL

DATE _October 27, 19--_   SHEET NO. _81_

RECEIPT NUMBER	DATE	DESCRIPTION-CODE	CHARGE	PAYMENT	ADJUSTMENTS	BALANCE	PREVIOUS BALANCE	NAME
1								
2								
3								
4								
5								
6								
7								
8								
9								
10								
11								
12								
13								
14								
15								
16								
17								
31								
32								
33								
34								
TOTALS			Column A	Column B	Column C	Column D	Column E	

◄ ALL RECEIPTS MUST BE IN NUMERICAL ORDER

PROOF OF POSTING

COLUMN E TOTAL $ _____
"PLUS" COLUMN A TOTAL $ _____
SUB TOTAL $ _____
"MINUS" COLUMN B TOTAL $ _____
EQUALS COLUMN D TOTAL $ _____

ACCOUNTS RECEIVABLE CONTROL

PREVIOUS BALANCE $ _____
"PLUS" COLUMN A $ _____
SUB TOTAL $ _____
"MINUS" COLUMN B TOTAL $ _____
PRESENT ACC'TS REC. BALANCE $ _____

DAILY CASH SUMMARY

OPENING CASH ON HAND
AT BEGINNING OF DAY $ _____
CASH RECEIVED DURING DAY $ _____
TOTAL $ _____

FORM NO. 210-1

Check 1

NO. 4700 $ 700 00/100
DATE 10/1   19 --
TO Reins Carpets, Inc.
FOR Carpeting

	DOLLARS	CENTS
BALANCE	3874	50
AMT. DEPOSITED	—	
TOTAL	3874	50
AMT. THIS CHECK	700	00
BALANCE	3174	50

MARK NEWMAN, M.D.
2235 South Ridgeway Avenue
Chicago, IL 60623-2240

NO. 4700   2—62/710

October 1   19 --

PAY TO THE ORDER OF Reins Carpets, Inc. $ 700 00/100

Seven hundred and 00/100   **DOLLARS**

First National Bank
Chicago, IL 60623-2791

⑆0710⑈0062 242⑈027720⑈

Check 2

NO. 4701 $ 25 45/100
DATE 10/1   19 --
TO Surgical Supplies, Inc.
FOR rubber gloves

	DOLLARS	CENTS
BALANCE	3174	50
AMT. DEPOSITED	—	
TOTAL	3174	50
AMT. THIS CHECK	25	45
BALANCE	3149	05

MARK NEWMAN, M.D.
2235 South Ridgeway Avenue
Chicago, IL 60623-2240

NO. 4701   2—62/710

October 1   19 --

PAY TO THE ORDER OF Surgical Supplies, Inc. $ 25 45/100

Twenty-five and 45/100   **DOLLARS**

First National Bank
Chicago, IL 60623-2791

⑆0710⑈0062 242⑈027720⑈

Check 3

NO. 4702 $ 10 07/100
DATE 10/1   19 --
TO Consumer Pharmacy
FOR normal saline

	DOLLARS	CENTS
BALANCE	3149	05
AMT. DEPOSITED	—	
TOTAL	3149	05
AMT. THIS CHECK	10	07
BALANCE	3138	98

MARK NEWMAN, M.D.
2235 South Ridgeway Avenue
Chicago, IL 60623-2240

NO. 4702   2—62/710

October 1   19 --

PAY TO THE ORDER OF Consumer Pharmacy $ 10 07/100

Ten and 07/100   **DOLLARS**

First National Bank
Chicago, IL 60623-2791

⑆0710⑈0062 242⑈027720⑈

Check 4

NO. 4703 $ 55 11/100
DATE 10/1   19 --
TO Consolidated Gas Co.
FOR gas

	DOLLARS	CENTS
BALANCE	3138	98
AMT. DEPOSITED	—	
TOTAL	3138	98
AMT. THIS CHECK	55	11
BALANCE	3083	87

MARK NEWMAN, M.D.
2235 South Ridgeway Avenue
Chicago, IL 60623-2240

NO. 4703   2—62/710

October 1   19 --

PAY TO THE ORDER OF Consolidated Gas Co. $ 55 11/100

Fifty-five and 11/100   **DOLLARS**

First National Bank
Chicago, IL 60623-2791

⑆0710⑈0062 242⑈027720⑈

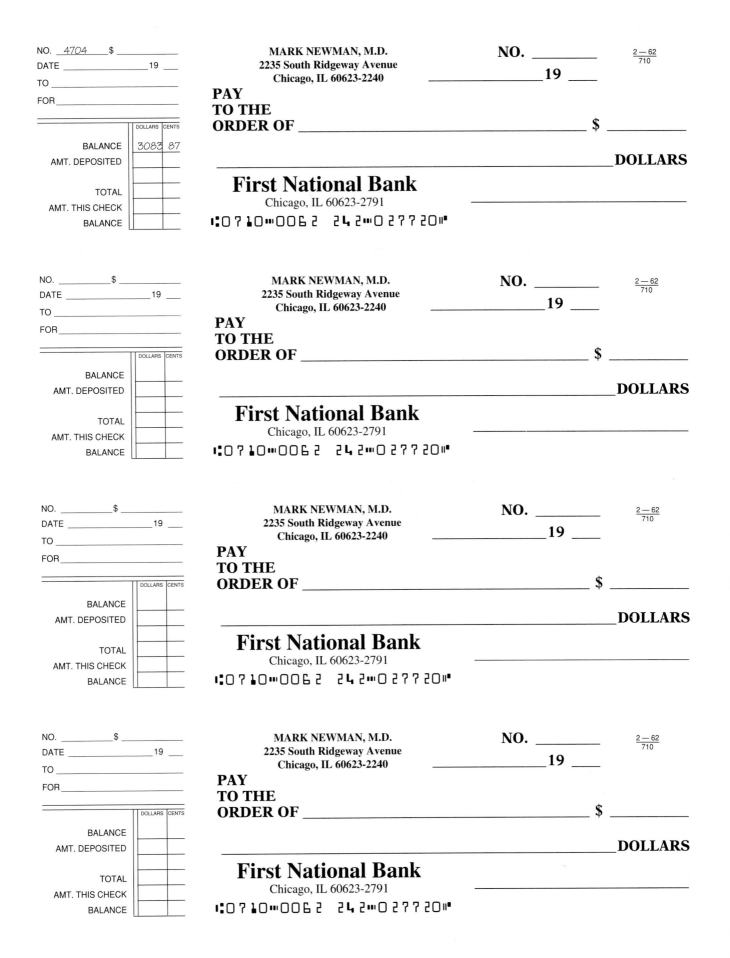

NO. _4704_ $ _____
DATE _____ 19 ___
TO _____
FOR _____

	DOLLARS	CENTS
BALANCE	3083	87
AMT. DEPOSITED		
TOTAL		
AMT. THIS CHECK		
BALANCE		

MARK NEWMAN, M.D.
2235 South Ridgeway Avenue
Chicago, IL 60623-2240

NO. _____   2 — 62
                 710
_____ 19 ___

PAY
TO THE
ORDER OF _____ $ _____

_____ DOLLARS

First National Bank
Chicago, IL 60623-2791

_____

⑆0710⑈0062 242⑈027720⑈

NO. _____ $ _____
DATE _____ 19 ___
TO _____
FOR _____

	DOLLARS	CENTS
BALANCE		
AMT. DEPOSITED		
TOTAL		
AMT. THIS CHECK		
BALANCE		

MARK NEWMAN, M.D.
2235 South Ridgeway Avenue
Chicago, IL 60623-2240

NO. _____   2 — 62
                 710
_____ 19 ___

PAY
TO THE
ORDER OF _____ $ _____

_____ DOLLARS

First National Bank
Chicago, IL 60623-2791

_____

⑆0710⑈0062 242⑈027720⑈

NO. _____ $ _____
DATE _____ 19 ___
TO _____
FOR _____

	DOLLARS	CENTS
BALANCE		
AMT. DEPOSITED		
TOTAL		
AMT. THIS CHECK		
BALANCE		

MARK NEWMAN, M.D.
2235 South Ridgeway Avenue
Chicago, IL 60623-2240

NO. _____   2 — 62
                 710
_____ 19 ___

PAY
TO THE
ORDER OF _____ $ _____

_____ DOLLARS

First National Bank
Chicago, IL 60623-2791

_____

⑆0710⑈0062 242⑈027720⑈

NO. _____ $ _____
DATE _____ 19 ___
TO _____
FOR _____

	DOLLARS	CENTS
BALANCE		
AMT. DEPOSITED		
TOTAL		
AMT. THIS CHECK		
BALANCE		

MARK NEWMAN, M.D.
2235 South Ridgeway Avenue
Chicago, IL 60623-2240

NO. _____   2 — 62
                 710
_____ 19 ___

PAY
TO THE
ORDER OF _____ $ _____

_____ DOLLARS

First National Bank
Chicago, IL 60623-2791

_____

⑆0710⑈0062 242⑈027720⑈

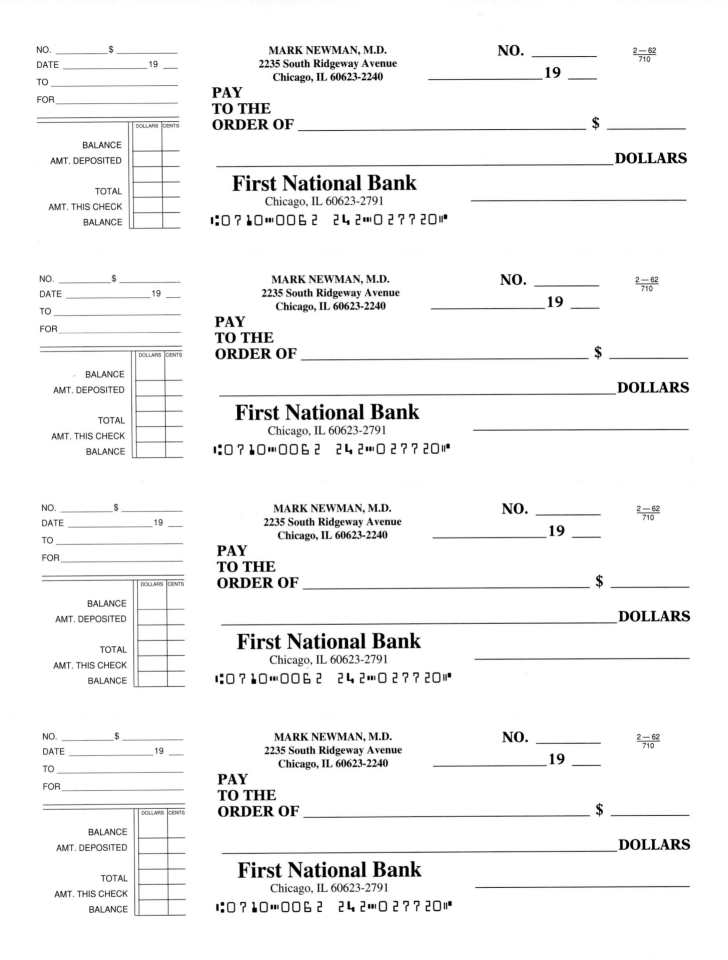

NO. _____ $ _____
DATE _____ 19 ___
TO _____
FOR _____

	DOLLARS	CENTS
BALANCE		
AMT. DEPOSITED		
TOTAL		
AMT. THIS CHECK		
BALANCE		

MARK NEWMAN, M.D.
2235 South Ridgeway Avenue
Chicago, IL 60623-2240

NO. _____

2—62
710

_____ 19 ___

PAY
TO THE
ORDER OF _____ $ _____

_____ **DOLLARS**

First National Bank
Chicago, IL 60623-2791

_____

⑆0710⑉0062 242⑈027720⑈

NO. _____ $ _____
DATE _____ 19 ___
TO _____
FOR _____

	DOLLARS	CENTS
BALANCE		
AMT. DEPOSITED		
TOTAL		
AMT. THIS CHECK		
BALANCE		

MARK NEWMAN, M.D.
2235 South Ridgeway Avenue
Chicago, IL 60623-2240

NO. _____

2—62
710

_____ 19 ___

PAY
TO THE
ORDER OF _____ $ _____

_____ **DOLLARS**

First National Bank
Chicago, IL 60623-2791

_____

⑆0710⑉0062 242⑈027720⑈

NO. _____ $ _____
DATE _____ 19 ___
TO _____
FOR _____

	DOLLARS	CENTS
BALANCE		
AMT. DEPOSITED		
TOTAL		
AMT. THIS CHECK		
BALANCE		

MARK NEWMAN, M.D.
2235 South Ridgeway Avenue
Chicago, IL 60623-2240

NO. _____

2—62
710

_____ 19 ___

PAY
TO THE
ORDER OF _____ $ _____

_____ **DOLLARS**

First National Bank
Chicago, IL 60623-2791

_____

⑆0710⑉0062 242⑈027720⑈

NO. _____ $ _____
DATE _____ 19 ___
TO _____
FOR _____

	DOLLARS	CENTS
BALANCE		
AMT. DEPOSITED		
TOTAL		
AMT. THIS CHECK		
BALANCE		

MARK NEWMAN, M.D.
2235 South Ridgeway Avenue
Chicago, IL 60623-2240

NO. _____

2—62
710

_____ 19 ___

PAY
TO THE
ORDER OF _____ $ _____

_____ **DOLLARS**

First National Bank
Chicago, IL 60623-2791

_____

⑆0710⑉0062 242⑈027720⑈

SUMMARY OF EXPENSE (From Reverse Side)

	AMOUNT
DRUGS AND PROFESSIONAL SUPPLIES	
LAB EXPENSE	
SALARIES	
OFFICE RENT AND MAINTENANCE	
LAUNDRY SERVICE	
ELECTRICITY, GAS, WATER	
TELEPHONE	
DUES AND MEETINGS	
OFFICE EXPENSES (SUPPLIES, ETC.)	
PROFESSIONAL INSURANCE	
BUSINESS TAXES	
INTEREST PAID	
ENTERTAINMENT	
TOTAL FOR PRESENT MONTH	
FORWARDED FROM PREVIOUS MONTH	45,182 31
GRAND TOTAL	

MONTHLY BALANCES	
For the Present Month	
TOTAL RECEIPTS (COL. B)	
TOTAL EXPENSE	
NET EARNINGS	
For the Year To Date	
GRAND TOTAL RECEIPTS	
GRAND TOTAL EXPENSE	
NET EARNINGS	
ACCOUNTS RECEIVABLE (FROM LAST DAY SHEET OF THE MONTH)	$
CHECKED BY	

SUMMARY FOR MONTH — October — YEAR 19—

DAY OF MONTH	CHARGES (COLUMN "A")	PAYMENTS (COLUMN "B")	ADJUSTMENT	MISCELLANEOUS SUMMARIES			
1	270 00	100 00					
2	—	150 00					
3	—	120 00					
4	—	—					
5	—	—					
6	301 75	300 00					
7	725 00	150 00					
8	285 50	200 00	75 00				
9	—	—					
10	—	—					
11	—	—					
12	65 00	—					
13	—	—					
14	415 50	—					
15	230 00	—					
16	125 00	—					
17	—	—					
18	—	—					
19	—	—					
20	20 00	—					
21	317 00	—					
22							
23							
24							
25							
26							
27							
28							
29							
30							
31							
TOTAL FOR MONTH							
BROUGHT FORWARD	75,540 25	64,921 75					
GRAND TOTAL							

WP 79

EXPENDITURES FOR THE MONTH

DRUGS AND PROFESSIONAL SUPPLIES

DAY	ITEM	AMOUNT
10/1	Surgical Supplies	25 45
	Consumer Phramacy	10 07
	TOTAL	

SALARIES

DAY	ITEM	AMOUNT
	TOTAL	

LAB EXPENSE

DUES AND MEETINGS

DAY	ITEM	AMOUNT
	TOTAL	

OFFICE EXPENSES (SUPPLIES, ETC.)

ENTERTAINMENT

DAY	ITEM	AMOUNT
	TOTAL	

OTHER

DAY	ITEM	AMOUNT
	TOTAL	

OFFICE RENT AND UPKEEP

DAY	ITEM	AMOUNT
10/1	Reins Carpets, Inc.	700 00
	TOTAL	

LAUNDRY SERVICE

TOTAL	

PROFESSIONAL INSURANCE

TOTAL	

ELECTRICITY, GAS, WATER

DAY	ITEM	AMOUNT
10/1	Consolidated Gas	55 11
	TOTAL	

BUSINESS TAXES

TOTAL	

TELEPHONE

TOTAL	

INTEREST PAID

TOTAL	

NONPROFESSIONAL EXPENSES

DAY	SOURCE	AMOUNT
	TOTAL	

NONPROFESSIONAL RECEIPTS

DAY	SOURCE	AMOUNT
	TOTAL	

TOTAL	

ALL TOTALS TO BE TRANSFERRED TO PART A

No. _____1214_____

To _____

Date _____

For _____

Amount _____

_____

No. _____1214_____

Received from _____

_____ *Dollars*

FOR _____

_____

$ _____

_____ *19* _____

No. _____

To _____

Date _____

For _____

Amount _____

_____

No. _____

Received from _____

_____ *Dollars*

FOR _____

_____

$ _____

_____ *19* _____

No. _____

To _____

Date _____

For _____

Amount _____

_____

No. _____

Received from _____

_____ *Dollars*

FOR _____

_____

$ _____

_____ *19* _____

No. _____

To _____

Date _____

For _____

Amount _____

_____

No. _____

Received from _____

_____ *Dollars*

FOR _____

_____

$ _____

_____ *19* _____

DAILY JOURNAL

DATE _October 28, 19--_   SHEET NO. _82_

RECEIPT NUMBER	DATE	DESCRIPTION-CODE	CHARGE	PAYMENT	ADJUSTMENTS	BALANCE	PREVIOUS BALANCE	NAME
1								
2								
3								
4								
5								
6								
7								
8								
9								
10								
11								
12								
13								
14								
15								
16								
17								
31								
32								
33								
34								
TOTALS			Column A	Column B	Column C	Column D	Column E	

◄ ALL RECEIPTS MUST BE IN NUMERICAL ORDER

PROOF OF POSTING

COLUMN E TOTAL $ _____
"PLUS" COLUMN A TOTAL $ _____
SUB TOTAL $ _____
"MINUS" COLUMN B TOTAL $ _____
EQUALS COLUMN D TOTAL $ _____

ACCOUNTS RECEIVABLE CONTROL

PREVIOUS BALANCE $ _____
"PLUS" COLUMN A $ _____
SUB TOTAL $ _____
"MINUS" COLUMN B TOTAL $ _____
PRESENT ACCT'S REC. BALANCE $ _____

DAILY CASH SUMMARY

OPENING CASH ON HAND
AT BEGINNING OF DAY $ _____
CASH RECEIVED DURING DAY $ _____
TOTAL $ _____

FORM NO. 210-1

DEPOSITED IN
First National Bank
Chicago, IL 60623-2791

THIS DEPOSIT ACCEPTED UNDER AND SUBJECT TO THE PROVISIONS
OF THE UNIFORM COMMERCIAL CODE.

DATE _____

Mark Newman, M.D.
2235 South Ridgeway Avenue
Chicago, IL 60623-2240

⑆0710⑈0062 242⑉027720⑉

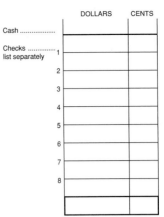

DEPOSITED IN
First National Bank
Chicago, IL 60623-2791

THIS DEPOSIT ACCEPTED UNDER AND SUBJECT TO THE PROVISIONS
OF THE UNIFORM COMMERCIAL CODE.

DATE _____

Mark Newman, M.D.
2235 South Ridgeway Avenue
Chicago, IL 60623-2240

⑆0710⑈0062 242⑉027720⑉

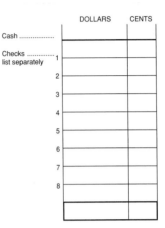

DEPOSITED IN
First National Bank
Chicago, IL 60623-2791

THIS DEPOSIT ACCEPTED UNDER AND SUBJECT TO THE PROVISIONS
OF THE UNIFORM COMMERCIAL CODE.

DATE _____

Mark Newman, M.D.
2235 South Ridgeway Avenue
Chicago, IL 60623-2240

⑆0710⑈0062 242⑉027720⑉

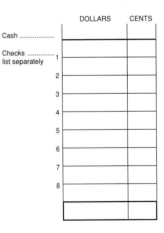

DEPOSITED IN
First National Bank
Chicago, IL 60623-2791

THIS DEPOSIT ACCEPTED UNDER AND SUBJECT TO THE PROVISIONS
OF THE UNIFORM COMMERCIAL CODE.

DATE _____

Mark Newman, M.D.
2235 South Ridgeway Avenue
Chicago, IL 60623-2240

⑆0710⑈0062 242⑉027720⑉

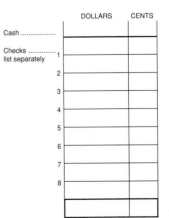

First National Bank
Chicago, IL 60623-2791

STATEMENT OF
ACCOUNT NUMBER

242 027720

CLOSING DATE ITEMS

10/24   5

MARK NEWMAN, M.D.
2235 SOUTH RIDGEWAY AVENUE
CHICAGO, IL 60623-2240

PERSONAL CHECKING ACCOUNT STATEMENT

BEGINNING BALANCE	(+) TOTAL CREDITS	(-) TOTAL DEBITS	(-) SERVICE CHARGE	(=) NEW BALANCE
3874.50	1020.00	1070.26		3824.24

CHECKS & OTHER DEBITS		DEPOSITS & OTHER CREDITS	DATE	BALANCE
700.00		370.00	10/3	3544.50
25.45		300.00	10/6	3819.05
55.11	18.50		10/7	3745.44
163.21		350.00	10/8	3932.23
32.99	75.00		10/22	3824.24

SYMBOLS

C = CORRECTION	DM = DEBIT MEMO	RI = RETURN ITEM	ST = SAVINGS TRANSFER
CM = CREDIT MEMO	OD = OVERDRAFT	SC = SERVICE CHARGE	

CHANGE OF ADDRESS ORDER

TO CHANGE YOUR ADDRESS PLEASE COMPLETE THIS FORM:

THEN CUT ALONG DOTTED LINE AND MAIL OR BRING TO THE BANK

NEW ADDRESS:

NUMBER
AND STREET _____

CITY _____ STATE AND
ZIP CODE _____ NEW PHONE
NUMBER _____

DATE _____ CUSTOMER'S SIGNATURE _____

- -

OUTSTANDING CHECKS

NUMBER	AMOUNT	
TOTAL		

TO RECONCILE YOUR
STATEMENT AND CHECKBOOK

1. DEDUCT FROM YOUR CHECKBOOK BALANCE ANY SERVICE OR OTHER CHARGE ORIGINATED BY THE BANK. THESE CHARGES WILL BE IDENTIFIED BY SYMBOLS AS SHOWN ON FRONT.

2. ARRANGE ENDORSED CHECKS BY DATE OR NUMBER AND CHECK THEM OFF AGAINST THE STUBS IN YOUR CHECKBOOK.

3. LIST IN THE OUTSTANDING CHECKS SECTION AT THE LEFT ANY CHECKS ISSUED BY YOU AND NOT YET PAID BY US.

TO RECONCILE YOUR
STATEMENT AND CHECKBOOK

LAST BALANCE SHOWN ON STATEMENT			
PLUS:	DEPOSITS AND CREDITS MADE AFTER DATE OF LAST ENTRY ON STATEMENT		
	SUBTOTAL		
MINUS:	OUTSTANDING CHECKS		
BALANCE:	WHICH SHOULD AGREE WITH YOUR CHECKBOOK		

INDIVIDUAL EMPLOYEE'S EARNINGS RECORD

Name _Linda Jenson_

Address _4815 N. Oak Park Avenue_

City _Chicago, IL 60634-3727_

Telephone _555-3672_

Social Security No. _095-37-4732_

Marital Status _Single_

No. of Allowances _1_

Birthdate _05/17/--_

Position _Medical Assistant_

Monthly Rate _____

Weekly Rate _$450_

Overtime Rate _____

Period Ending	Hours Worked	Gross Earnings			Deductions							Net Pay	Accumulated Earnings (Gross)
		Regular	Overtime	Total	FICA	Federal Withholding	State Withholding	City Withholding	Insurance	Other	Total		

DAILY JOURNAL

DATE __October 29, 19--__   SHEET NO. __83__

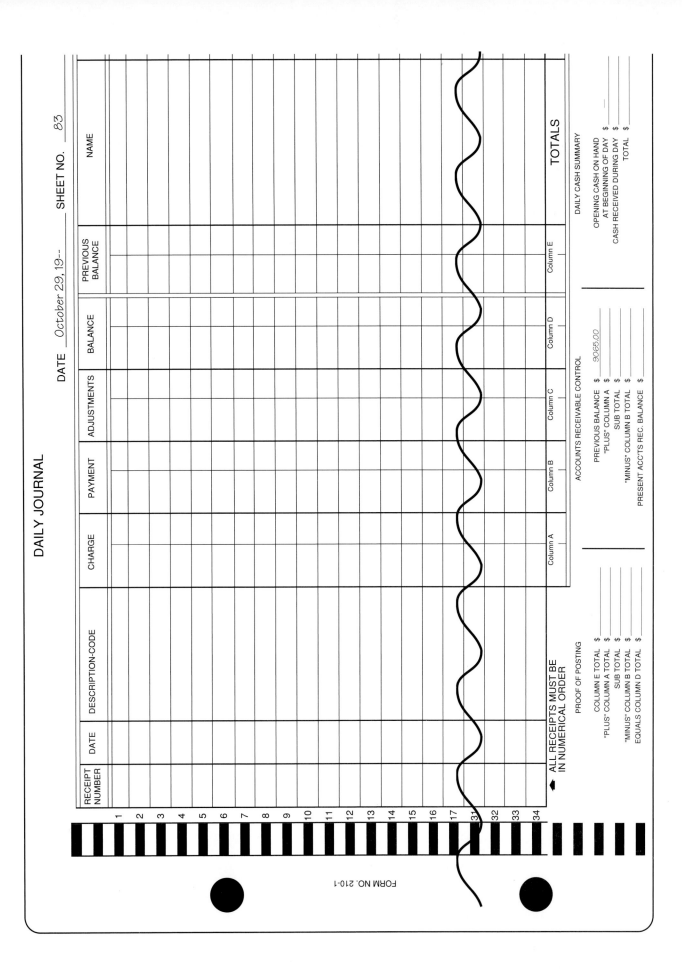

RECEIPT NUMBER	DATE	DESCRIPTION-CODE	CHARGE	PAYMENT	ADJUSTMENTS	BALANCE	PREVIOUS BALANCE	NAME
1								
2								
3								
4								
5								
6								
7								
8								
9								
10								
11								
12								
13								
14								
15								
16								
17								
31								
32								
33								
34								
TOTALS			Column A	Column B	Column C	Column D	Column E	

◀ ALL RECEIPTS MUST BE IN NUMERICAL ORDER

PROOF OF POSTING

COLUMN E TOTAL $ _____
"PLUS" COLUMN A TOTAL $ _____
SUB TOTAL $ _____
"MINUS" COLUMN B TOTAL $ _____
EQUALS COLUMN D TOTAL $ _____

ACCOUNTS RECEIVABLE CONTROL

PREVIOUS BALANCE $ _9065.00_
"PLUS" COLUMN A $ _____
SUB TOTAL $ _____
"MINUS" COLUMN B TOTAL $ _____
PRESENT ACC'TS REC. BALANCE $ _____

DAILY CASH SUMMARY

OPENING CASH ON HAND
AT BEGINNING OF DAY $ _____
CASH RECEIVED DURING DAY $ _____
TOTAL $ _____

FORM NO. 210-1

TO-DO LIST

DATE _____

RUSH	THINGS TO DO	DONE

TELEPHONE LOG

DATE _____

TIME	CALLER	TELEPHONE NUMBER	REASON	DONE

NAME Eugene Sinclair   **DATE** 10/29

Exam	Code	Charge
OVF	99212	
LAB:		
X RAY:		
OTHER:		
TOTAL		

Diagnosis: 707 ulcer/nose

NAME Randy Burton   **DATE** 10/29

Exam	Code	Charge
OVF	99212	
LAB:		
X RAY:		
OTHER:		
TOTAL		

Diagnosis: 052 varicella

NAME Cheng Sun   **DATE** 10/29

Exam	Code	Charge
CPE (OV Comprehensive)	99215	
LAB:		
X RAY:		
OTHER:		
TOTAL		

Diagnosis: V700 Health Care maintenance
272.0 Hypercholesterolemia

APPROVED OMB-0938-0008

CARRIER

PICA

HEALTH INSURANCE CLAIM FORM

PICA

PATIENT AND INSURED INFORMATION

| 1. MEDICARE (Medicare #)   MEDICAID (Medicaid #)   CHAMPUS (Sponsor's SSN)   CHAMPVA (VA File #)   GROUP HEALTH PLAN (SSN or ID)   FECA BLK LUNG (SSN)   OTHER (ID) | 1a. INSURED'S I.D. NUMBER   (FOR PROGRAM IN ITEM 1) |

2. PATIENT'S NAME (Last Name, First Name, Middle Initial)

3. PATIENT'S BIRTH DATE MM DD YY   SEX   M   F

4. INSURED'S NAME (Last Name, First Name, Middle Initial)

5. PATIENT'S ADDRESS (No., Street)

6. PATIENT RELATIONSHIP TO INSURED   Self   Spouse   Child   Other

7. INSURED'S ADDRESS (No., Street)

CITY   STATE

8. PATIENT STATUS   Single   Married   Other   Employed   Full-Time Student   Part-Time Student

CITY   STATE

ZIP CODE   TELEPHONE (Include Area Code)

ZIP CODE   TELEPHONE (INCLUDE AREA CODE)

9. OTHER INSURED'S NAME (Last Name, First Name, Middle Initial)

10. IS PATIENT'S CONDITION RELATED TO:

11. INSURED'S POLICY GROUP OR FECA NUMBER

a. OTHER INSURED'S POLICY OR GROUP NUMBER

a. EMPLOYMENT? (CURRENT OR PREVIOUS)   YES   NO

a. INSURED'S DATE OF BIRTH MM DD YY   SEX   M   F

b. OTHER INSURED'S DATE OF BIRTH MM DD YY   SEX   M   F

b. AUTO ACCIDENT?   PLACE (State)   YES   NO

b. EMPLOYER'S NAME OR SCHOOL NAME

c. EMPLOYER'S NAME OR SCHOOL NAME

c. OTHER ACCIDENT?   YES   NO

c. INSURANCE PLAN NAME OR PROGRAM NAME

d. INSURANCE PLAN NAME OR PROGRAM NAME

10d. RESERVED FOR LOCAL USE

d. IS THERE ANOTHER HEALTH BENEFIT PLAN?   YES   NO   **If yes**, return to and complete item 9 a-d.

READ BACK OF FORM BEFORE COMPLETING & SIGNING THIS FORM.
12. PATIENT'S OR AUTHORIZED PERSON'S SIGNATURE I authorize the release of any medical or other information necessary to process this claim. I also request payment of government benefits either to myself or to the party who accepts assignment below.

SIGNED _____ DATE _____

13. INSURED'S OR AUTHORIZED PERSON'S SIGNATURE I authorize payment of medical benefits to the undersigned physician or supplier for services described below.

SIGNED _____

PHYSICIAN OR SUPPLIER INFORMATION

14. DATE OF CURRENT: MM DD YY   ILLNESS (First symptom) OR INJURY (Accident) OR PREGNANCY(LMP)

15. IF PATIENT HAS HAD SAME OR SIMILAR ILLNESS. GIVE FIRST DATE MM DD YY

16. DATES PATIENT UNABLE TO WORK IN CURRENT OCCUPATION MM DD YY   FROM   TO   MM DD YY

17. NAME OF REFERRING PHYSICIAN OR OTHER SOURCE

17a. I.D. NUMBER OF REFERRING PHYSICIAN

18. HOSPITALIZATION DATES RELATED TO CURRENT SERVICES MM DD YY   FROM   TO   MM DD YY

19. RESERVED FOR LOCAL USE

20. OUTSIDE LAB?   YES   NO $ CHARGES

21. DIAGNOSIS OR NATURE OF ILLNESS OR INJURY. (RELATE ITEMS 1,2,3 OR 4 TO ITEM 24E BY LINE)

1. |___.___ 3. |___.___
2. |___.___ 4. |___.___

22. MEDICAID RESUBMISSION CODE   ORIGINAL REF. NO.

23. PRIOR AUTHORIZATION NUMBER

24. A DATE(S) OF SERVICE From / To MM DD YY / MM DD YY	B Place of Service	C Type of Service	D PROCEDURES, SERVICES, OR SUPPLIES (Explain Unusual Circumstances) CPT/HCPCS MODIFIER	E DIAGNOSIS CODE	F $ CHARGES	G DAYS OR UNITS	H EPSDT Family Plan	I EMG	J COB	K RESERVED FOR LOCAL USE
1										
2										
3										
4										
5										
6										

25. FEDERAL TAX I.D. NUMBER   SSN EIN

26. PATIENT'S ACCOUNT NO.

27. ACCEPT ASSIGNMENT? (For govt. claims, see back)   YES   NO

28. TOTAL CHARGE $

29. AMOUNT PAID $

30. BALANCE DUE $

31. SIGNATURE OF PHYSICIAN OR SUPPLIER INCLUDING DEGREES OR CREDENTIALS (I certify that the statements on the reverse apply to this bill and are made a part thereof.)

SIGNED _____ DATE _____

32. NAME AND ADDRESS OF FACILITY WHERE SERVICES WERE RENDERED (If other than home or office)

33. PHYSICIAN'S, SUPPLIER'S BILLING NAME, ADDRESS. ZIP CODE & PHONE #

PIN#   GRP#

(APPROVED BY AMA COUNCIL ON MEDICAL SERVICE 8/88)   **PLEASE PRINT OR TYPE**

FORM HCFA-1500 (12-90)
FORM OWCP-1500   FORM RRB-1500
FORM OP 050191

WP 89

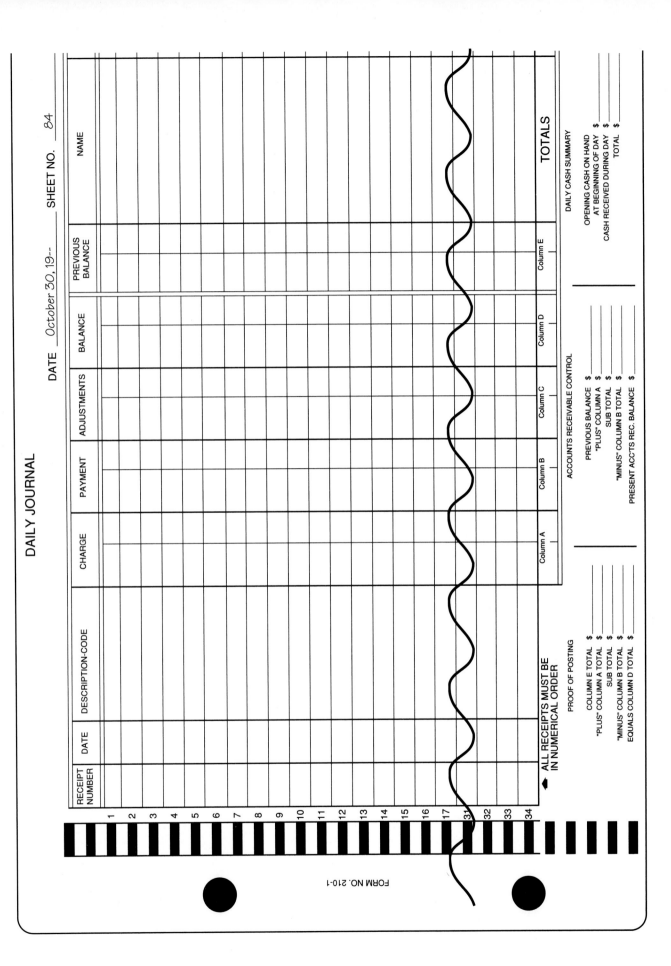

DAILY JOURNAL

DATE _October 30, 19--_   SHEET NO. _84_

RECEIPT NUMBER	DATE	DESCRIPTION-CODE	CHARGE	PAYMENT	ADJUSTMENTS	BALANCE	PREVIOUS BALANCE	NAME
1								
2								
3								
4								
5								
6								
7								
8								
9								
10								
11								
12								
13								
14								
15								
16								
17								
31								
32								
33								
34								
TOTALS			Column A	Column B	Column C	Column D	Column E	

◀ ALL RECEIPTS MUST BE IN NUMERICAL ORDER

PROOF OF POSTING

COLUMN E TOTAL $
"PLUS" COLUMN A TOTAL $
SUB TOTAL $
"MINUS" COLUMN B TOTAL $
EQUALS COLUMN D TOTAL $

ACCOUNTS RECEIVABLE CONTROL

PREVIOUS BALANCE $
"PLUS" COLUMN A $
SUB TOTAL $
"MINUS" COLUMN B TOTAL $
PRESENT ACCT'S REC. BALANCE $

DAILY CASH SUMMARY

OPENING CASH ON HAND
AT BEGINNING OF DAY $
CASH RECEIVED DURING DAY $
TOTAL $

FORM NO. 210-1

WP 90

Ridgeway Radiology
2248 South Ridgeway Avenue
Chicago, IL 60623-2240
312-555-7357

PATIENT: Cheng Sun
DOCTOR: Mark Newman, M.D.
DATE: 10/27/--

REPORT: Chest film

Normal chest X ray.

HWC

H. Wilson Campbell, M.D./pa

Ridgeway Radiology
2248 South Ridgeway Avenue
Chicago, IL 60623-2240
312-555-7357

PATIENT: Theresa Dayton
DOCTOR: Mark Newman, M.D.
DATE: 10/21/--

REPORT: Low-dose mammogram

No breast malignancy is identified with no
change since last mammogram.

HWC

H. Wilson Campbell, M.D./pa

HEMATOLOGY—CHEMISTRY *MN*

Name _Cheng Sun_ Doctor _Newman_

Test Results

5.1	WBC	92	Glucose
	Hematocrit	229	Cholesterol
14.6	Hemoglobin	13	BUN
	Differential	9.5	Calcium
64	PMN	3	Phosphorous
	Bands	0.5	Bilirubin
32	Lymphs	4	Uric acid
2	Mono	75	Alkaline phosphatase
3	Eos	4.2	Albumin
1	Baso	7	Protein, total
	Platelets	120	LDH
	Thyroid	15	SGOT

29 HDL

132 LDL

Date _10/15_

URINE—Miscellaneous *MN*

Name _Cheng Sun_ Doctor _Newman_

Color _pale yellow_ Pap Smear _____

pH _6_

Specific Gravity _1.0_

Protein _neg._ Vaginal Smear _____

Glucose _neg._

Ketone _____

WBCs/hpf _0-2_ Hemoccults _x3_

RBCs/hpf _0-1_ _negative_

Bacteria _____

Culture _____

Date _10/15_

URINE—Miscellaneous *MN*

Name _Theresa Dayton_ Doctor _Newman_

Color _____ Pap Smear _____

pH _____ _negative_

Specific Gravity _____

Protein _____ Vaginal Smear _____

Glucose _____

Ketone _____

WBCs/hpf _____ Hemoccults _____

RBCs/hpf _____

Bacteria _____

Culture _____

Date _10/21_

NO. 5321 $\frac{2-62}{710}$

October 24 **19** --

**PAY
TO THE
ORDER OF** Mark Newman $ 50 and no/100

Fifty and no/100 ——————————————— **DOLLARS**

First National Bank
Chicago, IL 60623-2791

Lawrence Lund

⑆0710⑈0062 0815⑈02249⑈

NO. 1909 $\frac{2-62}{710}$

October 24 **19** --

**PAY
TO THE
ORDER OF** Mark Newman, M.D. $ 100 no/100

One hundred and no/100 ——————————————— **DOLLARS**

First National Bank
Chicago, IL 60623-2791

Theresa Dayton

⑆0710⑈0062 242⑈046580⑈

NO. 1964 $\frac{2-62}{710}$

October 24 **19** --

**PAY
TO THE
ORDER OF** Dr. Mark Newman $ 75 and 00/100

Seventy-five and 00/100 ——————————————— **DOLLARS**

First National Bank
Chicago, IL 60623-2791

Suzanne Roberts

⑆0710⑈0062 202⑈056232⑈

NO. 2278 $\frac{2-62}{710}$

October 25 **19** --

**PAY
TO THE
ORDER OF** Mark Newman, M.D. $ 200 no/100

Two hundred and no/100 ——————————————— **DOLLARS**

Chicago Bank
Chicago, IL 60621

Alan Mitchell

⑆0710⑈0155 262⑈025592⑈

NO. _4392_ $\frac{2-62}{710}$

_____ October 25 19 _--_

PAY
TO THE
ORDER OF _Mark Newman, M.D._____ $ 105 00/100

One hundred five and no/100 _____ DOLLARS

First National Bank
Chicago, IL 60623-2791   _Todd Grant_

⑈0710⑈0062 242⑈046580⑈

NO. _1983_ $\frac{2-62}{710}$

_____ October 25 19 _--_

PAY
TO THE
ORDER OF _Dr. Mark Newman_____ $ 50 and no/100

Fifty and no/100 _____ DOLLARS

First National Bank
Chicago, IL 60623-2791   _Ana Mendez_

⑈0710⑈0062 202⑈056232⑈

NO. _2475_ $\frac{2-62}{710}$

_____ October 26 19 _--_

PAY
TO THE
ORDER OF _Mark Newman, M.D._____ $ 95 00/100

Ninety-five and no/100 _____ DOLLARS

Chicago Bank
Chicago, IL 60621   _Gary Robertson_

⑈0710⑈0155 262⑈025592⑈

NO. _7043_ $\frac{2-62}{710}$

_____ October 26 19 _--_

PAY
TO THE
ORDER OF _Mark Newman_____ $ 125 and no/100

One hundred twenty-five and no/100 _____ DOLLARS

Furst National Bank
Chicago, IL 60623-2791   _Clarence Rogers_

⑈0710⑈0062 0815⑈02249⑈

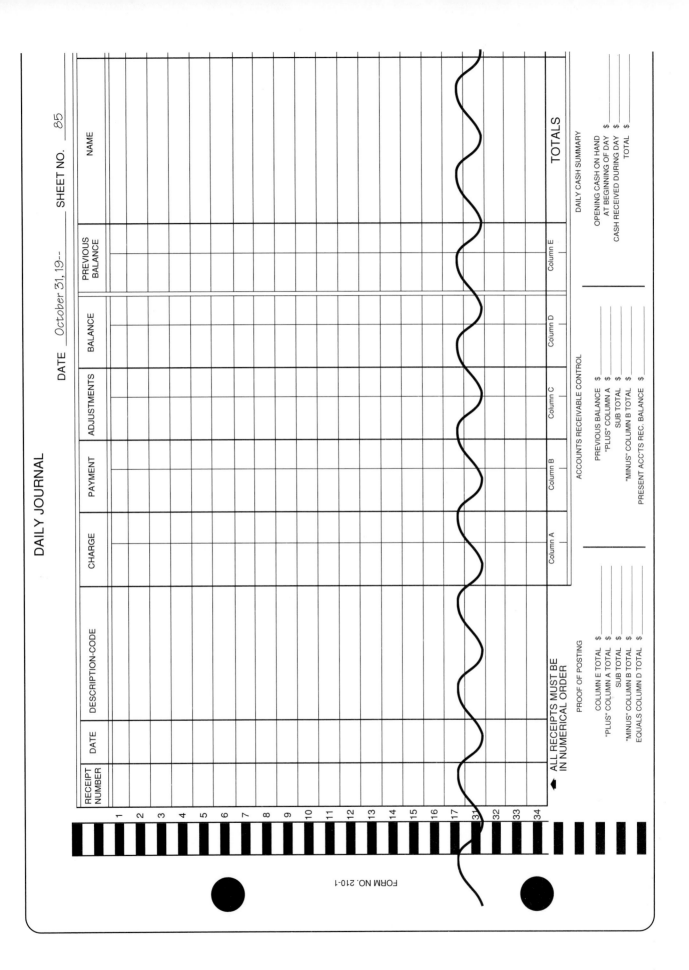

DAILY JOURNAL

DATE _October 31, 19--_   SHEET NO. _85_

RECEIPT NUMBER	DATE	DESCRIPTION-CODE	CHARGE	PAYMENT	ADJUSTMENTS	BALANCE	PREVIOUS BALANCE	NAME
1								
2								
3								
4								
5								
6								
7								
8								
9								
10								
11								
12								
13								
14								
15								
16								
17								
31								
32								
33								
34								
			Column A	Column B	Column C	Column D	Column E	TOTALS

◀ ALL RECEIPTS MUST BE
IN NUMERICAL ORDER

PROOF OF POSTING

COLUMN E TOTAL $ _____
"PLUS" COLUMN A TOTAL $ _____
SUB TOTAL $ _____
"MINUS" COLUMN B TOTAL $ _____
EQUALS COLUMN D TOTAL $ _____

ACCOUNTS RECEIVABLE CONTROL

PREVIOUS BALANCE $ _____
"PLUS" COLUMN A $ _____
SUB TOTAL $ _____
"MINUS" COLUMN B TOTAL $ _____
PRESENT ACCTS REC. BALANCE $ _____

DAILY CASH SUMMARY

OPENING CASH ON HAND
AT BEGINNING OF DAY $ _____
CASH RECEIVED DURING DAY $ _____
TOTAL $ _____

FORM NO. 210-1

To: Elizabeth Miller-Young   Re: Monica Armstrong

In the near future, you will be seeing one of my patients, Monica Armstrong. She is a 50-year-old woman with menopausal bleeding. I have completed a physical examination, and, basically, she is in good health.

I am enclosing a copy of ~~my~~ the exam done on October 28, ~~The Pap smear was returned today and is negative and the~~ a copy of the laboratory and X-ray reports I have performed in my office.

Please send me your evaluation. If you have any questions, please contact me.

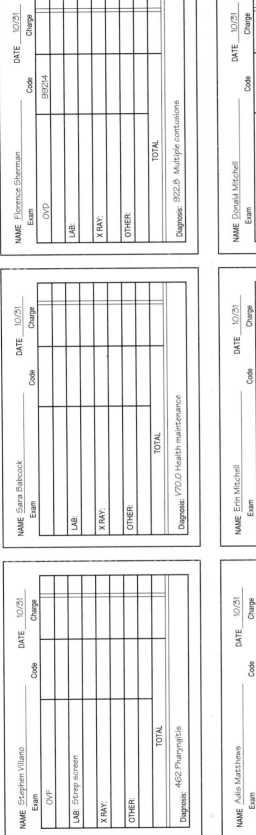

NAME Florence Sherman   **DATE** 10/31

Exam	Code	Charge
OVD	99214	
LAB:		
X RAY:		
OTHER:		
TOTAL		

Diagnosis: 922.8 Multiple contusions

NAME Donald Mitchell   **DATE** 10/31

Exam	Code	Charge
LAB:		
X RAY:		
OTHER:		
TOTAL		

Diagnosis:

NAME Sara Babcock   **DATE** 10/31

Exam	Code	Charge
LAB:		
X RAY:		
OTHER:		
TOTAL		

Diagnosis: V70.0 Health maintenance

NAME Erin Mitchell   **DATE** 10/31

Exam	Code	Charge
LAB:		
X RAY:		
OTHER:		
TOTAL		

Diagnosis:

NAME Stephen Villano   **DATE** 10/31

Exam	Code	Charge
OVF		
LAB: Strep screen		
X RAY:		
OTHER:		
TOTAL		

Diagnosis: 462 Pharyngitis

NAME Adis Matthews   **DATE** 10/31

Exam	Code	Charge
OVD	99214	
LAB:		
X RAY:		
OTHER:		
TOTAL		

Diagnosis: 784.0 Headache

CAFFEINISM INTOXICATION

Mark Newman, M.D.

Family Practice, University Hospital

There are two drugs we see so often that we sometimes forget they are drugs. Even though they be harmful, they are legal. They are sold in stores, and some can be purchased by children. These two drugs are nicotine and caffeine. However, caffeine is not as harmful or as addictive as some other dugs.

Caffeine is the most commonly used drug in the ~~states~~ world and may date from 4700 B.C. coffee is the largest source of caffeine in the american diet.

Effects

Caffeine is a stimulant. The following list tells what body systems are affected and what the effects are.

1. Affects the cardiovascular system by dilating blood vessels and increasing the pulse rate. Caffeine may also raise cholesterol levels.

2. Affects the digestive system by stimulating secretion of acid in the stomach and decreasing hungar.

3. Affects the entire CNS by increasing the feeling of alertness and gives a feeling of increased energy. Caffeine may make it more difficult to control precise fine motor movements. It also reduces fatigue and drowsiness and my speed reaction time, but it does <u>not</u> heighten the ability to think.

4. Affects the musculoskeletal system by promoting metabolism of fat during exercising and sparing the carbohydrates stored in the muscles, therefore possibly heightening performance. Caffiene may interfere with calcium absorption.

5. Affects the endocrine system by boosting the basal metabolic rate, thus burning more calories and assisting in wieght loss. Caffeine may also affect a diabetic's ability to burn sugar.

6. Affects the respiratory system by increasing the rate of breathing and causing bronchodilation, acting like an asthmatic drug.

7. Affects the reproductive system by negatively affecting fertility in women. Caffeine may be a factor in fibrocystic disease, and heavy use may increase the symptoms of PMS.

8. Affects the urinary system functions by increasing urination.

Several studies have been done, but the research was poorly controlled. These study have linked caffeine (especially coffee) to cancer, heart disease, digestive problems, and breast disease in women. Those that have link heavy coffee consumption, to a greater risk for heart disease (five or more cups a day) did not control the lifestyle or the diet of the group. At the present time, the link between coffee and heart disease is still controversial.

Although coffee drinkers have been found to have higher levels of cholesterol, the exact cause is not known. It may be the brewing process or even a substance other then caffeine causing high cholesterol in some coffee drinkers. There may be a substance in coffee that effects cholesterol metabolism and the length of brewing time may thus account for this higher incidence.

Even decaffeinated coffee is not problem-free. There is some concern about the chemical used to seperate the caffeine from coffee. It is feared that chemical may be as harmful (carcinogenic) as the coffee bean itself.

Caffeine does not lower blood alcohol levels and does not sober the person who drank to much alcohol. It also does not improve judgment or coordination.

3

At this time, there is no concrete evidence that caffeine causes heart disease, ulcers, bladder or other cancers, birth defects, or difficulties during pregnancy.

Nevertheless, moderation of caffeine consumption is recommended. *Moderation* is defined as the equivalent of about ② cup of coffee per day. Learn to be aware of how caffeine affects your body. If you are ac͡ustomed to drinking large quantities of coffee or other caffeine-containing drinks, you may experience withdrawal symptoms when you reduce the amount of caffeine in your diet. Some of these symptoms are tiredness, headaches, and irritability. Habitual use will build a tolerance, as with many drugs.

Sources

Natural sources if caffeine are tea, cocoa (from the cocoa plant--note the coca plant, which produces cocaine), and cola drinks, which use the kola nut in preparation. Chocolate is cocoa with the addition of sugar. Caffeine is also added to some foods (as a flavoring) such as soft candy, pudding, gelatin, and frozen dairy products. Caffeine is also used in many allergy medicines, decongestants, analgesics, and cough and cold preparations because of its stimulating effect. Common caffeine sources and estimates of the amount of caffeine are listed in the table taht follows:

Source	Amount	Caffeine
COFFEE		
brewed (perk/drip)	8 oz	100-150 mg
decaffeinated	8 oz	2-8 mg
TEA		
brewed	8 oz	20-100 mg
instant	8 oz	30-70 mg
SOFT DRINKS		
colas	12 oz	36-54 mg
others	12 oz	34-61
OTHER		
~~mild chocolate~~	~~1 oz~~	~~6 mg~~
semisweet chocolate	1 oz	14-25 mg
chocolate cake	1 slice	20-30 mg
No-Doz	1 tablet	100 mg
Excedrin	1 tablet	65-75 mg
Anacin	1 tablet	32 mgs
Dristan	1 tablet	16 mg

ANNUAL NATIONAL MEDICAL SOCIETY MEETING
Kon Tiki Hotel, 2364 E. Van Buren St., Phoenix, AZ 85006
606-555-9361

SUNDAY, NOVEMBER 16

3:00–5:00 p.m.	✓ Registration—Atrium
6:00–7:00 p.m.	✓ Reception: hors d'oeuvres, chamber music—Atrium
8:00 p.m.	✓ Dinner: Guest speakers, Drs. Gary Reinhart, Olaf Nielsen, and Anna Kapuscinski—Gold Room at Arizona Biltmore, 24th St. and Missouri.

MONDAY, NOVEMBER 17

7:30 a.m.	✓ Continental breakfast—Atrium
8:00–8:10 a.m.	✓ Announcements—Atrium
8:15–8:55 a.m.	✓ Manifestations of Ischemia, Dr. Robert Ballard—Oakwood Room
9:00 a.m.–6:00 p.m.	Exhibits open—Auditorium
9:00–9:40 a.m.	Pathophysiology of Myocardial Ischemia, Dr. Robert Ballard—Oakwood Room
	✓ HLA Typing and Renal Transplantation, Dr. Laurie Hudson—Shorewood Room
9:45–10:00 a.m.	✓ Break—Atrium
10:05–10:45 a.m.	✓ Silent Symptoms and Acute Ischemic Syndromes, Dr. Saul Katz—Fernwood Room
	Hyperlipidemia in Patients With Chronic Renal Failure, Dr. J. Harold Shanley—Lakewood Room
10:50–11:30 a.m.	Diagnostic Techniques of Noninvasive Modalities, Dr. Penny Beryl—Oakwood Room
	✓ Plasmapheresis: Indications in Symptomatic Illness, Dr. Paul Hutt —Shorewood Room
11:35 a.m. –12:15 p.m.	Noninvasive Diagnostic Techniques: Hands-On Workshop, Drs. Paul Hutt, Penny Beryl, and Laurie Hudson—Fernwood Room
12:30–1:45 p.m.	Lunch
1:45–2:30 p.m.	Committee meetings per arrangements
2:30–3:10 p.m.	✓ Acute MI Interventions, Dr. Hasson Sahni—Lakewood Room
3:15–3:55 p.m.	✓ Case Study: Manifestations of Ischemia, panel of Drs. Robert Ballard, Saul Katz, and Lee Young-Nam—Elmwood Plaza
4:30–6:00 p.m.	✓ Wine and Cheese Party—Atrium • Sign up for hospital tour, Tuesday from noon–4 p.m.

- Sign up for small-group discussions, Wednesday from 10:20–11 a.m.

✓ Dinner—Pinnacle Peak Patio, 10426 E. Pinnacle Peak Road, Scottsdale (555-7311): 45-minute drive (Reservations must be made.)

TUESDAY, NOVEMBER 18

7:30 a.m.	Continental breakfast—Atrium
8:00–8:40 a.m.	✓ Pain Management in Critical Care, Drs. Stanton Dorsey and Pattianne Davidson—Elmwood Plaza
8:45–9:25 a.m.	✓ Electrolyte Emergencies in Critical Care, Dr. Thomas F. Catchings—Candlewood Room
9:30–9:45 a.m.	✓ Break—Atrium
9:50–10:30 a.m.	✓ Advancements in Management of Sudden Death, panel of Drs. Stanton Dorsey, Pattianne Davidson, and Thomas F. Catchings—Elmwood Plaza
10:35–11:15 a.m.	Invasive Candidiasis, Dr. Alan E. Dunn—Fernwood Room
noon–4:00 p.m.	✓ Hospital tour, to include coronary unit, dialysis center, and diagnostic labs. (Sign up on Monday.)
noon–8:00 p.m.	✓ Exhibits open—Auditorium
7:00–8:30 p.m.	✓ Dinner (open to spouses)—The Totally Electronic Office, a multimedia presentation— Elmwood Plaza

WEDNESDAY, NOVEMBER 19

7:15 a.m.	Continental breakfast—Atrium
8:00– 9:55 a.m.	✓ Long-Term Care of Transplant Recipients, panel of Drs. Laurie Hudson, J. Harold Shanley, and Paul Hutt—Elmwood Plaza
10:00–10:15 a.m.	✓ Break—Garden
10:20–11:00 a.m.	Small-group discussions—sign-up roster and location in Atrium

- Coding differentials in ischemias
- Coding differentials in transplantations
✓ • Reimbursement—containments
- Donor transplant concerns
- Establishment of support groups for transplantations
- Patient awareness in chronic renal failure

11:15 a.m.	✓ Closing session and brunch—Atrium and Garden

November 15	Leave for Phoenix, 8:45 a.m.
15–18	Reservations Kon Tiki Hotel 2364 E. Van Buren Street, Phoenix, AZ 85006 (606–555–9361)
16–19	National Medical Convention
19	Leave early afternoon for Sedonna. Reservations at Cathedral Rock Lodge, Star Route 2, Box 856, Sedonna, AZ 86356 (606–555–5639)
20	Grand Canyon. Reservations at Dierken House, 423 West Cherry, Flagstaff, AZ 86001 (606–555–9833)
21	En route to Las Vegas (no reservations)
22–23	Reservations at Bed and Breakfast International, 6250 Pinewood Avenue, Las Vegas, NV 89103 (702–555–4569)
24	Lake Havasu City (no reservations)
25–26	En route to Phoenix (no reservations)
27–28	Staying in Phoenix with Mrs. Newman's brother, Dr. Stephen Gilman, 8514 West Sherman Avenue, Phoenix, AZ 85007 (606–555–2948).
29	Arrive back in Chicago, 2 p.m.

TELEPHONE LOG

DATE _____

TIME	CALLER	TELEPHONE NUMBER	REASON	DONE

TO-DO LIST

DATE _____

RUSH	THINGS TO DO	DONE
	Bring day sheet and ledgers up to date for 11/3 - 11/10.	
	Dr. Karen Larsen on call while Dr. Newman on vacation.	

ELIZABETH MILLER-YOUNG, M.D.
Practice limited to Obstetrics and Gynecology
2901 West Fifth Avenue, Suite 205
Chicago, IL 60612-9002
312-555-3500
Refill line: 312-555-3501

November 6, 19--

Mark Newman, M.D.
2235 South Ridgeway Avenue
Chicago, IL 60623-2240

Dear Dr. Newman:

RE: MONICA ARMSTRONG   DOB: 8/12/--

Recently, your patient Monica Armstrong came to see me. As you
may remember, she had complaints of menometrorrhagia, cervical
polyps, and a cervical erosion.

An endometrial sampling was performed in my office. Those
results are pending at the time of this dictation. She is
being treated with hormonal therapy while we await the report.
It is my plan to schedule her for a hysterectomy in the near
future. That will, of course, remedy several of her
gynecologic problems.

Thank you for referring this interesting patient to me.

Sincerely,

Elizabeth Miller-Young, M.D.

Elizabeth Miller-Young, M.D.

ru

Charles Jonathan III

NAME Charles Jonathan III		DATE 11/11
Exam	Code	Charge
OVF		
LAB: Synovial fluid		
X RAY:		
OTHER: Sterile tray		
Depo Medrol 80mg		
TOTAL		

Diagnosis: knee effusion 719.06

(blank)

NAME		DATE
Exam	Code	Charge
LAB:		
X RAY:		
OTHER:		
TOTAL		

Diagnosis:

Jeffrey Kramer

NAME Jeffrey Kramer		DATE 11/11
Exam	Code	Charge
OVF		
LAB:		
X RAY:		
OTHER:		
TOTAL		

Diagnosis: Otitis media with perforation, serous media 381, 382.01

Florence Sherman

NAME Florence Sherman		DATE 11/11
Exam	Code	Charge
OVF		
LAB:		
X RAY:		
OTHER:		
TOTAL		

Diagnosis: Vestibular neuronitis 386.12
contusion 922.1, 920, 923

Theresa Dayton

NAME Theresa Dayton		DATE 11/11
Exam	Code	Charge
OVF		
LAB:		
X RAY:		
OTHER:		
TOTAL		

Diagnosis: Headache 307.81

Clarence Rogers

NAME Clarence Rogers		DATE 11/11
Exam	Code	Charge
OVF		
LAB:		
X RAY:		
OTHER:		
TOTAL		

Diagnosis: consult V25.2

letterhead

Facsimile Transmittal Sheet

↓ ts

Fax Telephone No.

↓ ts

Date: _____   Time:_____

↓ ts

To: _____   From: _____

↓ ts

Location:_____

↓ ts

Number of Pages (Include cover sheet): _____

↓ ts

Message: _____

↓ ts
_____

↓ ts
_____

↓ ts
_____

↓ ts
_____

NO. 1900 $\frac{2-62}{710}$

November 7   **19** --

**PAY
TO THE
ORDER OF** Mark Newman, M.D. ——————————— $ 200⁰⁰/100

Two hundred and ⁰⁰/100 ————————————————— **DOLLARS**

First National Bank
Chicago, IL 60623-2791

Monica Armstrong

⑆0710⑈0062 613⑉017740⑈

NO. 2847 $\frac{2-62}{710}$

November 10   **19** --

**PAY
TO THE
ORDER OF** Dr. Mark Newman ——————————— $ 50⁰⁰/100

Fifty and ⁰⁰/100 ————————————————— **DOLLARS**

First National Bank
Chicago, IL 60623-2791

Joseph Castro

⑆0710⑈0062 327⑉025732⑈

NO. 2259 $\frac{2-62}{710}$

November 9   **19** --

**PAY
TO THE
ORDER OF** Mark Newman, M.D. ——————————— $ 80⁰⁰/100

Eighty and ⁰⁰/100 ————————————————— **DOLLARS**

First National Bank
Chicago, IL 60623-2791

Warren Richards

⑆0710⑈0062 211⑉023301⑈

DAILY JOURNAL

DATE 11/3 - 11/10/--   SHEET NO. 86

RECEIPT NUMBER	DATE	DESCRIPTION-CODE	CHARGE	PAYMENT	ADJUSTMENTS	BALANCE	PREVIOUS BALANCE	NAME
1	11/3	OVE/Sinus X ray	100 00	—		235 00	135 00	Ana Mendez
2		OVF/Strep	50 00			50 00	—	Stephen Villano
3								
4	11/4	OV Comprehensive Pap/wet prep	150 00			180 00	30 00	Sara Babcock
5								
6	11/5	OV Comprehensive	100 00			100 00		Ellen Stevens—NP
7								
8								
9	11/10	OVE	40 00	—		40 00	—	Doris Casagranda
10								
		TOTALS	Column A	Column B	Column C	Column D	Column E	

PROOF OF POSTING

COLUMN E TOTAL	$
"PLUS" COLUMN A TOTAL	$
SUB TOTAL	$
"MINUS" COLUMN B TOTAL	$
EQUALS COLUMN D TOTAL	$

IN NUMERICAL ORDER

ACCOUNTS RECEIVABLE CONTROL

PREVIOUS BALANCE	$ 9120.00
"PLUS" COLUMN A	$
SUB TOTAL	$
"MINUS" COLUMN B TOTAL	$
PRESENT ACC'TS REC. BALANCE	$

DAILY CASH SUMMARY

OPENING CASH ON HAND AT BEGINNING OF DAY	$
CASH RECEIVED DURING DAY	$
TOTAL	$

FORM NO. 210-1

To Do 11/11
① Need to balance and total
② Need to post to patients' ledgers

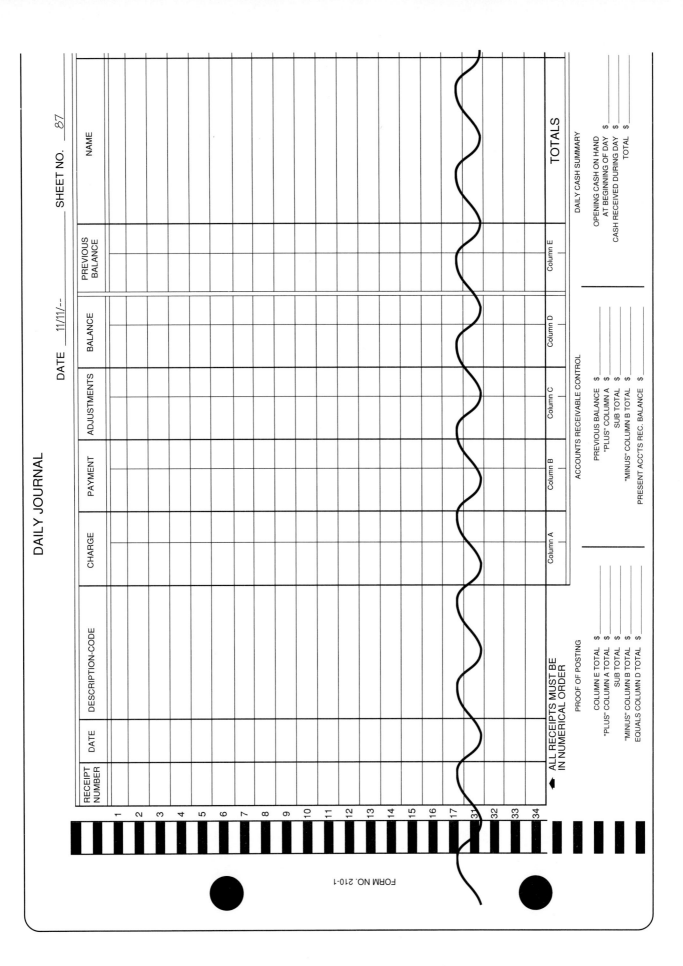

DAILY JOURNAL

DATE 11/11/--   SHEET NO. 87

RECEIPT NUMBER	DATE	DESCRIPTION-CODE	CHARGE	PAYMENT	ADJUSTMENTS	BALANCE	PREVIOUS BALANCE	NAME
1								
2								
3								
4								
5								
6								
7								
8								
9								
10								
11								
12								
13								
14								
15								
16								
17								
31								
32								
33								
34								
		Column A	Column B	Column C	Column D	Column E		TOTALS

◄ ALL RECEIPTS MUST BE
IN NUMERICAL ORDER

PROOF OF POSTING

COLUMN E TOTAL $ _____
"PLUS" COLUMN A TOTAL $ _____
SUB TOTAL $ _____
"MINUS" COLUMN B TOTAL $ _____
EQUALS COLUMN D TOTAL $ _____

ACCOUNTS RECEIVABLE CONTROL

PREVIOUS BALANCE $ _____
"PLUS" COLUMN A $ _____
SUB TOTAL $ _____
"MINUS" COLUMN B TOTAL $ _____
PRESENT ACCTS REC. BALANCE $ _____

DAILY CASH SUMMARY

OPENING CASH ON HAND
AT BEGINNING OF DAY $ _____
CASH RECEIVED DURING DAY $ _____
TOTAL $ _____

FORM NO. 210-1

PATIENT REGISTRATION

DATE ___11/5/--___

Patient Name	Stevens (Last)	Ellen (First)	A (Initial)	Birth Date	12/6/-- Age 59

Address 3234 North Central Park Avenue

City Chicago **State** IL **ZIP** 60618-3243

Telephone 555-5332 **Social Security No.** 580-18-6593

Responsible Person Ellen (Daniel) **Relationship** husband

Address Same **City** **State** **ZIP**

Employer Self-employed, Daycare

Address 3234 North Central Park Avenue **Work Phone** 555-5332

City Chicago **State** IL **ZIP** 60618-3243

NOTIFY IN CASE OF EMERGENCY

Name Lynda Stearns **Relationship** daughter

Address 7518 N. Central Ave. **Phone** 555-9903

City Chicago **State** IL **ZIP** 60634-2731

INSURANCE INFORMATION

	INSURANCE COMPANY	POLICY NO.	SUBSCRIBER
(1)	Blue Cross	580-18-6593	Ellen
(2)			

PLEASE DO NOT STAPLE IN THIS AREA

APPROVED OMB-0938-0008

PICA

HEALTH INSURANCE CLAIM FORM

PICA

1. MEDICARE	MEDICAID	CHAMPUS	CHAMPVA	GROUP HEALTH PLAN	FECA BLK LUNG	OTHER	1a. INSURED'S I.D. NUMBER	(FOR PROGRAM IN ITEM 1)
(Medicare #)	(Medicaid #)	(Sponsor's SSN)	(VA File #)	(SSN or ID)	(SSN)	(ID)		

2. PATIENT'S NAME (Last Name, First Name, Middle Initial)

3. PATIENT'S BIRTH DATE MM DD YY   SEX   M ☐ F ☐

4. INSURED'S NAME (Last Name, First Name, Middle Initial)

5. PATIENT'S ADDRESS (No., Street)

6. PATIENT RELATIONSHIP TO INSURED   Self ☐ Spouse ☐ Child ☐ Other ☐

7. INSURED'S ADDRESS (No., Street)

CITY   STATE

8. PATIENT STATUS   Single ☐ Married ☐ Other ☐

CITY   STATE

ZIP CODE   TELEPHONE (Include Area Code)

Employed ☐ Full-Time Student ☐ Part-Time Student ☐

ZIP CODE   TELEPHONE (INCLUDE AREA CODE)

9. OTHER INSURED'S NAME (Last Name, First Name, Middle Initial)

10. IS PATIENT'S CONDITION RELATED TO:

11. INSURED'S POLICY GROUP OR FECA NUMBER

a. OTHER INSURED'S POLICY OR GROUP NUMBER

a. EMPLOYMENT? (CURRENT OR PREVIOUS)   YES ☐ NO ☐

a. INSURED'S DATE OF BIRTH MM DD YY   SEX   M ☐ F ☐

b. OTHER INSURED'S DATE OF BIRTH MM DD YY   SEX   M ☐ F ☐

b. AUTO ACCIDENT?   PLACE (State)   YES ☐ NO ☐

b. EMPLOYER'S NAME OR SCHOOL NAME

c. EMPLOYER'S NAME OR SCHOOL NAME

c. OTHER ACCIDENT?   YES ☐ NO ☐

c. INSURANCE PLAN NAME OR PROGRAM NAME

d. INSURANCE PLAN NAME OR PROGRAM NAME

10d. RESERVED FOR LOCAL USE

d. IS THERE ANOTHER HEALTH BENEFIT PLAN?   YES ☐ NO ☐ **If yes**, return to and complete item 9 a-d.

READ BACK OF FORM BEFORE COMPLETING & SIGNING THIS FORM.
12. PATIENT'S OR AUTHORIZED PERSON'S SIGNATURE I authorize the release of any medical or other information necessary to process this claim. I also request payment of government benefits either to myself or to the party who accepts assignment below.

SIGNED   DATE

13. INSURED'S OR AUTHORIZED PERSON'S SIGNATURE I authorize payment of medical benefits to the undersigned physician or supplier for services described below.

SIGNED

14. DATE OF CURRENT: MM DD YY   ILLNESS (First symptom) OR INJURY (Accident) OR PREGNANCY(LMP)

15. IF PATIENT HAS HAD SAME OR SIMILAR ILLNESS. GIVE FIRST DATE MM DD YY

16. DATES PATIENT UNABLE TO WORK IN CURRENT OCCUPATION MM DD YY   FROM   TO   MM DD YY

17. NAME OF REFERRING PHYSICIAN OR OTHER SOURCE

17a. I.D. NUMBER OF REFERRING PHYSICIAN

18. HOSPITALIZATION DATES RELATED TO CURRENT SERVICES MM DD YY   FROM   TO   MM DD YY

19. RESERVED FOR LOCAL USE

20. OUTSIDE LAB?   YES ☐ NO ☐ $ CHARGES

21. DIAGNOSIS OR NATURE OF ILLNESS OR INJURY. (RELATE ITEMS 1,2,3 OR 4 TO ITEM 24E BY LINE)

1. └─ . ─┘   3. └─ . ─┘

2. └─ . ─┘   4. └─ . ─┘

22. MEDICAID RESUBMISSION CODE   ORIGINAL REF. NO.

23. PRIOR AUTHORIZATION NUMBER

24. A DATE(S) OF SERVICE						B Place of Service	C Type of Service	D PROCEDURES, SERVICES, OR SUPPLIES (Explain Unusual Circumstances) CPT/HCPCS MODIFIER	E DIAGNOSIS CODE	F $ CHARGES	G DAYS OR UNITS	H EPSDT Family Plan	I EMG	J COB	K RESERVED FOR LOCAL USE
From MM	DD	YY	To MM	DD	YY										
1															
2															
3															
4															
5															
6															

25. FEDERAL TAX I.D. NUMBER   SSN ☐ EIN ☐

26. PATIENT'S ACCOUNT NO.

27. ACCEPT ASSIGNMENT? (For govt. claims, see back)   YES ☐ NO ☐

28. TOTAL CHARGE $

29. AMOUNT PAID $

30. BALANCE DUE $

31. SIGNATURE OF PHYSICIAN OR SUPPLIER INCLUDING DEGREES OR CREDENTIALS (I certify that the statements on the reverse apply to this bill and are made a part thereof.)

SIGNED   DATE

32. NAME AND ADDRESS OF FACILITY WHERE SERVICES WERE RENDERED (If other than home or office)

33. PHYSICIAN'S, SUPPLIER'S BILLING NAME, ADDRESS. ZIP CODE & PHONE #

PIN#   GRP#

(APPROVED BY AMA COUNCIL ON MEDICAL SERVICE 8/88)   **PLEASE PRINT OR TYPE**

FORM HCFA-1500 (12-90)
FORM OWCP-1500   FORM RRB-1500
FORM OP 050191

WP 114

Name _Sara Babcock_ Doctor _Newman_

Test Results _____

____ WBC	____ Glucose
____ Hematocrit	_129_ Cholesterol
_13.5_ Hemoglobin	____ BUN
____ Differential	____ Calcium
____ PMN	____ Phosphorous
____ Bands	____ Bilirubin
____ Lymphs	____ Uric acid
____ Mono	____ Alkaline phosphatase
____ Eos	____ Albumin
____ Baso	____ Protein, total
____ Platelets	____ LDH
____ Thyroid	____ SGOT

HEMATOLOGY—CHEMISTRY
_MN_

Date _10/31_

Name _Sara Babcock_   Doctor _Newman_

Color _yellow_   Pap Smear _____

pH _6.0_   _____

Specific Gravity _1.010_   _____

Protein _0_   Vaginal Smear _____

Glucose _0_   _____

Ketone _____

WBCs/hpf _0-1_   Hemoccults _____

RBCs/hpf _0_   _____

Bacteria _0_

_____

Culture _____

_____

URINE—Miscellaneous

Date _10/31_

Name _Monica Armstrong_   Doctor _Newman_

Color _____   Pap Smear _negative_

pH _____   _____

Specific Gravity _____ _____

Protein _____   Vaginal Smear _____

Glucose _____   _____

Ketone _____

WBCs/hpf _____   Hemoccults _____

RBCs/hpf _____   _____

Bacteria _____

_____   _MN_

Culture _____

_____

URINE—Miscellaneous

Date _10/28_

WHEATON ORTHOPEDIC CLINIC
250 Main Street, Suite 100
Wheaton, IL 60187-4283

555-1879
Refill: 555-3384

NAME Sarah Morton   DATE 11/5/--

ADDRESS _____

Fracture going from shaft into epiphysis, metacarpal of index finger, left hand. Good alignment with evidence of rotation. Possible growth, dysfunction of epiphyseal injury. Short arm gutter. Splint applied. Index and middle fingers buddy-taped. To use ice and elevation. Recheck one week.

Tomas Reis, M.D.

NAME Thomas Baab   DATE 11/12

Exam	Code	Charge	
OVF			
LAB:			
X RAY:			
OTHER:			
TOTAL			

Diagnosis: Hypercholesterolemia 272

NAME Clarence Rogers   DATE 11/12

Exam	Code	Charge	
LAB: UA			
X RAY:			
OTHER:			
vasectomy	55250		
TOTAL			

Diagnosis: permament contraception V25.2

NAME Erin Mitchell   **DATE** 11/12

Exam	Code	Charge
OVF postpartum		
LAB:		
X RAY:		
OTHER:		
TOTAL		

Diagnosis: postpartum V24.2

NAME Warren Richards   **DATE** 11/12

Exam	Code	Charge
Initial HV 10/30		
12 HVs		
LAB:		
X RAY:		
OTHER:		
TOTAL		

Diagnosis: TIA 435.9

NAME Gary Robertson   **DATE** 11/12

Exam	Code	Charge
OVF		
LAB: UA		
X RAY:		
OTHER:		
TOTAL		

Diagnosis: pyelonephritis 590.1

NAME Sarah Morton   **DATE** 11/12

Exam	Code	Charge
OVF		
LAB:		
X RAY:		
OTHER:		
TOTAL		

Diagnosis: fracture metacarpal 815.03

NAME David Kramer   **DATE** 11/12

Exam	Code	Charge
LAB:		
X RAY:		
OTHER: DTP		
Oral Polio		
TOTAL		

Diagnosis: Vaccination V06.3

NAME Donald Mitchell   **DATE** 11/12

Exam	Code	Charge
OVE		
LAB:		
X RAY:		
OTHER:		
TOTAL		

Diagnosis: well-baby check V20.2

NO. 1982

November 8 19 --

2—62
710

PAY
TO THE
ORDER OF Dr. Mark Newman $ 105⁰⁰/100

One hundred five and ⁰⁰/100 ————————————————————— **DOLLARS**

First National Bank
Chicago, IL 60623-2791

Suzanne Roberts

⑈0710⑈0062 202⑈056232⑈

NO. 19642

November 7 19 --

2—62
710

PAY
TO THE
ORDER OF Dr. Mark Newman $ 100⁰⁰/100

One hundred and ⁰⁰/100 ————————————————————— **DOLLARS**

First National Bank
Chicago, IL 60623-2791

Raymond Murray

⑈0710⑈0062 375⑈043389⑈

NO. 5347

November 9 19 --

2—62
710

PAY
TO THE
ORDER OF Mark Newman $ 100⁰⁰/100

One hundred and ⁰⁰/100 ————————————————————— **DOLLARS**

First National Bank
Chicago, IL 60623-2791

Lawrence Lund

⑈0710⑈0062 815⑈022249⑈

PLEASE
DO NOT
STAPLE
IN THIS
AREA

APPROVED OMB-0938-0008

HEALTH INSURANCE CLAIM FORM

PICA | PICA

1. MEDICARE ☐ (Medicare #) MEDICAID ☐ (Medicaid #) CHAMPUS ☐ (Sponsor's SSN) CHAMPVA ☐ (VA File #) GROUP HEALTH PLAN ☐ (SSN or ID) FECA BLK LUNG ☐ (SSN) OTHER ☐ (ID)

1a. INSURED'S I.D. NUMBER (FOR PROGRAM IN ITEM 1)

2. PATIENT'S NAME (Last Name, First Name, Middle Initial)

3. PATIENT'S BIRTH DATE MM DD YY SEX M ☐ F ☐

4. INSURED'S NAME (Last Name, First Name, Middle Initial)

5. PATIENT'S ADDRESS (No., Street)

6. PATIENT RELATIONSHIP TO INSURED Self ☐ Spouse ☐ Child ☐ Other ☐

7. INSURED'S ADDRESS (No., Street)

CITY | STATE

8. PATIENT STATUS Single ☐ Married ☐ Other ☐ Employed ☐ Full-Time Student ☐ Part-Time Student ☐

CITY | STATE

ZIP CODE | TELEPHONE (Include Area Code)

ZIP CODE | TELEPHONE (INCLUDE AREA CODE)

9. OTHER INSURED'S NAME (Last Name, First Name, Middle Initial)

10. IS PATIENT'S CONDITION RELATED TO:

11. INSURED'S POLICY GROUP OR FECA NUMBER

a. OTHER INSURED'S POLICY OR GROUP NUMBER

a. EMPLOYMENT? (CURRENT OR PREVIOUS) YES ☐ NO ☐

a. INSURED'S DATE OF BIRTH MM DD YY SEX M ☐ F ☐

b. OTHER INSURED'S DATE OF BIRTH MM DD YY SEX M ☐ F ☐

b. AUTO ACCIDENT? PLACE (State) YES ☐ NO ☐

b. EMPLOYER'S NAME OR SCHOOL NAME

c. EMPLOYER'S NAME OR SCHOOL NAME

c. OTHER ACCIDENT? YES ☐ NO ☐

c. INSURANCE PLAN NAME OR PROGRAM NAME

d. INSURANCE PLAN NAME OR PROGRAM NAME

10d. RESERVED FOR LOCAL USE

d. IS THERE ANOTHER HEALTH BENEFIT PLAN? YES ☐ NO ☐ If yes, return to and complete item 9 a-d.

READ BACK OF FORM BEFORE COMPLETING & SIGNING THIS FORM.
12. PATIENT'S OR AUTHORIZED PERSON'S SIGNATURE I authorize the release of any medical or other information necessary to process this claim. I also request payment of government benefits either to myself or to the party who accepts assignment below.

SIGNED | DATE

13. INSURED'S OR AUTHORIZED PERSON'S SIGNATURE I authorize payment of medical benefits to the undersigned physician or supplier for services described below.

SIGNED

14. DATE OF CURRENT: MM DD YY ILLNESS (First symptom) OR INJURY (Accident) OR PREGNANCY(LMP)

15. IF PATIENT HAS HAD SAME OR SIMILAR ILLNESS. GIVE FIRST DATE MM DD YY

16. DATES PATIENT UNABLE TO WORK IN CURRENT OCCUPATION FROM MM DD YY TO MM DD YY

17. NAME OF REFERRING PHYSICIAN OR OTHER SOURCE

17a. I.D. NUMBER OF REFERRING PHYSICIAN

18. HOSPITALIZATION DATES RELATED TO CURRENT SERVICES FROM MM DD YY TO MM DD YY

19. RESERVED FOR LOCAL USE

20. OUTSIDE LAB? YES ☐ NO ☐ $ CHARGES

21. DIAGNOSIS OR NATURE OF ILLNESS OR INJURY. (RELATE ITEMS 1,2,3 OR 4 TO ITEM 24E BY LINE)
1. ____ . ____   3. ____ . ____
2. ____ . ____   4. ____ . ____

22. MEDICAID RESUBMISSION CODE | ORIGINAL REF. NO.

23. PRIOR AUTHORIZATION NUMBER

24. A DATE(S) OF SERVICE From MM DD YY To MM DD YY	B Place of Service	C Type of Service	D PROCEDURES, SERVICES, OR SUPPLIES (Explain Unusual Circumstances) CPT/HCPCS MODIFIER	E DIAGNOSIS CODE	F $ CHARGES	G DAYS OR UNITS	H EPSDT Family Plan	I EMG	J COB	K RESERVED FOR LOCAL USE
1										
2										
3										
4										
5										
6										

25. FEDERAL TAX I.D. NUMBER SSN ☐ EIN ☐

26. PATIENT'S ACCOUNT NO.

27. ACCEPT ASSIGNMENT? (For govt. claims, see back) YES ☐ NO ☐

28. TOTAL CHARGE $ | 29. AMOUNT PAID $ | 30. BALANCE DUE $

31. SIGNATURE OF PHYSICIAN OR SUPPLIER INCLUDING DEGREES OR CREDENTIALS (I certify that the statements on the reverse apply to this bill and are made a part thereof.)

SIGNED | DATE

32. NAME AND ADDRESS OF FACILITY WHERE SERVICES WERE RENDERED (If other than home or office)

33. PHYSICIAN'S, SUPPLIER'S BILLING NAME, ADDRESS, ZIP CODE & PHONE #

PIN# | GRP#

(APPROVED BY AMA COUNCIL ON MEDICAL SERVICE 8/88)   **PLEASE PRINT OR TYPE**

FORM HCFA-1500 (12-90)
FORM OWCP-1500   FORM RRB-1500
FORM OP 050191

WP 119

PLEASE DO NOT STAPLE IN THIS AREA

APPROVED OMB-0938-0008

CARRIER

PICA

HEALTH INSURANCE CLAIM FORM

PICA

1. MEDICARE (Medicare #) MEDICAID (Medicaid #) CHAMPUS (Sponsor's SSN) CHAMPVA (VA File #) GROUP HEALTH PLAN (SSN or ID) FECA BLK LUNG (SSN) OTHER (ID)

1a. INSURED'S I.D. NUMBER (FOR PROGRAM IN ITEM 1)

2. PATIENT'S NAME (Last Name, First Name, Middle Initial)

3. PATIENT'S BIRTH DATE MM DD YY SEX M F

4. INSURED'S NAME (Last Name, First Name, Middle Initial)

5. PATIENT'S ADDRESS (No., Street)

6. PATIENT RELATIONSHIP TO INSURED Self Spouse Child Other

7. INSURED'S ADDRESS (No., Street)

CITY STATE

8. PATIENT STATUS Single Married Other

CITY STATE

ZIP CODE TELEPHONE (Include Area Code)

Employed Full-Time Student Part-Time Student

ZIP CODE TELEPHONE (INCLUDE AREA CODE)

9. OTHER INSURED'S NAME (Last Name, First Name, Middle Initial)

10. IS PATIENT'S CONDITION RELATED TO:

11. INSURED'S POLICY GROUP OR FECA NUMBER

a. OTHER INSURED'S POLICY OR GROUP NUMBER

a. EMPLOYMENT? (CURRENT OR PREVIOUS) YES NO

a. INSURED'S DATE OF BIRTH MM DD YY SEX M F

b. OTHER INSURED'S DATE OF BIRTH MM DD YY SEX M F

b. AUTO ACCIDENT? PLACE (State) YES NO

b. EMPLOYER'S NAME OR SCHOOL NAME

c. EMPLOYER'S NAME OR SCHOOL NAME

c. OTHER ACCIDENT? YES NO

c. INSURANCE PLAN NAME OR PROGRAM NAME

d. INSURANCE PLAN NAME OR PROGRAM NAME

10d. RESERVED FOR LOCAL USE

d. IS THERE ANOTHER HEALTH BENEFIT PLAN? YES NO *If yes*, return to and complete item 9 a-d.

READ BACK OF FORM BEFORE COMPLETING & SIGNING THIS FORM.

12. PATIENT'S OR AUTHORIZED PERSON'S SIGNATURE I authorize the release of any medical or other information necessary to process this claim. I also request payment of government benefits either to myself or to the party who accepts assignment below.

SIGNED _____ DATE _____

13. INSURED'S OR AUTHORIZED PERSON'S SIGNATURE I authorize payment of medical benefits to the undersigned physician or supplier for services described below.

SIGNED _____

14. DATE OF CURRENT: MM DD YY ILLNESS (First symptom) OR INJURY (Accident) OR PREGNANCY(LMP)

15. IF PATIENT HAS HAD SAME OR SIMILAR ILLNESS. GIVE FIRST DATE MM DD YY

16. DATES PATIENT UNABLE TO WORK IN CURRENT OCCUPATION MM DD YY MM DD YY FROM TO

17. NAME OF REFERRING PHYSICIAN OR OTHER SOURCE

17a. I.D. NUMBER OF REFERRING PHYSICIAN

18. HOSPITALIZATION DATES RELATED TO CURRENT SERVICES MM DD YY MM DD YY FROM TO

19. RESERVED FOR LOCAL USE

20. OUTSIDE LAB? $ CHARGES YES NO

21. DIAGNOSIS OR NATURE OF ILLNESS OR INJURY. (RELATE ITEMS 1,2,3 OR 4 TO ITEM 24E BY LINE)

1. ___.___ 3. ___.___

2. ___.___ 4. ___.___

22. MEDICAID RESUBMISSION CODE ORIGINAL REF. NO.

23. PRIOR AUTHORIZATION NUMBER

24. A DATE(S) OF SERVICE From To MM DD YY MM DD YY	B Place of Service	C Type of Service	D PROCEDURES, SERVICES, OR SUPPLIES (Explain Unusual Circumstances) CPT/HCPCS MODIFIER	E DIAGNOSIS CODE	F $ CHARGES	G DAYS OR UNITS	H EPSDT Family Plan	I EMG	J COB	K RESERVED FOR LOCAL USE
1										
2										
3										
4										
5										
6										

25. FEDERAL TAX I.D. NUMBER SSN EIN

26. PATIENT'S ACCOUNT NO.

27. ACCEPT ASSIGNMENT? (For govt. claims, see back) YES NO

28. TOTAL CHARGE $

29. AMOUNT PAID $

30. BALANCE DUE $

31. SIGNATURE OF PHYSICIAN OR SUPPLIER INCLUDING DEGREES OR CREDENTIALS (I certify that the statements on the reverse apply to this bill and are made a part thereof.)

SIGNED _____ DATE _____

32. NAME AND ADDRESS OF FACILITY WHERE SERVICES WERE RENDERED (If other than home or office)

33. PHYSICIAN'S, SUPPLIER'S BILLING NAME, ADDRESS, ZIP CODE & PHONE #

PIN# GRP#

PATIENT AND INSURED INFORMATION

PHYSICIAN OR SUPPLIER INFORMATION

(APPROVED BY AMA COUNCIL ON MEDICAL SERVICE 8/88)

PLEASE PRINT OR TYPE

FORM HCFA-1500 (12-90) FORM OWCP-1500 FORM RRB-1500 FORM OP 050191

WP 120

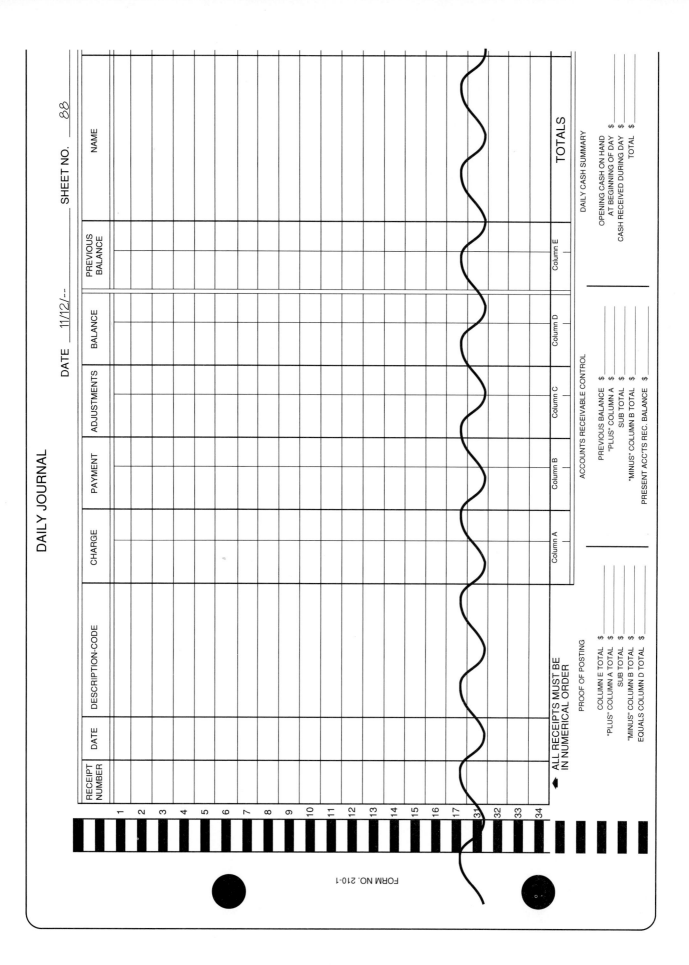

DAILY JOURNAL

DATE 11/12/--   SHEET NO. 88

RECEIPT NUMBER	DATE	DESCRIPTION-CODE	CHARGE	PAYMENT	ADJUSTMENTS	BALANCE	PREVIOUS BALANCE	NAME
1								
2								
3								
4								
5								
6								
7								
8								
9								
10								
11								
12								
13								
14								
15								
16								
17								
31								
32								
33								
34								
			Column A	Column B	Column C	Column D	Column E	TOTALS

◄ ALL RECEIPTS MUST BE
IN NUMERICAL ORDER

PROOF OF POSTING

COLUMN E TOTAL $ _____
"PLUS" COLUMN A TOTAL $ _____
SUB TOTAL $ _____
"MINUS" COLUMN B TOTAL $ _____
EQUALS COLUMN D TOTAL $ _____

ACCOUNTS RECEIVABLE CONTROL

PREVIOUS BALANCE $ _____
"PLUS" COLUMN A $ _____
SUB TOTAL $ _____
"MINUS" COLUMN B TOTAL $ _____
PRESENT ACCT'S REC. BALANCE $ _____

DAILY CASH SUMMARY

OPENING CASH ON HAND
AT BEGINNING OF DAY $ _____
CASH RECEIVED DURING DAY $ _____
TOTAL $ _____

FORM NO. 210-1